Study Guide to Accompany

Pharmacology
FOR NURSING CARE

Study Guide to Accompany

RICHARD A. LEHNE

Pharmacology
FOR NURSING CARE

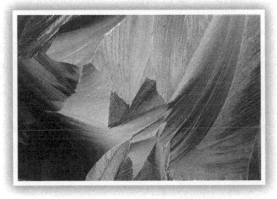

FIFTH EDITION

PREPARED BY

MARSHAL SHLAFER, PhD

Professor of Pharmacology
University of Michigan Medical School
Ann Arbor, Michigan

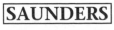

An Imprint of Elsevier

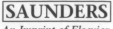

An Imprint of Elsevier

11830 Westline Industrial Drive
St. Louis, Missouri 63146

Previous editions copyrighted 2000, 1999

International Standard Book Number 0-7216-0128-6

Acquisitions Editor: Lee Henderson
Developmental Editor: Celia Cruz
Publishing Services Manager: Gayle May
Project Manager: Joseph Selby
Designer: Teresa Breckwoldt

KI/MVB

Printed in the United States of America

Last digit is the print number: 9 8 7 6 5 4 3 2

Preface

This *Study Guide,* developed to accompany *Pharmacology for Nursing Care*, fifth edition, was prepared for three main reasons: (1) to assist you in learning and understanding and applying the most important material presented in the text; (2) to help and guide your integration of related or otherwise pertinent material that may be presented in chapters that are far apart in the book; and (3) to get you to *think*, not just *memorize*, things that are important in the realms of pharmacology and drug therapy.

You'll find *Key Terms* and *Objectives* in each chapter of this Study Guide. You'll also find one or both of *Critical Thinking and Study Questions* and *Case Studies*.

KEY TERMS

These are words or phrases that should become familiar to you in terms of their meaning and implications. You should be able to recognize (with some degree of accuracy) the correct definition or meaning of the words and terms; and you should be able to provide some reasonable definition or explanation of what they mean on your own.

Most are "new" and specific to pharmacology and therapeutics. You will also have to have some knowledge of the terms and language from the realms of basic physiology, pathophysiology, biochemistry, and nursing fundamentals. Quite simply, you need to be able to understand and speak the language.

OBJECTIVES

Objectives focus on facts and concepts you should know and understand (and be able to describe) after completing each chapter. The stated objectives are limited to what one might reasonably expect a student who is new to the discipline of pharmacology and drug therapy to meet. Meeting the objectives should, therefore, serve you well if you are, for example, enrolled in a survey course or preparing for exams.

Without a doubt, there is far more good information in the text that is of a more specific or advanced nature, and generally such issues have not been included in the *Objectives* list. Ultimately, however, at some time in your career (or now, with the expectation of your instructors), your objectives may increase in scope and depth.

Some objectives are so broad or general that they are not listed in each chapter because they apply to virtually every drug-oriented chapter, every drug or every drug group. They are fundamentally important for your learning and the eventual application of your knowledge, whether to an exam or to clinical practice. These include the following examples:

- Being able to define or recognize the definitions of the key terms
- Stating how drugs are classified (whether pharmacologically, chemically, by body system or clinical use, etc.)
- Stating the main actions and mechanisms of actions of drugs in the chapter
- Stating the clinical uses of specified drugs or drug groups
- Identifying the main side effects, adverse responses, precautions, contraindications, and interactions of/for named drugs

In other instances, I've added learning objectives that are quite specific (and relevant) to the topic(s) at hand. You should challenge yourself to meet those objectives. Doing so will pay off in the long run.

CRITICAL THINKING AND STUDY QUESTIONS

Most of the *Critical Thinking and Study Questions* are pretty straightforward, and you can find the answers almost verbatim in Dr. Lehne's textbook.

Others require you to do a bit more creative thinking, assimilation of information and knowledge, and application of that knowledge to the case at hand. Still others ask for your personal or professional opinions. This is where you have to think, not just recall facts or concepts.

In the early parts of this Study Guide, most of the questions are basically focused on the chapter being considered. But as you progress through the text and your course, many of the *Critical Thinking and Study Questions* force you to call up, integrate, and apply knowledge that you should have gained earlier.

This is, after all, how drug therapy really is: integrated and of necessity linked. You can't, for example, think only about "which drug is best for my hypertensive patient (and why)" without realizing that he or she may have glaucoma, asthma, or some other medical condition that may be helped – or harmed – by a particular drug or drug class.

Finally, those of you who have seen an earlier edition of this book will see that we have changed the terminology for our follow-ups to *Critical Thinking and Study Questions*, and the *Case Studies*, from "Answers" to "Comments." For many of the questions in this workbook there are answers, and rather clear-cut ones at that. However, in many cases (here and in the real world too), there is no one absolutely right or wrong answer. Some therapeutic choices are better than others, some worse, but the final decision is a judgment call. You need to be able to think things through, weigh pros and cons and various other alternatives, and come up with some reasonable conclusion or interpretation. That's what we do here.

Please feel free to write your answers in the space provided beneath each question and use a separate piece of paper if necessary. To check your answers, go to http://evolve.elsevier.com/Lehne/ for Study Guide Comments from the author.

CASE STUDIES

You'll find *Case Studies* in many later chapters of this study guide because to put your knowledge of drug action and drug therapy to a real test in the *Case Study* context, you need to get a certain amount of basic information about specific drugs under your belt.

In addition, some later chapters do not include *Case Studies*. That is usually because the drugs that are the focus of a particular chapter are often used with drugs discussed elsewhere. Rather than formulating a very focused but rather narrow and contrived *Case Study*, we'll refer you to another chapter where you'll have to pull together relevant information from several chapters.

Similar to the *Critical Thinking and Study Questions*, some of the *Case Studies* focus on the material in a particular chapter or the unit in which the chapter is presented. That's the approach I take when I think it's appropriate. After that, as we progress through the book (and you progress through your course), *Case Studies* can become more expansive, encouraging you to apply your knowledge from other areas. In fact, I'll force you to integrate.

You may expect the *Case Study* scenarios to describe a patient with just one disease—a medication plan that is simple, logical, straightforward, and done "by the book"—and clinical outcomes in which the patient lives happily ever after. If that's your expectation, you may be surprised.

Treating real patients often isn't that simple. Sometimes there may be many approaches, some of which may be equally acceptable and some of which are not; and sometimes drug therapy causes more problems than it solves. (On average, we spend more money to undo the problems caused by drugs than we spend on the drugs that caused the problems.)

Drug therapy isn't simple or straightforward; sometimes there are several "right" ways to treat a patient; sometimes there are clearly wrong (or at least problematic) management approaches, yet they are used every day, and sometimes the outcomes are not happy.

So in this Study Guide, I include treatment approaches that may not be optimal or appropriate. I identify problems that arise and urge you to comment on them. I describe situations in which a medication plan is implemented but is inappropriate. You will have to deal with these situations eventually, and so I think considering some of them now is appropriate and important.

Some may say that these lines of thinking are "up to the MD." I disagree. Excellent health care involves valued contributions from not just physicians, but also from nurses (whether that is someone with an associate's degree, bachelor's degree, or such specialization as a nurse-practitioner has). It is a checks-and-balances system, ideally. It is, in my opinion, your responsibility to have some idea of "What was the MD thinking in terms of Mrs. A?" or "What was the doctor's rationale for doing thus and so for Mr. B?"

WHAT'S NOT HERE?

Proper dosages and dosing calculations
Although your instructors may feel differently, I do not ask any questions or require you to have any knowledge of the "right" dose of drug A for Mr. B, and how often it should be given. I will not ask you to calculate how many milliliters of drug C you need to inject if Ms. D. requires 10 mg of drug C and drug C is available as a 100 mg/mL solution.

Such knowledge and skills needed to be able to memorize the information or calculate the right answer are important. However, knowing the right dose, the right route, or how to calculate the right number of tablets or the correct dilution is not sufficient for proper, safe, drug therapy. In fact, knowing this involves little more than rote memorization and the use of some basic math skills. You'll learn that information and those skills elsewhere or later on (we hope). Besides, you should always look up and double-check dosing information and other facts before you give a drug.

What may set you apart from other colleagues— what I try to stress—is your broader knowledge of pharmacology and therapeutics—your ability to think, understand, question, and explain. You memorized the right dose of a drug. You can do all the math to figure out how many tablets or milliliters to give. But you have no clue about what the drug does (good and bad), what to expect, when not to give it, how to assess responses, what to educate the patient about, and the like. That's not good enough in the long run.

Every drug or drug product that's discussed in Dr. Lehne's text

In this Study Guide, I've had to be selective in terms of what I ask of you. I can't address everything that's in Dr. Lehne's text. I can't address everything your instructor may think is crucially important. I can, however, be reasonably assured that if you can correctly answer or comment on what is presented in this Study Guide, you'll have a reasonably good and adequate knowledge of the overall subject matter and all that it encompasses.

Every drug or drug product that exists

You will never be able to learn all you eventually need to know about every drug or drug product that exists. Not with one pharmacology course or a dozen. Not with decades of clinical practice. There's just too much information (some of which is more important than the rest), and it changes too quickly.

You will learn best and in a more meaningful way, now, by focusing your studying on drug classes, their prototypes, and properties that apply to them. You should gain enough information from that learning effort to be able to apply that knowledge to drugs that are classified similarly and that are, largely, more like the prototype than significantly different from them.

In this Study Guide, I've tried to focus on the big stuff—that which is usually in "big type" in your text. That should serve as a solid foundation of knowledge, understanding, and application of knowledge. Learn that well and learning and understanding the rest should be much easier.

Multiple-choice questions

It's obvious that most of your learning during your education, and as you apply for licensure, will be assessed by your answers to multiple-choice questions. I have not included any of those "bubble-in-the-answer" questions or matching or short-answer items.

But, as you go through the text, and especially as you go though this Study Guide, think and look closely. Information provided in the *Critical Thinking and Study Questions* and in the *Case Studies* are goldmines of information that can (and almost certainly will) be turned into good test items. No doubt, your instructor will be using this resource to make some of his or her tests or quizzes. Spend the effort to go through the contents of this book and understand the answers (and why they are correct or wrong), and you should do just fine.

And if things aren't clear or understandable, ask your instructors for clarification. That's why they are there.

Good luck.

Marshal Shlafer, Ph.D.
Ann Arbor, Michigan
October, 2003

Table of Contents

Orientation to Pharmacology

KEY TERMS

clinical pharmacology
drug
pharmacology
pharmacy (as a
   discipline)

selectivity (as it applies
   to a drug's effects)
side effect(s) (of a drug)
therapeutics

OBJECTIVES

After reading and studying this chapter you should
be able to:

1. Define the following terms: *drug, pharmacology,
   clinical pharmacology,* and *therapeutics.*
2. List the three "most important" properties of an
   ideal drug, as well as others that are important,
   and state several ways that many drugs fail to
   possess those traits.

CRITICAL THINKING AND STUDY QUESTIONS

1. Describe the differences among pharmacology,
   clinical pharmacology, and therapeutics (pharmacotherapeutics).

2. What are three *most* important characteristics or
   properties of an "ideal" drug? List at least four
   other important properties, and explain in general
   how drugs do– or don't–have these characteristics.

3. What is the overall goal of drug therapy, regardless of the drug or the purposes for which it is
   given?

evolve To check your answers, go to http://evolve.elsevier.com/Lehne/ for Study Guide Comments from the author.

1

Application of Pharmacology in Nursing Practice

OBJECTIVES

After reading and studying this chapter you should be able to:

1. Describe how the nursing process (assessment, analysis, planning, implementation, and evaluation) applies to the understanding and administration of drugs to patients.
2. Discuss the goals of preadministration assessment related to drug administration and patient teaching.
3. Discuss the analysis of the data and develop a diagnosis for using drugs in the plan of care.
4. List the steps in a plan of care to meet a patient's needs.
5. Analyze the way evaluation of drug administration and teaching are conducted and documented.

CRITICAL THINKING AND STUDY QUESTIONS

1. State and briefly describe the five steps of the nursing process as they apply to medication administration.

2. State several factors that might negatively influence a patient's compliance in taking medications (i.e., his or her adherence to the medication plan).

3. In drug therapy, one objective of the analysis phase of the nursing process is to judge the likelihood that the proposed treatment will be safe and effective. Discuss four factors that might suggest that the proposed treatment will *not* be safe and effective. What should you do if any of these factors apply to your patient?

4. What's the difference between a contraindication and a precaution with regard to adverse drug reactions and to the decision about whether to give the drug?

5. Epinephrine (adrenalin) is generally contraindicated for people with hypertension, hyperthyroidism, and certain types of glaucoma. However, it is also considered a "drug of choice" for managing an anaphylactic reaction. Your patient, who has a history of all the conditions for which epinephrine is contraindicated, experiences an anaphylactic reaction that almost certainly will be fatal without proper drug treatment. What do you do, and what does this tell you about contraindications?

2

6. Patient education must be well planned and properly executed. What are the central elements a nurse must keep in mind with respect to drug interactions when planning a patient's education?

7. Discuss some useful and usually effective measures to evaluate a patient's compliance with (adherence to) a drug regimen.

evolve To check your answers, go to http://evolve.elsevier.com/Lehne/ for Study Guide Comments from the author.

Drug Regulation, Development, Names, and Information

KEY TERMS

approved use (of a drug or product) chemical name (of drug)
generic name (of drug)
new drug application (NDA)

off-label (unlabeled) use (of drug)
postmarketing surveillance
proprietary name (of drug)

OBJECTIVES

After reading and studying this chapter you should be able to:

1. Describe the key legislation that has had significant implications for pharmacology and nursing care. (Memorizing which law was passed when is not a profitable exercise; you should devote your studying to more important matters.)
2. State what generally is involved in Phases I, II, III, and IV of clinical testing of new drugs.
3. State the important information that can be gained from Phase IV (postmarketing surveillance) of clinical drug testing, and state the nurse's (and physician's) roles and responsibilities in gathering and reporting data.
4. Give a brief description of what chemical, generic, and proprietary (trade or brand) names of drugs indicate (or don't). Summarize the pros and cons of referring to drugs by these names.
5. Identify appropriate resources for pharmacologic information and patient care, as well as several reasons that some sources may be more suitable than others for a specific purpose (e.g., a specific type of information you are looking for).

CRITICAL THINKING AND STUDY QUESTIONS

1. How does Phase IV (postmarketing surveillance) of drug testing differ from Phases I, II, and III?

Since drugs are approved after a favorable review of Phase III trials, why is the postmarketing surveillance phase so important? What new and essential information is likely to come out of postmarketing surveillance, and why might that information not be gained in previous phases? What are the roles and responsibilities of healthcare providers in Phase IV?

2. Until recently, what groups of potential patients basically have been excluded from preclinical drug testing, so that we have very little information on how they may respond to drugs once those drugs are approved for use?

3. A 13-year-old boy with headache, fever, and mild GI upset is taken to the doctor's office by his mom. The doctor diagnoses the problem as a mild viral illness that should resolve in 3 days. In the meantime, the doctor instructs the mother to give the boy one Tylenol tablet every 4 hours for 2 days. That should alleviate the symptoms.

What are some likely reasons that the doctor specifically recommended Tylenol, which is a brand-name product? What could have been recommended instead? What are the potential problems with simply recommending Tylenol, even though the number of tablets and duration of administration were specified?

Answer this in the context of discussing the main disadvantages of referring to drugs (or writing medication orders for them) by proprietary

4

names. What are some of the problems with proprietary names (compared with generics)?

4. Take a trip to a retail pharmacy or grocery store. Head to the over-the-counter medicine section. Locate a package of Benadryl® brand of allergy medicine. Make note of the active ingredient(s) and amount (dose) per tablet or capsule, and instructions for the user (including warnings and precautions). Bring the package to the sleep-aid section and find a box of Nytol® brand sleep aid. Compare the information on the two packages—not just the "what's it for" on the front of the box, but also information on the other sides, including ingredients, doses, cautions, and the like. If there are store-brand alternatives to these two medications on the shelves, take a look at their package labels too.

What did you find?

What might happen if a person with an allergy and a touch of insomnia takes a dose of both medications at the same time?

Could a person with mild allergy symptoms take Nytol® if it were available and there were no Benadryl® handy? Would the outcome of taking Nytol(R) be any different than taking Benadryl(R), and if so, how or why?

What potentially problematic side effect is likely to occur if the allergy sufferer took some Benadryl® in the morning before heading off to school or work?

5. In your text, in a drug reference book, or on the Internet, look up the generic name, dose, and indications for the brand-name product Serafem, which is labeled as indicated for managing premenstrual dysphoric disorder. Do the same for the proprietary drug, Prozac, for which the main label use (but not the only use) is management of depression.

What does this tell you about how some drugs are marketed and about how some drug manufacturers can find not only new uses for "old" drugs,

but also legitimate ways to keep a revenue stream by patenting new uses for existing medications? (See also item 6, right below.)

6. Apropos item 5, what are "unlabeled uses" for a drug? Any idea how many unlabeled uses there are for the active ingredient in the brand-name product Prozac?

7. Here are three brand-name drugs: Celexa, Cerebyx, Celebrex. Pronounce them out loud. Imagine you are taking an oral order for one of these from a physician who doesn't speak clearly or who has just as much trouble pronouncing them as you may. Imagine that your hearing is "just a little off."

Write the names in script, perhaps trying to use the notoriously poor penmanship that is typical of many people (healthcare providers included).

Now, using your preferred information source (the text, a drug handbook the Web), look up the generic names of each of these products and the main approved uses for each.

What potential problems do you see? What steps could be avoided to eliminate, or at least drastically reduce, the problem(s)?

8. Pick any drug handbook and grab a copy of the *Physician's Desk Reference (PDR)* too. It makes no difference which year. Flip through the pages. What do you find? Give your thoughts about whether these are good tools for a "newbie" learning about pharmacology and drug therapy, and why.

Pharmacokinetics

KEY TERMS

absorption
bioavailability
bioequivalence
bound (or unbound or "free") drug
cytochrome P450 system
distribution
enteric-coated (drug preparation)
enterohepatic recirculation
excretion
first-pass effect
half-life
hydrophilic (and hydrophobic)
induction (of drug metabolism)
infusion (of drug)
lipophilic
maintenance dose (of drug)
metabolism
minimum effective concentration (of drug in plasma or blood)
parenteral
pharmacokinetics
plateau (of drug effect or plasma/blood level)
polar (and nonpolar)
prodrug
quaternary
therapeutic range (of drug concentration in plasma or blood)

OBJECTIVES

After reading and studying this chapter you should be able to:

1. List and briefly describe the four main processes that make up pharmacokinetics, and state why knowing about the pharmacokinetics of a drug is clinically useful.
2. Identify the advantages and disadvantages of the various techniques of drug administration as they relate to pharmacokinetics. Focus on oral, intramuscular, intravenous, and topical administration.
3. Discuss the main process by which most drugs move across cell membranes and the characteristics of drug molecules that either facilitate or hinder their ability to do that.
4. Describe the ultimate goal of drug metabolism, the general processes that are involved in it, and where (anatomically) most of the body's drug metabolizing activity goes on.
5. Given the half-life of a drug, state how you can estimate how long it will take blood levels of that drug to reach a steady state with repeated admin-

istration at specified dosages and intervals; state how you can calculate how much of a drug is left in the bloodstream at specified intervals once administration of that drug is stopped. State the other conditions that must be met for your estimate or calculations to be reasonably correct.
6. Explain the consequences of drug blood levels that fluctuate considerably, or erratically, between doses; be able to describe how to assess for the likely cause(s) of such fluctuations and how we might modify the therapeutic plan to eliminate or at least reduce them.

CRITICAL THINKING AND STUDY QUESTIONS

1. Your patient has just begun treatment with a new drug that has a half-life of 12 hours. If he takes the same dose every day, about how long will it taker average plasma drug levels to reach a plateau, or what is also known as a steady state blood levels? Besides taking the same dose each day, what conditions must be met in order for the way that you calculate your answer to apply?

2. Mr. Smith, who is an efficiency expert at a major corporation, is started on a new medication having a half-life of 12 hours. The instructions advise him to take 2 tablets every 12 hours. Assume (pretend) that all the drug is absorbed instantaneously after it is ingested.

   Wanting to be more efficient, he decides to take 4 tablets every 24 hours, which makes it the same total dose per 24 hours. What are the likely impacts of this change on the time it will take average plasma drug levels to reach a plateau, peak blood levels (those measured right after the dose is taken), and trough

6

(minimum) blood levels (those measured right before the next dose)?

3. Assume blood levels of a drug have reached a steady state, the reason for giving the drug is no longer there (the patient is "cured" or the signs and symptoms for which the drug was originally given are gone), and so drug administration is stopped. How much drug will be left in the system at the end of three half-lives? To make your life simpler, assume that at the time the drug is stopped the blood concentration is 100 fg/mL (micrograms/milliliter), and the drug has a half-life of 6 hours.

4. State and describe some of the most common factors that affect drug absorption. To simplify things, focus on oral administration.

5. Compare and contrast some risks and benefits associated with the various routes of administration of a drug. To simplify things, focus on intravenous, intramuscular, and oral administration routes.

6. A patient is having blood levels tested at specified intervals to follow the plasma levels of a drug he is taking. The results show that the levels are not remaining stable. What could be done with dosing amounts or times to help control wide fluctuations?

7. Explain the clinically significant difference between a narrow (or small) and a wide (or large) therapeutic range (margin of safety) for drugs.

8. The bioavailability of Drug X, taken orally, is 10%. What does that mean, and what factors can affect the bioavailability of this, or just about any other, drug.

9. What is one way to "guarantee" that a drug is 100% bioavailable?

10. Imagine you are helping with a pharmacokinetics study of a new drug. Assume your study subject (who is absolutely healthy and normal) will first receive an oral dose of the agent. Then, at some later time when all the effects of the initial dose have disappeared permanently (and all of the previous dose has been eliminated), the pharmacokinetics of the same dose of the same drug is evaluated after intravenous injection.

   For the following, assume that the drug must enter the bloodstream to cause an effect, and realize that the concentration of drug in the bloodstream is related to the intensity of its effects. You pick the hypothetical effect, so long as it's something you can measure easily and accurately.

   Now, comparing oral and IV administration, which of the following will differ depending on the administration route, and why?

A. Time to the onset of the measurable effect

F. The drug's plasma half-life

B. The intensity of the effect and how long it will take to occur

11. A test subject is given an IV injection of a drug that is eliminated by renal excretion. It is filtered and undergoes tubular secretion, and in the normally acidic urine most of the drug molecules are nonionized (because of local pH). Some time after the injection is given the urine is collected and the concentration of drug is measured. It is found to be 100 units per milliliter of urine.

The experiment is repeated. This time, however, the subject ingests some sodium bicarbonate (baking soda), which alkalinizes the urine and shifts urine pH to the alkaline range. Now, because of the pH change, most of the drug molecules in the urine are in the ionized form.

Assuming nothing else changes, will the concentration of the drug in the urine be equal to, less than, or more than the "control" value of 100 units per milliliter of urine. Why? What might the results of this experiment tell you about how this hypothetical drug is "handled" by the kidneys?

C. The drug's minimum effective concentration

D. Therapeutic range

E. How the drug is eliminated from the body (e.g., metabolized or excreted) *after* it has reached the systemic circulation

evolve To check your answers, go to http://evolve.elsevier.com/Lehne/ for Study Guide Comments from the author.

Pharmacodynamics

KEY TERMS

affinity
agonist
antagonist, antagonism
competitive
    (surmountable)
dose-response
    relationship (or dose-
    response curve)
ED_{50}
Efficacy
intrinsic activity

LD_{50}
noncompetitive
    antagonist/antagonism
pharmacodynamics
potency
receptor
safety
selectivity (of drug
    action)
therapeutic index

OBJECTIVES

After reading and studying this chapter you should be able to:

1. Discuss the mechanisms of pharmacodynamics.
2. Describe the reason that the typical dose-response curve looks the way it does.
3. Explain the differences among affinity, efficacy, and potency.
4. Describe how receptors function in response to many drugs and physiologic processes, such as activity of the nervous and endocrine systems.
5. Explain the differences among drugs that are agonists, partial agonists, or antagonists.
6. List the four primary families of receptors.
7. Define ED_{50} and LD_{50}.
8. Explain the differences among desensitization ("down-regulation") and hypersensitivity ("up-regulation" or supersensitivity) as they apply to the responses to drugs and the receptors they act on.
9. State how you would translate the concept of a drug's therapeutic index into practical use, such as the relationships between the dose of a drug and its effects—whether it's subtherapeutic (inadequate), therapeutic (desired responses), or toxic (adverse effects related to excessive dosage).

CRITICAL THINKING AND STUDY QUESTIONS

1. Define **pharmacodynamics.**

2. You have two patients who are obtaining equal pain relief from two different drugs. The first patient is receiving Drug X ordered at 50 mg, and the second patient is receiving Drug Y ordered at 5 mg. What does this probably tell you about the two drugs?

3. Describe the relationships among affinity, efficacy, intrinsic activity, and potency. How do these terms relate to whether a drug is an agonist or an antagonist?

4. What are the differences and similarities among an agonist, an antagonist, and a partial agonist if they all act on the same type of receptor?

9

5. Define ED_{50} as it applies to agonists.

Which drug is most efficacious?
Which is most potent?
Which has the greatest therapeutic index (or margin of safety)?
Which is safer to administer?
Which causes the fewest side effects?

6. Here are data for two pain-relieving drugs used to manage severe postoperative pain. Both are able to relieve pain completely, provided the proper dosage is given.

Drug A ED_{50} = 10 mg LD_{50} = 500 mg
Drug B ED_{50} = 1 mg LD_{50} = 20 mg

7. Identify some clinical implications of interpatient variations (variations from one patient to another) with regard to drug responses.

evolve To check your answers, go to http://evolve.elsevier.com/Lehne/ for Study Guide Comments from the author.

Drug Interactions

KEY TERMS

cytochrome P450
  (CYP) system
grapefruit juice effect
induction (of drug
  metabolism)

pharmacodynamic drug
  interaction
pharmacokinetic drug
  interaction

OBJECTIVES

After reading and studying this chapter you should
be able to:

1. Recognize the term *cytochrome P450 (CYP...)
   system* as the liver's main drug-metabolizing
   enzyme system and one that is a main target of or
   participant in many drug-drug interactions.
2. State succinctly the main role(s) of drug metabolism. Focus on the liver as an example of a drug-
   metabolizing system, and explain why it is such a
   critical participant in many drug-drug interactions.
3. Differentiate between pharmacokinetic and pharmacodynamic drug-drug interactions.
4. Give some examples of drug interactions that are
   dangerous or unwanted and some that are actually beneficial. Although you might need a little
   more pharmacologic knowledge under your belt,
   you can probably come up with some examples
   based on your own experiences if you really
   think about it.
5. State the expected roles of the physician, the
   nurse, and the pharmacist in a "checks and bal-
   ances" system to reduce the likelihood of drug-
   drug interactions and increase the likelihood that
   they are detected early enough and don't become
   big problems. Does ultimate responsibility to
   avoid problems rest with any one of those healthcare professionals?

At this time it is probably not necessary to memorize
all the sample drugs that interact by the various

mechanisms noted in this chapter. You'll learn about
them in more detail as you work through the text. For
now, all you may need to do is simply understand the
concepts behind the mechanisms so that when specific drugs are discussed later you will understand
what is meant. Be sure to check with your instructor
for his or her expectations.

CRITICAL THINKING AND STUDY QUESTIONS

1. A drug reference you are reading states that one
   drug (Drug X) your patient is taking induces the
   liver's cytochrome P450 (CYP) drug-metabolizing enzyme. Your patient has just had a second
   drug ordered. It has a low therapeutic index and is
   completely dependent on metabolism by the liver
   for its elimination from the body. What might you
   expect from the interaction of these two drugs? If
   it is necessary for the patient to take both drugs,
   what might be done to change the therapeutic
   plan?

2. Describe four basic mechanisms by which drugs
   interact.

3. Your patient just started taking an oral antibiotic and has developed diarrhea of 5 days' duration. He also takes an oral anticonvulsant to control his seizure disorder (epilepsy). Should you be concerned about his drug levels and seizure activity as a result of the diarrhea? Once the diarrhea is controlled, what else do you need to be thinking about?

4. Your patient receives a prescription for a new oral medication, and the pharmacist has attached a label stating "Do not take with grapefruit juice." Your patient asks what that means. Explain it.

5. What's generally meant when instructions for an oral medication say "Take on an empty stomach"?

6. Some oral medications should be taken on an empty stomach, and instructions (e.g., on the prescription label) will state that. Sometimes administration instructions are more focused, saying "Don't take with milk or dairy products." On the flip side, instructions for other medications advise taking the drug with a meal or with milk. Why the differences?

7. Is it correct to say that clinically significant drug-drug interactions involve only two or more *prescription* drugs? Just about anyone can purchase over-the-counter (OTC) drugs (which, we assume, must be perfectly safe if we can get them without a doctor's OK). So, is it safe to assume that if OTCs interact with other drugs, those interactions aren't important? Can you make a reasonable argument to support the notion that, in some ways, interactions involving an OTC drug are more problematic than those involving only prescribed drugs?

8. You've learned in this chapter that antacids can interact with many orally administered drugs if they're administered within a certain time of one another or if they're taken together. One mechanism involves the high mineral (calcium, aluminum, magnesium) content of the antacids, which binds many drugs in the gut and reduces absorption. There's a recent trend in "modifying" many foods and beverages we can buy in the supermarket, and it may cause precisely the same interaction problem, perhaps to a greater degree than applies to antacids. Can you think of what that may be and make some conclusions about what might be done about it?

9. Can just one drug interact with itself?

evolve To check your answers, go to http://evolve.elsevier.com/Lehne/ for Study Guide Comments from the author.

Adverse Drug Reactions and Medication Errors

KEY TERMS

adverse drug reaction
allergic reaction
carcinogenic (effect)
iatrogenic
idiosyncratic effect
  (idiosyncrasy)

MedWatch
physical dependence
side effect
teratogenic (effect)
toxicity (of a drug)

OBJECTIVES

After reading and studying this chapter you should be able to:

1. Describe the groups of people who are at increased risk for adverse drug events.
2. Explain how and why adverse drug reactions occur, given the facts that (a) in order for a prescription drug to be approved for use it must have demonstrated and documented safety and (b) there is rather explicit printed information about such facts as doses, routes, interactions, and so on.
3. State the typical relationship between the dose of a drug to which a patient is allergic and the intensity of the reaction the patient is likely to experience if he or she receives that drug.
4. Discuss the measures that can be used to minimize adverse drug events.

CRITICAL THINKING AND STUDY QUESTIONS

1. The same dose of the same drug is administered once in the morning and again in the evening to the same patient. There is no change in the patient's overall health between the doses, and no other drugs (or anything else) that can alter the responses of this drug have been taken. Is it possible that one of the drug's side effects can be unwanted when taken at one of those times and desirable when taken at the other?

2. Two patients are receiving two regular strength (325 mg each) aspirin tablets by mouth every 4 hours for headache. One patient develops gastric distress, and the other develops shortness of breath and respiratory distress. Identify the type of reaction each patient is experiencing.

3. Your patient tells you that she was treated in the emergency room once for a "terrible reaction" to an antibiotic. What additional information do you need, and why is it important to get it?

4. Are the adverse effects of drugs confined to the structures or systems on which they exert their main therapeutic effects or to the organs mainly responsible for eliminating them (e.g., the liver, in terms of the site of metabolism, or the kidneys, the main organs of drug excretion)? In answering this, ignore allergic reactions as a type of adverse drug response.

5. A patient has signs and symptoms of toxicity (overdose) in response to a particular drug, but there's abundant proof that the dosage that was administered was well within recommended guidelines. What can explain this?

6. Many experienced healthcare professionals will say, "Don't be the first person to prescribe, or take, a new drug that has just been approved for use." What might they mean by this, and why do they believe it?

7. Virtually all hospitals, and many other healthcare agencies, have a formulary of approved drugs. Although there may be a dozen different drugs in a therapeutic class, prescribers working in that agency can write orders for perhaps only two or three of those many alternatives. Aside from cost, why is this done? What are the advantages to both the prescriber and the patient?

evolve To check your answers, go to http://evolve.elsevier.com/Lehne/ for Study Guide Comments from the author.

Individual Variation in Drug Responses

KEY TERMS

bioavailability
idiosyncrasy,
  idiosyncratic response
metabolic tolerance
pharmacodynamic
  tolerance

placebo and placebo
  effect
tachyphylaxis

OBJECTIVES

After reading and studying this chapter you should be able to:

1. Explain why the average effective dose of a drug for a population (i.e., the "recommended dose" that you'll find listed in many drug references) may not be the "right" drug for a given individual.
2. Differentiate between pharmacokinetic and pharmacodynamic tolerance.
3. Describe what bioavailability of a drug is and how it affects the actions of the medication.
4. Identify the major causes of individual (person-to-person) variations in responses to drugs, that is, differences in how various people respond to the same dose of the same drug given by the same route at the same time.

CRITICAL THINKING AND STUDY QUESTIONS

1. State at least four ways in which the very young (e.g., neonates and infants) and the very old differ in the way they "handle" drugs (pharmacokinetic aspects). Why do their responses to some drugs differ in intensity (e.g., unusually diminished or excessive responses to a given dose)?

2. What are the differences between pharmacodynamic ("functional") and metabolic ("drug-dispositional") *tolerance* to drugs? What is their common feature, aside from the fact that they, too, are variable from person to person?

3. How might **achlorhydria,** a condition in which there is a significant lack of gastric acid production, vary the effects of a drug that is administered orally?

4. Your healthcare agency is conducting a clinical study to evaluate the effects of a new drug. Your patient reads the informed consent form and notices that the control group will receive a placebo. He asks what this means. What is your response?

15

5. Three patients are given the same medication in three oral dosage forms: liquid, enteric coated tablets, and sustained-release tablets. Will the bioavailabilities of the forms differ, and if so, why?

6. The active ingredients for generic and brand-name drugs may be exactly alike and they may be present in exactly the same amount (dose); however, the bioavailability may be different because of the inert substances used in the medication. For some drugs this difference is significant. For drugs with a very narrow therapeutic index, what would you recommend if a patient asked to change from the generic to the brand name when it was time for the prescription to be refilled?

CASE STUDY

We do a clinical study with a new drug that is supposed to elevate blood pressure (BP). (Whether it is an old one or a new one makes no difference.) We have 500 people in our study. Their ages range from 21 to 71 years. Everyone gets the same dose of the same drug.

1. Two men, who happen to be identical twins, experience a 30 mm Hg fall of BP. For all the rest, BP changes range from no change to a 50 mm Hg increase.

   What is the most likely explanation for the responses of the two brothers? What is this very unusual or atypical response usually called?

Now for the remaining 498 people in the study:

2. Why did their responses to the same dose of the same drug vary from no change of BP to a 50 mm Hg rise? What *didn't* we account for in this study, based on the information we provided?

3. We now tell you that all the subjects in the study received the drug orally either 3 hours before or 3 hours after eating or drinking anything. Why is this important? Would eating right before or after taking the drug *necessarily* affect the intensity of the response to the test drug?

4. We look at our results again and find that half the people in the study were men. However, the average responses to the drug by men and women weren't statistically significantly different. What does this tell you, and is it surprising?

5. We average the BP responses of the 498 people (all participants but the identical twins) and find that the average BP change for all is 16 mm Hg, with a standard deviation of 2 mm Hg. We find that the few people who incurred no BP change, or as little as 7 mm Hg change (less than 4 standard deviations below the mean), were all very obese. What might this tell you? (You don't have to be a statistician to appreciate that being so many standard deviations below or above a mean for a group is a big difference.)

6. We look even more closely at our data, this time eliminating the responses of the twin brothers and the obese patients. We now evaluate the data and find that subjects older than 65 years have, on average, greater BP changes in response to the drug than subjects aged 20 through 40 years. What other age-related physiologic changes would you want to know about to help figure out why older people had a greater response to the drug?

7. You get the information you want about the elderly group and learn that all the elderly patients who have had excessive drug responses have normal liver and kidney function, even when compared with those of 21-year-old subjects. What might you conclude from that?

8. We look at our data even more closely and find that all the hyper-responders have low serum albumin levels. What should this mean to you?

9. If we were to continue investigating the possible clinical usefulness of this drug, would we want to keep the few people who had a 50 mm Hg rise of blood pressure in the study? I say no. Tell me why you agree or disagree.

10. We eliminate at-risk subjects from the study and give repeated doses (same doses) of the drug to our subjects once a day for 2 weeks. Gradually, their responses become less and less. What is this called? What might we conclude from this?

evolve To check your answers, go to http://evolve.elsevier.com/Lehne/ for Study Guide Comments from the author.

Drug Therapy During Pregnancy and Breast-Feeding

KEY TERMS

FDA pregnancy
classification
placental barrier

teratogen, teratogenic
effect

OBJECTIVES

After reading and studying this chapter you should be able to:

1. Determine why dosage adjustments for some drugs may need to be made once a woman becomes pregnant, as pregnancy proceeds, and possibly after delivery.
2. Make reasonable statements about whether or how well lipid-soluble and ionized drug molecules cross the placental barrier.
3. Discuss risks to the neonate and infant from breast-feeding from a mother who is taking drugs. Consider the health and well-being of both the mother and the fetus.
4. Distinguish among the categories (A, B, C, D, X) established by the FDA to classify drug risks to the fetus. Comment on what each category means in terms of fetal risks, the reasons medications are placed in one of the various categories, and the types of evidence upon which the classifications are assigned for each drug.

Note: This chapter contains examples of drugs that may necessitate therapy changes during pregnancy. At this point in your studies it may be premature to expect you to know all the nuances of the pharmacokinetic and pharmacodynamic properties of these drugs. You will learn that later. Therefore, in the questions below we focus on general pregnancy-related concepts and avoid asking specific questions that require more thorough knowledge of specific drugs.

CRITICAL THINKING AND STUDY QUESTIONS

1. You are administering a drug that is excreted unchanged by the kidneys to a woman who is 8 months pregnant. The drug is not teratogenic. Her dosage has remained the same since she started this medication 4 years ago. Given this late stage of the pregnancy, are there specific things related only to the actions of this drug that you should be anticipating and looking for?

2. The drug you are giving to your 2-month-pregnant patient is highly lipid soluble. What should this piece of general information mean to you when you consider administering this agent to the pregnant woman? Along the lines of therapeutic modification, what things might you discuss with the prescriber?

3. Of what should you be aware, in general, when a drug described as highly ionized, very polar, or highly bound to plasma protein (e.g., albumin) is to be given to a pregnant woman?

4. Your patient is breastfeeding a 2-year-old child. Her physician has prescribed a lipid-soluble drug for back pain. She did not tell the physician that she is still breast-feeding. What would you do in this situation?

5. Your patient, 7 weeks pregnant, comes in for her first prenatal visit. In the course of assessment you ask what medications she is taking. She tells you she is taking a blood pressure medicine. What additional information do you need in order to make a proper recommendation about this drug in light of her pregnancy?

6. Describe the main events in fetal development and maturation during the three main stages of gestation (pregnancy). How can each stage of pregnancy be affected by teratogens or other drugs that, as far as we know, don't have teratogenic effects?

7. Are teratogenic effects of a drug the only adverse effects we should be concerned about regarding drug administration during pregnancy?

CASE STUDY

Although this case study is hypothetical, it concerns a common problem encountered during pregnancy. We do not expect you to know all the answers at this point in your studies (so early in the text), we hope that when you look at the comments you will learn useful information that you can apply later.

Carol Smith, a 28-year-old woman with a history of severe epilepsy, is taking an antiepileptic (anticonvulsant) drug. She has been seizure-free for a full year on this medication. She becomes pregnant. Her neurologist and obstetrician consult and decide to continue it during pregnancy. You check a reference book and learn the drug is FDA Pregnancy Risk Category D.

1. You politely ask the physician about use of this Category D drug throughout pregnancy. He acknowledges the risk but says it's necessary to continue the drug. What might lead to his decision?

2. Now the obstetrician says that he's having Mrs. Smith visit her neurologist monthly during pregnancy to monitor serum levels of the drug. "It's necessary," he says, "to ensure that things are going well. Besides," he adds, "the neurologist will be putting Mrs. Smith on folic acid supplements to reduce fetal risks further." Why might this be done?

3. You do some further checking. You find that the overall risk of some sort of birth defect occurring in the entire population of children of healthy, drug-free pregnant women is 2% (2 per 100 births). With the drug Mrs. Smith will be taking, the risk is 3% with proper perinatal care. Is the 50% increase in the incidence a big and worrisome increase?

4. Now you're really interested and start reading avidly. You ponder whether Mrs. Smith might become hypertensive during pregnancy and require antihypertensive drug therapy. You see that a group of drugs called angiotensin-converting enzyme (ACE) inhibitors are widely used to manage hypertension. You learn that they're

wonderful drugs for persons with diabetes mellitus too, and you start wondering whether Mrs. Smith might develop gestational diabetes. It seems that an ACE inhibitor would be wonderful for her in two respects. However, you see that the ACE inhibitors are Pregnancy Category X. What does that classification mean? You ask the physician whether Mrs. Smith needs an ACE inhibitor or if there's something else we can give her to reduce the teratogenic risk—sort of along the lines of giving folic acid supplements along with the anticonvulsant. He says no.

6. Once mom reaches the third trimester the neurologist advises giving vitamin K supplements to the mom and wants to make sure the obstetrics team gives the baby a vitamin K injection ASAP upon delivery. You look up vitamin K and the antiepileptic drug, and you see that the anticonvulsant can cause bleeding disorders in the newborn, but it's not a known teratogen under the circumstances we'll be using it. Giving vitamin K as we described is a routine and important prophylactic measure. Why didn't we give the vitamin K from the outset of pregnancy, along with the folic acid?

5. Mrs. Smith remains seizure-free during pregnancy. She's taking her anticonvulsant. You now learn that the neurologist recommends increasing the dosage as she enters her third trimester. What might that tell you?

7. Mrs. Smith gives birth to a happy, healthy baby. She needs to continue her anticonvulsant, but wishes to breastfeed her baby. You look at Table 9-1 (*Drugs That Should Be Avoided During Pregnancy*) and see that Mrs. Smith's drug isn't listed. She's been advised to take her anticonvulsant (2 times a day) right after she breastfeeds. Since the drug isn't listed in the table, what's the need for this advice?

evolve To check your answers, go to http://evolve.elsevier.com/Lehne/ for Study Guide Comments from the author.

Drug Therapy in Pediatric Patients

OBJECTIVES

After reading and studying this chapter you should be able to:

1. Identify the main age-associated physiologic, pathophysiologic, and pharmacologic factors that contribute to the different ways neonates, infants, and children respond to drugs, and state how those differences could (or likely will) affect drug responses.
2. Summarize the main reasons that we might say very young patients are highly sensitive to drugs. In your summary, consider both pharmacokinetic (absorption, distribution, elimination) factors and pharmacodynamic factors that affect this apparent sensitivity.
3. Identify several classes of drugs that cause qualitatively unique adverse effects in children. (Here we are talking about different or unique types of adverse effects, not the general concept of increased sensitivity to a given dose of a particular medication.)
4. Given several pieces of information about such age-related factors as body water content, body fat content, lean body mass, and serum albumin levels, and state the properties of a drug that would make its actions, time-course of action, or other important properties, different from what you might expect in, say, a 20-year-old person.
5. Explain some of the ways that drug dosages are calculated (or estimated) for pediatric patients. State what is most likely the best source of advice and guidance on dosage adjustments for young or very young patients.

Note: The textbook chapter contains examples of specific drugs that may necessitate therapy changes for the pediatric patient. At this point in your studies it may be premature to expect you to know all the nuances of the pharmacokinetic and pharmacodynamic properties of these drugs. You will learn that later. Therefore, in the questions below we focus on general concepts that apply to the young or very

young patient, and we avoid asking specific questions that require more knowledge of specific drugs.

You will find identical or similar objectives and critical thinking and study items in Chapter 11, which deals with older adults. It's important to make comparisons between very young and very old patients. So, if you're pondering a particular question or issue in this chapter dealing with the pediatric population, think about the same question as it might apply to the elderly, and *vice versa.*

CRITICAL THINKING AND STUDY QUESTIONS

1. For each of the following physiologic changes, which are typically found in neonates, infants, and children, state the properties of drugs (chemical or physical) that make those medications particularly susceptible to the age-related differences. At this point in your studies you need not state specific drugs or drug groups; just focus on drug properties in a global sense. Assume we're giving drugs orally.

   A. Prolonged and irregular gastric emptying time

   B. Relative lack of gastric acid–secreting activity

C. Lower body fat content

Age (yr)	Dose (per 24 hr)
0.5–9	24 mg/kg
9–12	20 mg/kg
12–16	18 mg/kg
≥ 16	13 mg/kg

D. Higher total body water content

A. What information do you need to explain and apply these dosage recommendations in the clinical setting?

E. Reduced amount of serum albumin and of albumin's drug-binding capacity

B. Assume the dosages apply only to oral administration of the drug, not to intravenous administration. Assume further that they apply only to patients who are receiving no other drugs and who have normal kidney and liver functions.

   How might you explain why, for example, a child aged 6 months to 9 years should get nearly twice the dose of an adult when the dose is expressed in terms of milligrams per kilogram of body weight?

F. Immature activity of hepatic drug-metabolizing enzymes

G. Low glomerular filtration rates and renal blood flow

C. What might you conclude if the *intravenous* dosages for these drugs for the various age ranges listed in the table were equal when expressed in mg/kg body weight?

2. Why or how is the statement, "Very young patients are highly sensitive to some drugs" rather imprecise, if not naïve?

D. Without doing lab tests, how might you figure out whether age-related differences in elimination are results of changes in metabolism, excretion, or both?

3. A drug handbook lists the following age-related maximum maintenance doses of a drug that is sometimes used to manage asthma or other instances of bronchospasm. The total daily (24-hour) dose is to be administered as 3 or 4 doses.

E. The dose recommendation of 24 mg/kg/24 hours applies to a rather broad age range (9 months–6 years). Based on the general principles you should have learned in this and previous chapters (see Chapters 4, 5, and 8), is it reasonable to conclude that the differences are due to immaturity of drug-metabolizing or -excreting processes?

F. What is the "take-home" message that you ought to get by just looking at the data table we provided? What myth does it debunk? But do the data really say that, for example, if you have a 1-year-old child you give him or her a bigger dose of the drug than you'd give to an 18-year-old?

4. Probably the most widely used over-the-counter (OTC) medication for managing mild pain and fever in children of all ages is acetaminophen. Most of you know it by its most recognized brand name, Tylenol. In fact, most of you have heard the phrase "Take Tylenol" from a healthcare provider; perhaps that was said to your parents or guardians as a medication for you to take.

Although you'll learn much about the pharmacology of acetaminophen, for now let's ask a few basic questions that apply to administering this drug to the pediatric patient and that relate to the general problems of drug administration to children by their parents or other caregivers.

You'll find that many OTC products contain acetaminophen, both brand-name (in addition to the familiar Tylenol) and "no-name" or store brands. Look in your local pharmacy or consult a comprehensive drug reference book or website to see just how many acetaminophen-containing products there are (or how many there are on the pharmacy shelves).

Look carefully at the labels, especially as they apply to use for children of various ages. Check the strengths (concentrations, drug in mg/mL or mg/5 mL, for example) of drug in the liquid formulations. Look at the dosages in tablets or capsules. Jot the down numbers.

Now...

A. Can having so many different products and so many different formulations actually make it difficult for some parents or other caregivers to administer these products optimally and safely?

B. Virtually all these products give explicitly instructions about what dose to give, and how often, based on the child's age. But a more general guideline is to administer 10–15 mg/kg of body weight per dose, repeated every 4 hours, up to 5 doses per 24-hour period. Calculate the dose (mg) of acetaminophen to administer to a 15-kg child.

C. State why telling a parent or guardian to "administer acetaminophen, 10–15 mg/kg every 4 hours up to 5 doses per 24 hours" might be giving very *explicit and precise* yet totally meaningless or useless instructions.

D. So why is just telling a parent to "give your child Tylenol" not a wise or safe instruction?

5. We look up the dosage of Drug X, which is to be administered by slow intravenous injection (over 5 minutes) for a specific disorder. According to several references we consult (package insert, *PDR*, etc.) we find that it is 10 mg/kg of body weight for patients of all ages.

A. We need to administer this drug to a 10-kg child. Will the proper dose for him or her be 10 mg/kg? Why or why not?

B. The plasma half-life for an adult (≥ 18 years old), according to the reference books, is 8 hours, and we're advised to administer this dose every 8 hours. Can you assume that the half-life of this drug will be the same in the 10-kg child? After all, the dosage for everyone, of every age, is 10 mg/kg. What are the implications if we ignored a different age-related half-life? For the purpose of answering this question, assume that we have to give the drug repeatedly for 2 weeks.

6. Drugs do not readily cross into an adult's central nervous system (CNS). This is not true in neonates. What difference between the adult and the neonate makes drug characteristics more of a concern in neonates than in adults?

evolve To check your answers, go to http://evolve.elsevier.com/Lehne/ for Study Guide Comments from the author.

Drug Therapy in Geriatric Patients

OBJECTIVES

After reading and studying this chapter you should be able to:

1. Identify the main age-related physiologic, patho-physiologic, and pharmacologic, factors that contribute to how elders respond differently to drugs, and state how those differences could (or likely will) affect drug responses.
2. Describe common reasons for noncompliance or nonadherence that are particularly relevant to elders, and state some approaches to minimize those problems and improve compliance.

CRITICAL THINKING AND STUDY QUESTIONS

1. Why do we have to be particularly careful when using the term *normal* to describe physical findings, drug dosages, and responses to drugs by older adults? How can something that many people would call normal be abnormal?

2. Why are there more and more frequent (if not serious) drug-drug interactions with older adults than with any other age group?

3. You should already know (from studying previous chapters) some of the key properties of drugs and how they depend on or are affected by the main determinants or processes related to pharmacokinetics. For each of the following changes that are typical in older adults, state how responses to drugs (in general) may change; as needed, state the characteristics of a drug that would make it most susceptible to those changes. At this point in your studies you need not state specific drugs or drug groups; just focus on drug properties in a global sense.

A. Increased percent of body fat

B. Decreased lean body mass

C. Decreased total body water

D. Reduced concentration of serum albumin and of albumin's drug-binding capacity

4. A 75-year-old man who is taking no other medications receives an oral dose of a drug that is normally completely (100%) excreted by the kidneys. It undergoes no metabolism before it is eliminated, and so hepatic function is not at all important to how, how quickly, or how well this drug gets out of the patient's body. Moreover, and remarkably, this patient has renal function on par with that of a healthy 25-year-old! We have reliable creatinine clearance, urea nitrogen, and other pertinent lab test results to prove just how healthy his kidneys are.

   Will the plasma half-life of this drug be the same as (or very similar to) the half-life we'd find in the 25-year-old?

   Will giving this 75-year-old man a "25-year-old's dose" of this drug cause exactly (or approximately) the same response(s)—type, intensity, onset, duration, and so on—that we'd see in a 25-year-old? Give some reasons for your answers.

5. Which one pharmacokinetic process is altered in the elderly such that it accounts for more adverse drug effects (including excessive effects) than changes in any of the other three main processes?

6. Your 73-year-old patient brings in bottles of 20 different prescription and OTC medications and tells you she takes them every day exactly as her doctors ordered. How can we ensure that the desired (therapeutic effects) of each drug will be optimal and that no significant adverse effects or drug-drug interactions will occur? After all, the patient is following doctor's orders precisely.

7. Refer to the hypothetical elderly patient taking 20 different medications, as described in question 6, above. What would you do to lessen the problems that almost certainly will occur? Answer this question wearing two hats: (1) the professional nurse who has the legal responsibility to care for this patient, who is *your* patient and (2) the nurse who knows this individual not as a patient but as a family member, and you are giving her advice because she or someone in the family asked for it.

8. In an effort to improve compliance by simplifying the drug regimen, it may be possible for the physician to prescribe fixed-dose combination products: two (sometimes three) different drugs combined in one tablet, capsule, or other dosage form. Aside from simplifying the regimen, what are some other advantages of prescribing in this manner? When should this approach not be used, and what is one main limitation of doing this?

9. An elderly woman with very poor eyesight and a significant loss of taste (dysgeusia) is prescribed nitroglycerin for her angina pectoris. When this drug is prescribed in oral or sublingual forms and excessive dosages are taken, it can cause profound hypotension and reflex stimulation of the heart. But this woman is being treated with nitroglycerin ointment, which is meant to be applied to the skin (topically). She comes to the emergency department with profound hypotension and tachycardia one evening after brushing her teeth before going to bed? What happened?

Basic Principles of Neuropharmacology

KEY TERMS

neuropharmacologic drug   receptor
neurotransmitter   synaptic transmission

OBJECTIVES

After reading and studying this chapter you should be able to:

1. Describe the general steps involved in neurotransmission (synaptic transmission); state the elements or processes that need to occur, no matter where in the nervous system, for synaptic transmission to work.
2. Summarize general or specific ways in which drugs can modify the responses normally caused by neurotransmitters.

As you work your way through this unit, pay special attention to the various roles of specific neurotransmitters in some important and common neurologic and neuropsychiatric disorders. Get a good appreciation for how, for some functions, there must be a balance between the effects of one neurotransmitter and another that tends to cause opposing effects, and understand how altering one neurotransmitter imbalance with drugs that help a particular disorder may actually cause the development of others.

CRITICAL THINKING AND STUDY QUESTIONS

1. What must a substance "do" in order to be called or classified as a neurotransmitter?

2. List and succinctly describe the steps of synaptic transmission and activation of target structures by a neurotransmitter.

3. Given the overall organization of the nervous systems (central and peripheral) and what you ought to know about the various processes of synaptic transmission, how selective (or not) might the following pharmacologic interventions be in terms of causing their effects? Explain how you came up with your answers.

   A. Giving a drug that inhibits the ability of axons to conduct an action potential

   B. Giving a drug that inhibits synthesis of a specific neurotransmitter

C. Giving a drug that blocks release of a specific neurotransmitter

D. Giving a drug that blocks specific receptors that are normally activated by a neurotransmitter

4. Neurotransmitters are endogenous substances; they're made in our own bodies. Are there any or many endogenous substances that block the ability of those neurotransmitters to cause their effects on target structures—"anti-neurotransmitters," so to speak? For example, is that how ACh, which slows heart rate, counteracts the effects of epinephrine to speed up heart rate?

5. Acetylcholine and norepinephrine are great examples of neurotransmitters. Are their effects stopped, physiologically, in the same way? That is, is there one common process that stops or turns off the effects of all neurotransmitters?

6. Are there any neurotransmitters that do *not* work by binding to and acting on specific receptors?

7. We've talked about the need for neurotransmitters to be synthesized and released, to activate specific receptors on target structures, and to have their actions on those targets stopped by some process. Aside from giving or doing "something" to affect the nerves where we find the neurotransmitters or the receptors on which they act, are there other things that might happen to alter this signal-response process?

evolve   To check your answers, go to http://evolve.elsevier.com/Lehne/ for Study Guide Comments from the author.

Physiology of the Peripheral Nervous System

KEY TERMS

adrenergic (nerve, drug, effect)
afferent (neuron)
$alpha_1$, $alpha_2$
autonomic tone
baroreceptor reflex
$beta_1$, $beta_2$
catecholamine
central nervous system
cholinergic (nerve, drug, effect)
efferent (neuron)
muscarinic
nicotinic
parasympathetic nervous system
peripheral nervous system
post (pre)-junctional
pre (and post)-ganglionic
reuptake (as applied to fate of norepinephrine)
somatic nervous system
sympathetic nervous system

OBJECTIVES

After reading and studying this chapter you should be able to:

1. Identify the two major divisions of the peripheral nervous system.
2. Differentiate between the somatic (motor) nervous system and the sympathetic and parasympathetic branches of the autonomic nervous system (ANS) in terms of:

    Overall anatomic organization (numbers, types of nerves)

    Neurotransmitters made and released by the nerves

    The targets of (effectors) their actions, whether those structures are innervated by one or both branches of the ANS, and the effects of activating those structures
3. Describe the differences among the four main subtypes of adrenergic receptor—$alpha_1$, $alpha_2$, $beta_1$, and $beta_2$—in terms of where (on what structures) they are found and the types of responses they cause when activated.

4. Describe the differences between the two main subtypes of cholinergic receptor—nicotinic (both N_N and N_M) and muscarinic—in terms of where (on what structures) they are found and the responses they cause when activated.
5. Identify the basic processes by which the main ANS neurotransmitters are terminated (stopped) physiologically.

CRITICAL THINKING AND STUDY QUESTIONS

1. Figure 13-3 in your text is a schematic diagram of the basic anatomy of the parasympathetic, sympathetic, and somatic (motor) nervous systems. All the neurons shown are efferent neurons. What does *efferent* mean?

    In contrast, what are *afferent* neurons, and what roles do they play in control of the autonomic nervous system? (*Hint:* Look at Figure 13-2 and nearby text on page 99 related to feedback regulation.)

2. Look at Figure 14-4 in your text—the schematic diagram of the peripheral nervous systems (autonomic and somatic)—but hide the summary in the legend. Now, answer the following questions.
    A. How many neurons make up these various pathways (in the schematic), and what are their names?

B. Which are cholinergic (synthesize and release ACh as their neurotransmitter), and which are adrenergic (synthesize and release norepinephrine as their neurotransmitter)?

4. How is the way in which the ANS controls the activity of most body structures similar to the way you control the temperature of the water when you want to take a bath or shower? (This may seem like a silly question, but think about it.)

3. Read the following general statements and decide whether they're true. If not, state at least one major exception that justifies your conclusion.

5. You may be able to get a better grasp of how the two main branches of the autonomic nervous system—parasympathetic and sympathetic—exert control over key body structures and functions by combining *selected information* from Table 13-2 and Table 13-3 into one table. We've set that up for you here; in the table on the next page, fill in the blanks (and check the website for the answers to make sure they're correct). Then you can answer a few questions.

A. All preganglionic neurons are cholinergic.

B. All postganglionic parasympathetic neurons are cholinergic.

After you've completed the table, look at it and decide if the following statements are true. If they're not true, state why.

C. All postganglionic sympathetic neurons are adrenergic.

A. *All* the responses of target structures (effectors such as the heart, lungs, GI tract, bladder, glands, etc.) to parasympathetic nervous system activation involve activation of muscarinic receptors by ACh.

D. Epinephrine is the neurotransmitter released from the adrenal gland when the sympathetic nervous system is activated.

Structure (Location)	Cholinergic–Parasympathetic Control		Adrenergic–Sympathetic Control	
	Receptor on Target Structure	Response to Activation	Receptor on Target Structure	Response to Activation
Eye, pupil size	Muscarinic	Miosis (decreased pupil diameter; pupil constriction)	Alpha$_1$	Mydriasis (increased pupil diameter; pupil dilation)
Eye, ciliary muscle/focus of the lens of the eye				
Heart rate (spontaneous depolarization of the sino-atrial (SA) node [normal pacemaker])				
Heart, force of contraction				
Heart, rate of electrical impulse conduction through myocardium, nodal tissues				
Arterioles and veins				
Lungs (airway smooth muscle)				
Bladder and urinary tract				
GI tract tone and motility				
Secretion of tears (lacrimal glands), mucus (e.g., mucous glands in respiratory tract)				

B. *All* the responses of target structures to parasympathetic activation (i.e., the effects of ACh on muscarinic receptors) can be called "inhibitory." That is, when those receptors are activated the level of activity of the effector is reduced.

C. For all structures under control by the ANS, the effects of parasympathetic activation are the opposite of, and equal in intensity to, the effects of sympathetic activation.

D. Blood vessels (e.g., arterioles) will dilate if you activate the parasympathetic nervous system or inject ACh (which, as we know by now, is a good agonist for muscarinic receptors).

E. *A*drenergic nerves release *a*drenalin (epinephrine), which activates only the *a*lpha subtype of *a*drenergic receptor.

F. You can think of the beta$_1$ subtype of adrenergic receptor as the "cardiac" beta receptor.

G. As shown in Table 13-4 of your text, the sympathetic neurotransmitter, norepinephrine, stimulates alpha-adrenergic and beta$_1$-adrenergic receptors. Therefore, it would be a good drug to dilate a patient's bronchi (relax bronchial smooth muscle).

6. A. Think about what you do every day, and make a list of some autonomic reflexes—or other cases of autonomic activation—that occur. For the purposes of this exercise, focus on parasympathetic responses.

B. Looking at the list, what can you conclude about whether the parasympathetic nervous system is activated all at once or in a way that causes certain localized responses? Compare that with how your body acts in the fight-or-flight response that occurs with activation of the sympathetic nervous system.

7. Compare and contrast alpha$_1$-adrenergic and alpha$_2$-adrenergic receptors in terms of where they are and what they do when they're activated.

8. If you were to administer a drug that activated alpha$_2$ receptors (and did nothing else), would it look like the activity of the sympathetic nervous system was increased or decreased?

Muscarinic Agonists and Antagonists

KEY TERMS

anhidrosis
anticholinergic
   (drug or effect)
belladonna alkaloid(s)
cholinergic (drug or effect)
direct-acting agonist
exocrine gland

miosis
muscarinic agonist
parasympatholytic
parasympathomimetic
photophobia
xerostomia

OBJECTIVES

After reading and studying this chapter you should be able to:

1. State the responses that a muscarinic agonist would be expected to cause through direct activation of muscarinic cholinergic receptors. (Keep bethanechol in mind when thinking about this.) You should focus on the main "targets" of parasympathetic nervous system (PNS) activity: the eye, the respiratory system, the heart and blood vessels, the GI and urinary tracts, and secretory activity of exocrine glands (lacrimal, mucous, etc.).
2. State what cholinergic responses are *not* normally caused when usual therapeutic doses of a muscarinic agonist are administered; and state why those effects do not occur.
3. State the main side effects of a muscarinic agonist (e.g., bethanechol) and related precautions for or contraindications to its use.
4. Give several reasons that acetylcholine itself is not used for producing selective muscarinic-activating effects and why we generally turn to other drugs instead.
5. Describe the signs and symptoms of muscarinic antagonist (e.g., atropine) poisoning, how it is managed, and how and where such a syndrome can occur without actually administering any therapeutic product to the patient.

CRITICAL THINKING AND STUDY QUESTIONS

1. On the table on the next page, list the expected effects of bethanechol on the structures listed. Name the receptor type(s) on which bethanechol is acting to cause these effects.

2. You are preparing to administer a subcutaneous dose of bethanechol to a postoperative patient with urinary retention. What other medical problems should you attempt to rule out before giving the drug? What should you assess for in the way of adverse responses once it is given?

   NO PHYSICAL BLOCKAGE, TO URINE FLOW, NO BLADDER WEAKNESS, INCREASE BOWEL SOUNDS AFTER GIVEN. RULE OUT ASTHMA, CHECK BP NOT HYPOSESATIVE IF BLADDER IS FULL, URINE SHOULD COME OUT. ASSES FOR BREATHING OR WHEEZING.

3. What is the *direct* effect of bethanechol on heart rate—the one that occurs when it directly activates muscarinic receptors on the heart's pacemaker (the sinoatrial node)? What are the potential effects on heart rate of injecting bethanechol into an intact human being?

   A SLOWING HEART RATE. WHEN INJECTED THE EFFECTS DEPEND OF MANY FACTORS. IT CAN DIALAE ARTERIOLES, CAUSING ↓ BP, UNPREDICTIBLE HEART RATE RESPONSE.

4. Make a table or list showing the expected responses to an effective dose of atropine or another drug that has atropine-like muscarinic antagonist activity. State simply why they occur. Write your answer on a separate piece of paper.

Structure	Response to Bethanechol	Receptor Type That's Activated
Eye, pupil size	CONTSRICT (MIOS)	
Eye, lacrimation	INCREASED	
Bronchial smooth	INCREASED CONTRACTION BRONCHOCONSTRICTION	
Muscle tone	DECREASED ?	
Mucous secretions in airways	INCREASE	All RESPONSES REQUIRE ACTIVATION
Sweat gland secretions	INCREASED	OF MUSCARINIC SUBTYPE OF
Heart rate	DECREASED	CHOLINERGIC RECPT.
Heart, force of contraction	DECREASED SLIGHTLY NOT AS IMPORTANT	
Tone of arterioles	DECREASED RELAXATION/VASODIALATION	
Activity of the urinary tract and bladder	INCREASE TONE RELAXATION OF SPHINCTER	
Activity of the GI tract	INCREASE TONE OF LONG MUSCLES; RELAX SPHINCTER	
Skeletal muscle tone	NO EFFECTS.	NICOTINIC RECEPTORS BETHANECH CANT DO

5. Sometimes we use the terms *parasympath-omimetic drug* and *muscarinic agonist* interchangeably. In most cases that's OK because giving a muscarinic agonist causes all the effects you'd expect to see if the PNS were stimulated, that is, if we mimicked the effects of the PNS.

   However, can you state a response that *is* caused by giving a muscarinic receptor agonist that is *not* caused by PNS activation?

   Can you name a response caused by giving a muscarinic agonist that's actually a normal response to *sympathetic* nervous system activation?

   DIALATION OF SOME BLOOD VESSELS,
   ARTERIOLES HAVE RECEPTORS FOR MUSCARINIC

   INCREASE SWEAT GLAND SECRETIONS
   ARE AN AGONISTS NORMAL RESPONSE.

6. Why is it *not* entirely correct to make the general statement, "Atropine and other muscarinic antagonists block only parasympathetic effects and have no effect on functions controlled by the sympathetic nervous system"?

   ACH & ITS ACTIVATION OF MUSCARINIC
   RECEPTORS. ITS CORRECT THAT MUSCARINIC
   ANTAGONISTS BLOCK MAINLY PARASYMPATHETIC
   RESPONSE, BUT NOT ONLY.

7. Giving bethanechol, the muscarinic agonist, may lower blood pressure. Giving atropine, the muscarinic antagonist (muscarinic-receptor blocker), usually does not change blood pressure. Why?

   THERE ARE NO PARA SYMPATHETIC
   NERVES SUPPLYING ARTERIOLES.

8. All patients who are about to receive a muscarinic-blocking drug (or any drug for that matter) should be assessed thoroughly to ensure there are no other conditions that may put them at increased risk for adverse drug effects. But why should the elderly—and elderly men in particular—be considered at even greater risk for adverse antimuscarinic effects?

   MA DIALATES
   ↑ PREVALENCE OF GLAUCOMA, PUPILS √DIALATE PUPIL.
   ↑PROSTATE HYPERTROPHY   BLOCKING URINARY
   FLOW.

9. Given the sometimes unpleasant side effects of antimuscarinics, and even the possible dangers of those drugs for some patients, should you be concerned that your patient may find (and take) nonprescription (OTC) drugs with atropine-like properties? In what sorts of OTC products will you find drugs with muscarinic antagonist activity? Are drugs with muscarinic agonist activity found in OTC products too?

   ANTI HISTAMINES,
   MUSCARINIC AGONIST —
   NONE ARE AVAILABLE OTC.

10. The diagram below (you'll see it again in Chapter 17) shows the baroreceptor reflex arc that is activated to reduce cardiac stimulation (i.e., to reduce heart rate and contractility) when we give a drug that quickly and significantly increases blood pressure. What drug, discussed in this chapter, can reduce that reflex cardiac inhibition yet have no effect on the blood pressure rise that triggers the reflex change? ***Hint:*** Look at step 4 in the diagram.

    ATROPINE, OR ANOTHER
    ANTIMUSCARNIC DRUH.

CASE STUDY

Judy Jones was born in Southeast Asia 38 years ago while her parents were working in the Peace Corps. When she was 3, she returned to the United States with her folks. After college she earned her master's degree. For the last 4 years she has lived in a small rural town, quite far from a major city or academic medical center, where she runs the business offices in the local school district.

Seven years ago she began developing progressive symmetrical weakness and paresis (incomplete paralysis) of her legs, with greatest involvement below the knees. There is no sensory nerve dysfunction.

CV Control Center in Brain
PNS Activity Increases   SNS Activity Decreases
2
(+)   3   (−)
Baroreceptors React
1
4
Vasoconstrictor (α–agonist) raises BP
Heart Rate Slows Reflexly

1. Does paralysis of skeletal muscle (partial or complete) usually reflect overstimulation or understimulation of muscarinic receptors on the skeletal muscle cells?

SKELETAL MUSCLE CONTRACTION INVOLVES ACTIVATION OF NICOTIN RECEPTORS.

There were two initial possible diagnoses by her family physician. One, based on where she was born, was that she had had a mild case of polio that went undiagnosed and she now is developing post-polio syndrome. Another diagnosis that was entertained was myasthenia gravis. Both eventually were ruled out.

Ms. Jones's leg dysfunction affected her gait progressively, such that she required canes, then crutches, to get around with some ease. Then a new problem developed: urinary incontinence.

2. A. What are the main bladder muscles that activate micturition (voiding)?

DETRUSOR MUSCLE CONTRACTS TO INCREASE PRESSURE IN BLADDER. BLADDER SPHINCTER MUST RELAX TO ALLOW URINE TO PASS THROUGH

B. What are the effects of sympathetic and parasympathetic nervous influences on them, and which receptors are involved?

ACTIVATION OF DETRUSOR/SPINCTER INVOLVE PARASYMPATHETIC INFLUENCES.

C. Which branch of the autonomic nervous system normally exerts predominant tone (influence)?

PNS EXERTS THE MAIN RESTING CONTROL OVER BLADDER FUNCTION.

ALPHA ADRENIC RECEPTORS.

3. What are the main symptoms that fall under the general term *urinary incontinence* and what drugs are used to manage them?

OR (ALPHA ADRENIC BLOCKER)
RETENTION - CANT USE MUSCLE (MUSCARIC AGONISTS)
INADEQUITE CONTROL OF SPHICTOR (ANTIMUSCARINC)
DETROL

Ms. Jones moves to a large city for a better opportunity for employment that might meet her lifestyle and disability. Concerned about worsening leg function, and particularly about her bladder difficulty, she gets an appointment with another specialist. Although the leg paralysis progressed, there was no involvement of her torso or upper extremities.

The physician orders a magnetic resonance imaging (MRI) scan. It reveals that Ms. Jones has a type of spina bifida that often goes undiagnosed because its symptoms aren't apparent (i.e., they are occult, or hidden) until later in life.

Ms. Jones's bladder dysfunction presents mainly as an inability to retain urine—coughing, stress, and other common events trigger urine leakage. The MD suggests that Ms. Jones learn how to catheterize herself. She asks if there are drugs that she could try first. The physician orders a long-acting preparation of oxybutynin chloride (Ditropan XL).

4. How is this drug classified, and what drug presented in Chapter 14 might be considered oxybutynin's prototype?

OXYBUTYNIN IS AN ANTIMUSCARINK DRUG. ATROPINE COULD REASONABLY BE CONSIDERED.

The specialist referred Ms. Jones to an orthotist for fitting of lower leg braces, which should make walking safer and easier. She tried them for a while, but eventually stopped. She said, "Well, I could probably benefit from wearing ankle braces because my ankles are not very strong and my left foot turns in when I walk. However, I've been unable to find braces that are cosmetically acceptable to me and that I would be able to wear with decent-looking shoes. Ultimately she chose to use an electric wheelchair nearly all the time. She rarely ambulates. Realizing she doesn't exercise much, she doesn't eat much in order to keep her caloric intake, and so her weight, from rising.

5. Given the actions of the oxybutynin (or the prototype you identified in item 4, above), what other problems (side effects) might arise? Which would be a potential problem for any patient? Which would be inapplicable to Ms. Jones, or unlikely to occur, due to her age and/or sex? Which might be especially problematic for Ms. Jones?

↑ SWEATING, ↓ HEAT LOSS, GI SIDE EFFECTS, ↑ CONSTIPATION

6. You are working with a student nurse in the clinic where Ms. Jones is being seen. In reviewing the case with the student, you ask her whether the oxybutynin might actually worsen Ms. Jones's paresis, given its anticholinergic mechanism of action. What correct answer do you hope your student nurse will give?

SKELETAL MUSCLE ACTIVATION INVOLVES ACTIVATION OF NICOTINIC CHOLINERGIC RECEPTOR. ANTIMUSCARINICS WILL BE NO EFFECT ON MS. JONES LEGS OR SKELETAL MUSCLE.

7. Let's assume that Ms. Jones's diagnosis were myasthenia gravis instead of the spina bifida occulta. Would the oxybutynin have any desired or adverse effects on skeletal muscle function in that disorder?

INSUFFICIENT ACTIVATION OF SKELETAL MUSCLE ONCE AGAIN, THAT INVOLVES NICOTINIC RECPT & DRUGS WITH MUSCARINIC AGONIST OR ANTAGONIST ACTIVITY WILL HAVE NO EFFECT.

8. Do antimuscarinic drugs play *any* role in management or diagnosis of myasthenia gravis? How is that disorder normally treated?

ACETYLCHOLINESTERASE INHIBITORS PLAY A MAJOR ROLE IN MANAGING IT SKELETAL ACTIVATION AFFECTS.

evolve To check your answers, go to http://evolve.elsevier.com/Lehne/ for Study Guide Comments from the author.

Cholinesterase Inhibitors and Their Use in Myasthenia Gravis

KEY TERMS

(acetyl) cholinesterase
  inhibitor
cholinergic crisis
irreversible
  cholinesterase
  inhibitor

myasthenic crisis
organophosphate
  cholinesterase
  inhibitor
quaternary (chemical
  structure)

OBJECTIVES

After reading and studying this chapter you should be able to:

1. Describe the main effects of cholinesterase inhibitors on structures controlled by the autonomic nervous system (ANS) and on skeletal muscle; state the general mechanism by which these effects occur.
2. Compare and contrast the effects of the cholinesterase inhibitors with those of bethanechol, which was described as the most representative muscarinic agonist (see Chapter 14).
3. State the main clinical uses of cholinesterase inhibitors; state precautions for and contraindications to their use.
4. Recognize the meaning and importance of the term **quaternary** when applied to the structure of a drug; compare and contrast the actions of neostigmine and physostigmine in the context of whether they are quaternary compounds.
5. Simply describe (compare and contrast) the cholinergic crisis and the myasthenic crisis in a hypothetical patient with myasthenia gravis; be able to describe simple assessments that would help you distinguish between (diagnose) the two conditions; and state the rationale for using cholinesterase inhibitors to help confirm the diagnosis.
6. Describe the signs and symptoms associated with cholinesterase inhibitor overdose and the general approaches to managing it.

7. State the rationales for administering a cholinesterase inhibitor to a patient who has been paralyzed intentionally (e.g., for surgery) with a neuromuscular blocking drug; state which class of neuromuscular blockers causes effects that can be reversed by the cholinesterase inhibitor; state the other main drug that is given as part of the post-op reversal procedure, and explain when and why it is given.

Be sure to integrate content in this chapter with Chapters 14 and 16, the other two chapters in the *Cholinergic Drugs* section of this unit. You will find study questions about the use of cholinesterase inhibitors as a means to reverse intentional skeletal neuromuscular blockade in the next chapter (Chapter 16). Also be sure to revisit this chapter when you study Chapter 100 (*Drugs for the Eye*), particularly the sections on drugs for glaucoma.

CRITICAL THINKING AND STUDY QUESTIONS

1. In the table on the following page, write the expected responses to a muscarinic agonist (e.g., bethanechol, Chapter 14) and to a cholinesterase inhibitor. (Don't worry about specific doses; just assume that each drug would be given at a dose sufficient to cause the expected responses.) State why there are (or aren't) differences in effects caused by the two classes of drugs.

THEY ARE IDENTICAL
THE ONLY DIFF IS HOW EFFECTS OCCUR

BETHANECHOL - DIRECTLY
CHOLINESTERASE ← INDIRECTLY.

Structure	Response to Bethanechol (Muscarinic Agonist)	Response to Cholinesterase Inhibitor
Eye, pupil size	CONSTRICTED	CONSTRICTED
Lacrimal, salivary, sweat gland secretions	INCREASE	↑
Bronchial smooth muscle tone	INCREASE CONTRACTION BROCHIOS	↑
Heart rate	↓	↓
Activity of the urinary tract and bladder	CONTRACTION of BLADDER	⁀⁀
Activity of the GI tract	CONTRACTION OF LONG MUSLE	⁀⁀
Skeletal muscle tone	NO EFFECT	CONTRACTION BECAUSE ACh RELEASED FROM SOMATIC MOTOR NERVES.

2. Explain why this statement is correct: "Acetylcholinesterase inhibitors cause many effects, but they don't activate any receptors."

THEY ARE INDIRECT, HAVE NO ABILITY TO DIRECTLY STIMULATE (OR BLOCK) ANY OF THE RECP.

3. Neostigmine, and most other clinically useful cholinesterase inhibitors, has chemical structures that are called quaternary. Physostigmine is not a quaternary compound. What does this mean, and what are the clinical implications of this difference?

THE STRUCTURE MAKES THEM DIFF TO CROSS THE BLOOD BRAIN BARRIES. PHYSOST OMINE MORE EASILY ABSORBED.

4. Why is physostigmine useful for managing muscarinic antagonist ("atropine") poisoning, but neostigmine (and most other cholinesterase inhibitors) is not?

CHOLINESTERASE INHIBITOR WILL CAUSE ENOUGH ACH TO ACCUMULATE IN ANS & OVERCOME SIGNS & SYMPTOMS.

5. Assume you're not very physically fit and you attempt to run 2 miles as fast as you can. What will soon happen to the strength of your leg muscles? Why? How does this phenomenon apply to the effects of excessive doses of cholinesterase inhibitors on skeletal muscle?

YOUR LEGS WONT MOVE ANYMORE IF TOO MUCH ACH RELEASED MOTOR NERVES CANT HANDEL MORE.

6. Since myasthenia gravis signs and symptoms reflect what amounts to dysfunctional receptors for ACh, why do we not see what appears to be a reduction in overall levels of activity of the parasympathetic nervous system, which depends on activation of smooth muscle, cardiac muscle, and glands by the very same neurotransmitter?

PARASYMPATHETIC RESPONSE ↓ ACTIVATION OF SWEAT GLANDS VIA SYMPATHETIC NERVOUS SYSTEM

7. What is probably the most important contraindication to administration of a cholinesterase inhibitor, regardless of the purpose of giving it? To be a bit provocative, assume we're going to administer just one drop of an ophthalmic formulation of a cholinesterase inhibitor on one glaucomatous eye for the purpose of constricting the pupil and increasing aqueous humor outflow so that intraocular pressure falls.

ASTMA MOST IMPORTANT CONTRANDICTION TO USING CHOLINESTERASE INHIBITOR.

CASE STUDY

Jane Allen is a 25-year-old with complaints of fatigue and muscular weakness that get worse as the day continues and get better with rest. She also says that she chokes frequently while eating and that she has developed ptosis (drooping eyelids). Jane has a positive antibody test (AChRab), confirming the diagnosis of myasthenia gravis. She is placed on oral neostigmine (a reasonable dose of 30 mg 3 times daily), with instructions to come back for a follow-up evaluation in 4 weeks and to call the physician's office at once if any severe side effects occur.

1. Ms. Allen isn't quite sure which medication she should be taking. She only recalls the physician mumbling something about a "stigmine." In lay terms, explain what the drug is and how it works to modify the disease.

MED MAKE MORE OF THE CHEMICAL AVAILABLE IN ATTEMPT TO OVERCOME THE REDUCED ABILITY OF MUSCLES.

2. Ms. Allen wants to know what "bad" effects the drug might cause, and which might be the earliest indication that her dose is too much. How would you reply?

DIARRHEA, ↑ URINATION, WHEEZING, ↑ SWEATING, TEARING.

3. The MD told Ms. Allen that you would be providing her with a diary. She wants to know what kind of information she should record in it and how compulsive she should be in keeping that information. "Why?" she asks.

SHE SHOULD BE AS FREQUENT AS POSSIBLE. INCLUDE TIME OF MUSCLE WEAKNESS.

Ms. Allen's condition had been stable for 6 months and then she skipped routine evaluations for another 6 months. Then one day her husband calls the physician's office to report that she has become progressively weak over the past week; she doesn't have enough strength to go to work or shop, and even gets "tired" walking around the house. She's coughed many times trying to swallow her food, and she's "not breathing too well."

Mr. Allen brings his wife to a nearby hospital's emergency department for immediate evaluation. She hasn't kept a diary to help determine what might be going on.

Given Ms. Allen's history, she's probably experiencing either a myasthenic crisis or a cholinergic crisis.

4. Would merely assessing skeletal muscle function (tone, strength, etc.) give you any meaningful clues about whether Ms. Allen is experiencing a myasthenic crisis rather than a cholinergic crisis? Why or why not?

   NO, CHOLINERGIC CRISIS MUSCLE
   FUNCTION IS REDUCED BECAUSE
   OF OVEDOSE OF INHIBITOR.

5. What other clinical findings should you assess for to help make the differential diagnosis, and why?

   PUPILS CONSTRICTED, EXSESS SALIVATION
   LACRIMATION, SWEATING

   WHEEZING, ↓ HR, ↑ BOWEL SOUNDS.

In talking to Mr. Allen, you learn that his wife has been self-medicating for hay fever signs and symptoms with OTC diphenhydramine several times a day for the last 2 weeks.

6. How is diphenhydramine classificd? What is the significance of that medication in terms of Ms. Allen's present condition, or your attempts to make a differential diagnosis between myasthenic and cholinergic crisis?

   ANTI/HISTAMINE OTC, EFFECT
   SKELETAL FUNCTION, MAKES IT
   DIFFICULT TO MAKE A
   PIFFERENTIAL DIAGNOSE.

7. What pharmacologic tool is used to help finalize the differential diagnosis betwccn myasthenic and cholinergic crises?

   A RAPID - ACTING OR SHORT ACTING
   CHOLINESTERASE INHIBITOR, eg EDROPHONIUM
   IS GIVEN INTRAVENOUSLY AS DIAGNOSTIC
   TOOL

8. What response(s) would indicate a myasthenic crisis when this drug is given? Why would they occur?

   PROMP IMPROVEMENT OF SKELETAL MUSCLE FUNCT.
   ↑ ACH LEVELS, RESP OF EVE/GUT, BLADDER,
   AIRWAYS, SWEAT GLANDS

9. What is the main risk of giving this drug if it turned out that, indeed, Mrs. Allen was experiencing a cholinergic crisis? Why? What related precautions or preparations need to be taken before the drug is given? Will Mrs. Allen's recent use of diphenhydramine prevent making the diagnosis?

   ACUTE WORSENING OF SKELETAL MUSCLE.
   POSSIBLE TOTALY
   PARAYLSIS.

evolve To check your answers, go to http://evolve.elsevier.com/Lehne/ for Study Guide Comments from the author.

CHAPTER

16

Neuromuscular Blocking Agents and Ganglionic Blocking Agents

KEY TERMS

curare
depolarizing
　(neuromuscular
　blocker)
ganglionic blockade
malignant hyperthermia
neuromuscular blocker
　(blockade)

neuromuscular junction
nondepolarizing
　(neuromuscular
　blocker)
pseudocholinesterase
quaternary

OBJECTIVES

After reading and studying this chapter you should be able to:

1. Describe the anatomy of the somatic nervous system, the key transmitter and type of receptor involved in skeletal muscle activation, and what happens physiologically when those cell receptors are activated. Compare and contrast those characteristics with cholinergic and parasympathetic neural control of smooth muscle and cardiac muscle.
2. Compare and contrast the mechanisms of actions of nondepolarizing and depolarizing neuromuscular blocking agents, and state how these actions affect using one class, rather than the other, in specified clinical situations.
3. Identify three specific uses for neuromuscular blocking agents and describe monitoring and other measures that are necessary when they are used.
4. Discuss the main risks and main cause of death as a result of administering neuromuscular blocking agents; describe steps to manage potentially fatal responses.
5. Identify the class of drugs used to reverse the effects of nondepolarizing neuromuscular blockers, and describe the mechanism by which they cause that reversal; explain why pharmacological

reversal is not used when succinylcholine is the neuromuscular blocker.
6. Describe the etiology, signs, and symptoms of malignant hyperthermia, the drugs associated with a high risk of that condition, and interventions to be implemented should it develop.

CRITICAL THINKING AND STUDY QUESTIONS

1. What will usual pharmacologic doses of atropine, the prototype muscarinic-receptor blocker, do to activation of skeletal muscle? Why?

2. What are the likely *direct* effects of giving tubocurarine in usual pharmacologic doses on airway smooth muscle tone, heart rate, and motility of the GI and urinary tracts? Why?

3. Why is it essential to ensure, as best as possible, that a patient who is going to receive a neuromuscular blocker have normal serum electrolyte levels, particularly potassium and magnesium?

42

4. Some texts describe the effects of tubocurarine and similarly classified neuromuscular blockers as "stabilizing" skeletal muscle cell membranes and membrane potential. In contrast, succinylcholine destabilizes them. Can you envision how these descriptions relate to the mechanisms of action of these two distinct classes of drug, both of which paralyze skeletal muscle?

5. Explain the basic biochemical process that enables skeletal muscle to contract and then relax normally, and what becomes abnormal such that it contributes to many of the consequences of malignant hyperthermia. Identify the drug used as an adjunct, and explain in simple terms how it works on abnormal skeletal muscle metabolism.

6. A patient with no history of cancer has had abdominal surgery and develops malignant hyperthermia in response to an interaction between succinylcholine and halothane. She has to be admitted directly to the ICU. Given the negative history for cancer, how can she develop *malignant* hyperthermia?

7. A patient with a genetic deficiency in serum cholinesterase activity is given an "otherwise correct" dose of succinylcholine to facilitate endotracheal intubation. How would the response to this neuromuscular blocker be different from normal? What drug would be administered to reverse the succinylcholine's effect, and would that approach be used only for a cholinesterase-deficient patient?

CASE STUDY

We'll integrate material from this chapter (and several others) into the case study in Chapter 26 (General Anesthetics), just to give you an opportunity to "put it all together."

evolve To check your answers, go to http://evolve.elsevier.com/Lehne/ for Study Guide Comments from the author.

17

Adrenergic Agonists

KEY TERMS

adrenergic

anaphylaxis,
    anaphylactic shock

catecholamines

ma huang

mydriasis

reuptake (as applies to
    norepinephrine)

sympathomimetic

OBJECTIVES

After reading and studying this chapter you should
be able to:

1. Recall (e.g., from Chapter 13) the sites (effectors)
   where you will find alpha$_1$-, beta$_1$-, and beta$_2$-adren-
   ergic receptors, and state the expected responses
   from their activation by a suitable agonist.
2. Classify the following agonists in terms of the
   adrenergic receptors they activate, and the
   responses they will cause as a result of direct
   receptor activation:
       Epinephrine
       Norepinephrine
       Phenylephrine
       Isoproterenol
       Terbutaline
       Dobutamine
3. Explain the difference between direct cardiac
   (beta$_1$) effects of adrenergic agonists and reflex
   (baroreceptor reflex–mediated) effects of those
   same drugs, using norepinephrine, phenylephrine, and isoproterenol as examples.
4. Explain how each of the following causes effects
   on structures controlled by the sympathetic nervous system, comparing how they work with how
   a direct-acting agonist like epinephrine works;
   and state one or more clinical uses for each:
       Ephedrine
       Amphetamines
       Cocaine
       Monoamine oxidase (MAO) inhibitors
5. Identify the effects that are wanted or needed
   when a therapeutic dose of epinephrine is given
   for anaphylaxis—the actions of the drug that earn
   it the label "drug of choice" for anaphylaxis.

CRITICAL THINKING AND STUDY QUESTIONS

1. Compare and contrast the terms **sympathomimetic, adrenergic agonist,** and **catecholamine.** Do they all mean the same thing?

   [handwritten: 1.) ONE OR MORE EFFECTS]
   [handwritten: 2.) DIRECTLY EFFECTS]
   [handwritten: 3.) SPECIFIC BASES]

2. Sometimes we can use the terms *sympathomimetic drug* (meaning a drug that causes one or
   more of the effects caused by activating the
   sympathetic nervous system) and *adrenergic
   agonist* interchangeably. However, there's at
   least one instance in which sympathetic nervous
   system activation will cause a certain effect, *but
   administering an adrenergic agonist (of any
   type) will not.* What is that response?

   [handwritten: SWEAT GLANDS - (EXCEPTION)]
   [handwritten: SNS ACTIVATION WILL ↑ SWEAT]
   [handwritten: GLAND EXCRETION]

3. Giving atropine or another antimuscarinic drug
   blocks many of the effects caused by parasympathomimetic drugs or by activation of the
   parasympathetic nervous system. Since many
   structures are controlled by both the SNS and
   the PNS, blocking sympathetic influences
   would cause what looks like activation of the
   SNS. Can we then call an antimuscarinic drug a
   sympathomimetic?

   [handwritten: NO, MUST EXERT]
   [handwritten: ITS EFFECTS BY SOME PROCESS]
   [handwritten: THAT ACTS ON ADRENERGIC]
   [handwritten: NERVES;]

4. On the table below, write the names of the adrenergic receptors involved in altering the activity of the following structures and functions, such as when the SNS is activated or a suitable adrenergic agonist is administered.

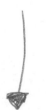

5. In the table below, put a check mark or X to indicate which adrenergic receptor types are activated by direct effects of the named adrenergic agonists.

6. Epinephrine can be used as a bronchodilator for patients with asthma, but drugs such as terbutaline and albuterol are used far more often, especially for outpatient therapy. Why might that be? Asthma-like bronchoconstriction is certainly a component of an anaphylactic reaction (e.g., a severe allergic reaction to a bee sting), so why is epinephrine the drug of choice for that? What are the other major life-threatening signs and symp-

Structure	Adrenergic Receptor That's Activated	Response to Direct Activation of That Receptor
Eye, pupil size	ALPH 1 ✓	MYDRASI PUPIL DILATION.
Bronchial smooth muscle tone	BETA 2 ✓	↓ SMOOTH MUSCLE
Heart rate	BETA 1	↑
Heart, force of contraction	BETA 1	↑
Heart, speed of electrical impulse conduction (e.g., through AV node)	BETA 1	↑
Tone of arterioles, veins	ALPH 1 ✓ BETA 2	ALPH ↑ BETA ↓
Kidneys (renin release)	BETA 1	↑
Liver, glycogen metabolism	BETA 2	

	Both Alpha₁ and Alpha₂	Beta₁	Beta₂	Dopamine
Epinephrine	✓	✓	✓	
Norepinephrine	✓	✓		
Phenylephrine	✓			
Isoproterenol		✓	✓	
Terbutaline			✓	
Dobutamine		✓		
Dopamine	✓	✓		✓

toms in an anaphylactic reaction—those that account for epinephrine's clearly being the drug of choice for managing them?

ASTHMA — BRONCHODILATION

ACTIVATION OF BETA₂

7. What are the expected effects of administering a drug that activates only alpha₁ receptors (e.g., phenylephrine) on blood pressure and heart rate? Briefly explain how these effects occur. (Don't worry about exact doses; just assume the dose is "enough" and assume we give the drug intravenously, so we don't have to worry about problems with how much drug is absorbed.)

BY DIRECTLY ACTIVATING

ALPHA 1 RECEPTORS ON

SMOOTH MUSLE OF ATERIOES

PHENYLEPHRINE CAUSE VASCONSTRICTION.

8. A friend who feels she needs to "lose a little weight" and get "a little more pep" asks for your opinions about taking a nonprescription product that contains ephedrine. Explain in simple terms what ephedrine is, what effects it causes (autonomic and in the CNS) and how those effects occur, and the possible side effects and related contraindications of taking such a product. (*Note:* There's not much coverage of ephedrine in this chapter, but what there is should be more than ample for you to be able to answer this question.)

EPHEDRINE, BEING

A NONCATECHOME

EFFECTIVE ORALLY.

9. Which class(es) or type(s) of cholinergic receptors (nicotinic, muscarinic) are activated by the following adrenergic agonists: epinephrine, norepinephrine, isoproterenol, and phenylephrine?

NONE OF ADRENTIC AGONISTS

ACTIVATE CHOLINERGIC RECPT.

10. In what types of over-the-counter (OTC) drugs are you likely to find that have adrenergic agonist (sympathomimetic) activity? Which of them include alpha agonists? Beta agonists?

DECONGESTANTS, ADRENIL, PESUDOPHEPINE-LIKE

11. A patient has a history of hypertension. He develops a cold and a profuse and bothersome runny nose. He'd like to take an OTC decongestant for a couple of days, and the ones that contain an adrenergic agonist certainly work well. Should he avoid such products "no matter what?"

THERE ARE SEVERAL ANSWERS TO THE QUESTION, SHOULD SOMEONE WITH HISTORY OF ↑ BP.

12. Take a trip to your local retail pharmacy or the OTC medicine aisles of your favorite supermarket. Look for several rather new products that are advertised as relieving nasal congestion, but labeled "for people with high blood pressure." (These may have such initials as HBP, high blood pressure, on the label.) What is the active ingredient in those products? While the medication in them may be OK for people who shouldn't take an adrenergic agonist (e.g., people with hypertension), it may not be good for people with other common disorders. What is the ingredient in those products? For whom might this ingredient pose risks, and why?

THE YOUNG & THOSE WITH ↑ BP.

CASE STUDY

Joan Armstrong, 23, was recently diagnosed with "mild" asthma, which seems to cause problems (periodic wheezing) only in the cold winter months. She also has an allergy to bees and wasps.

The physician prescribes an oral inhaler containing albuterol, for use "as needed" for her wheezing.

1. How is albuterol classified?

Ms. Armstrong has her prescription filled and begins using it quite often "just to get a good grip" on some flare-ups of bronchoconstriction she "knows are coming soon." In fact, she's using twice as many puffs of her inhaler each time, several times a day. That would be considered excessive.

2. What responses might Ms. Armstrong experience in the way of side effects—effects other than bronchodilation and the ability to breather easier?

Worried about side effects from the drug, Ms. Armstrong goes to her physician. She has no respiratory problems, but is obviously experiencing adverse cardiovascular effects. She's so stressed about yet another doctor's appointment that she takes many puffs of her inhaler right before arriving at the MD's office.

3. What would you expect to find in the way of Ms. Armstrong's heart rate and blood pressure (systolic and diastolic), and why do they occur, based on how the albuterol is classified?

Ms. Armstrong listens closely this time to her physician's instructions and pledges to follow them to avoid excessive use of her albuterol inhaler. She keeps her promise. A few weeks later, in the early spring, Ms. Armstrong goes camping. She's stung by a bee and develops all the signs and symptoms of what might turn into an anaphylactic reaction. She starts taking many puffs of her inhaler to help her breathe.

4. What are the main signs and symptoms of anaphylaxis? (Focus on the airways and cardiovascular system to keep things simple.) What beneficial or harmful effects might arise from Ms. Armstrong's use of her albuterol inhaler to combat this acute reaction?

A friend rushes Ms. Armstrong to the hospital. The physician considers Ms. Armstrong to be having a "mild" anaphylactoid (anaphylaxis-like) reaction.

5. What drug will be administered in the hospital to help normalize her signs and symptoms? How does it work differently from or better than Ms. Armstrong's albuterol inhaler?

Ms. Armstrong quickly recovers but becomes frustrated and concerned over her doctor's prescribing of albuterol for her periodic asthma signs and symptoms and the inconveniences of having to take so much time off from work to visit the MD.

6. If Ms. Armstrong goes to her local pharmacy to look for an inhaled asthma med that's classified exactly the same as her albuterol, will she find one?

Ms. Armstrong goes to her pharmacy and finds a nonprescription inhaler, advertised for asthma symptoms. Eureka! It contains exactly the same drug that she got in the emergency room when she had her bee sting. She buys it and begins using it, saying to herself, "If it worked so well when I had that horrible bee sting, it's gotta be perfect for me to use for my asthma."

7. Comment on the likely beneficial and adverse effects of this drug, knowing Ms. Armstrong's history and her specific plan to use it for her asthma on a long-term self-medication basis.

evolve To check your answers, go to http://evolve.elsevier.com/Lehne/ for Study Guide Comments from the author.

Adrenergic Antagonists

KEY TERMS

cardioselective (type of beta blocker)

chronotropic (e.g., positive or negative chronotropic effect of a drug)

inotropic (e.g., positive or negative inotropic effect of a drug)

intrinsic sympathomimetic

activity (ISA; of certain beta blockers)

orthostatic hypotension

partial agonist activity

pheochromocytoma

Raynaud's disease

rebound cardiac excitation

OBJECTIVES

After reading and studying this chapter you should be able to:

1. Summarize the main adrenergic receptor subtypes that mediate the ocular, cardiovascular, pulmonary, and uterine responses to sympathetic nervous system (SNS) activation.
2. Describe the main direct and indirect effects of alpha- and beta-adrenergic blockers (antagonists) on the above structures or on stated sympathetic and adrenergic responses. For each effect, state applicable precautions or contraindications to using such antagonists and explain the possible outcome if a stated blocker is administered to a patient for whom the antagonist ought not to be used.
3. Describe the physiologic changes that affect blood pressure and other aspects of cardiovascular function as the patient goes from the supine to standing position; explain the impact of alpha- and beta-adrenergic blockers on those compensatory processes.
4. Explain the practical clinical implications of classifying some adrenergic blockers as cardioselective and others as having intrinsic sympathomimetic activity. Describe when and why they may be suitable (or possibly better) alternatives to nonselective beta blockers (e.g., propranolol) overall and in particular for patients who may

experience adverse responses to the nonselective blockers.

CRITICAL THINKING AND STUDY QUESTIONS

1. When the entire sympathetic nervous system is activated, two adrenergic subsystems are basically activated at once: (a) the neural component, namely, increased activity of sympathetic nerves; and (b) an endocrine component in which the hormone, epinephrine, is released into the bloodstream. Are the two systems basically redundant? That is, are the ultimate effects of these two components—are the activities of the sympathetic neurotransmitter and the sympathetic hormone—identical throughout the body?

SEE THE ANSWERS FOR ADRENERGIC SUBSYSTEMS #14.

2. Sweating (increased sweat gland secretions) is one of the classic responses to widespread activation of the sympathetic nervous system. (Do *your* palms sweat when you start an exam you're not completely prepared for?) Since most of the responses to sympathetic activation involve activation of adrenergic receptors, which adrenergic-blocking drug would inhibit the sweating?

NO (AB) WILL INHIBIT SWEATING, ALTHOUGH THE RESPONSE IS SYMPATHETIC, HAVE TO GIVE ATROPINE

3. You are providing discharge instructions for a patient who has started taking prazosin for hypertension. How is prazosin classified? What side effects would you expect—those you should forewarn the patient about? Why do they

49

occur? What nursing assessments are involved in follow-up?

ORTHOSTATIC HYPERTENSION, REFLEX TACHYCARDIA, NASAL CONGESTION INHIBITED EJACULATION,

4. Where are the alpha$_2$-adrenergic receptors (in the peripheral autonomic nervous system)? What is the expected response when they are stimulated by an agonist, and what is the physiologic (endogenous, naturally occurring) agonist for them?

If we were to give a drug that selectively blocked the alpha$_2$ receptors (and did nothing to the alpha$_1$ receptors), what might the response look like in terms of overall activity of the SNS?

Now, how might this relate to the reflex cardiac stimulation caused by selective alpha$_1$ blockers such as prazosin compared with that caused by a nonselective alpha$_1$ or alpha$_2$ blocker such as phentolamine? Can you see why one blocker tends to cause less reflex cardiac stimulation than the other?

PERIPHERAL AUTONOMIC NERVOUS SYSTEM, ALPHA RECEPT.

5. A 73-year-old patient with benign prostatic hypertrophy (BPH) is prescribed an alpha-blocking agent. By what mechanism is this drug expected to cause symptom relief? Since it is given for its effects on the prostate, what if any side effects related to alpha-adrenergic blockade would you expect, and why?

↓ CONTRACTION OF SMOOTH MUSCLE IN THE BLADDER. ↓ PROSTATIC CAPSULE.

6. A patient starts oral beta-blocker therapy (whether it's for hypertension, angina, or a host of other indications makes no difference for this question). You do your teaching before sending the patient home, going over all the essential information including the name of the drug, the purpose for its use, the dose and how often to take it, expected side effects, and so on. What one other instruction *must* you give to this patient—one that is particularly important for beta blockers, perhaps more so than any other drugs—and why?

DONT STOP TAKING YOUR MEDS WITHOUT DOCTORS KNOWLEDGE. ↑ BP

7. Patient 1 has a routine eye exam, which reveals increased intraocular pressure in the right eye. The diagnosis is chronic open-angle glaucoma. This patient also has asthma that isn't controlled as well as it should be. Topical ophthalmic preparations (eye drops) of some beta blockers would be considered primary therapy for glaucoma. For patients with this mildly increased pressure, the dose would be 1 drop in the affected eye 2 times a day. Is a beta blocker a good approach for *this* patient, given his history? After all, the dose of the beta blocker couldn't get any smaller than 1 drop, and it's being applied directly to just one eye at 12-hour intervals. Explain your answer.

AIRWAYS OF ASTHMA ARE DEPENDANT ON BRONCHODIALATION EFFECTS.

8. Patient 2 has asthma too, but he has hypertension, for which oral beta blockers normally are a reasonable choice (see Chapter 44). Knowing that nonselective beta blockers are the ones that block bronchodilation, because of their beta$_2$-blocking activity, would you question a medication order calling for a cardioselective beta blocker (e.g., atenolol)? Why?

NO BETA BLOCKER SHOULD EVER BE USE ON ASTHMA PATIENT, UNLESS ABSOLUTELY NO ALTERNATIVE

9. Patient 3 has diabetes mellitus that is "reasonably well controlled." He recently had a heart attack (myocardial infarction), for which beta blockers are often prescribed long-term because they reduce the risk of a second (and possibly fatal) MI. What are the specific and general concerns for using beta blockers (e.g., for hypertension or angina) in patients with diabetes? Do those concerns depend on whether the beta blocker is nonselective, or cardioselective, or has intrinsic sympathomimetic activity? If so, how?

BETA BLOCKERS CAN ↓ BP GLUCOSE LEVELS.

10. A patient presents in the emergency department with severe hypertension and tachycardia. Unknown to the medical team, the problems are to the result of a massive overdose of ephedrine (ma huang; see Chapter 17), a mixed-acting sympathomimetic that under these conditions can cause extreme activation of both alpha- and beta-adrenergic receptors.

A. Knowing that beta blockers have antihypertensive effects and can slow heart rate, the physician orders an injection of a nonselective (beta₁ and beta₂) beta blocker (e.g., propranolol). What is the likely outcome? Why?

ACUTE HEART FAILURE

B. Would the outcome be significantly different if the physician chose a cardioselective beta blocker (e.g., atenolol or metoprolol)?

OUTCOME NOT SIG DIFF IF TO ADMINISTER A CARDIO SELECTIVE BETA BLOCKER

C. Would the outcome be significantly different if we used a combined alpha and beta blocker such as labetalol?

A MUCH BETTER OUTCOME. ↓ BP.

CASE STUDY

Jesse James is a 45-year-old man who is being treated for hypertension. His physician has decided to prescribe propranolol, 40 mg 2 times a day.

1. Mr. James wants to know what side effects he might experience from the propranolol. What will you tell him?

2. Why should patients be discouraged from abruptly stopping propranolol? Is this warning specific to propranolol or to any particular class of beta blockers?

3. You learn that Mr. James also has diabetes mellitus. What special consideration must be made when he is taking propranolol?

4. You learn that Mr. James has a history of asthma. Would metoprolol be a better choice of beta blocker for him? If so, why?

5. If Mr. James had undiagnosed hypothyroidism, how might the response to a beta blocker differ? Why?

6. Mr. James gets the message that losing a little weight will help lower his blood pressure. He asks about taking one of the popular OTC weight loss aids. You look up information about the product and see that it contains a fairly large dose of ephedrine. What advice would you give to Mr. James, considering he's taking a beta blocker for his blood pressure? What response(s) might he (and you) expect if he took that product?

7. The physician has considered the use of prazosin (Minipress) to control Mr. James's blood pressure. How is it classified? Is it likely to aggravate asthma, or diabetes, especially in comparison with a beta blocker? Why might this drug be considered for this patient? Do you think it would be a good choice for him?

Indirect-Acting Antiadrenergic Agents

KEY TERMS

adrenergic neuron-
   blocking drug
catecholamine depletion
centrally acting alpha
   agonist

Coombs' test
hemolytic anemia
rauwolfia alkaloid(s)
rebound hypertension

OBJECTIVES

After reading and studying this chapter you should
be able to:

1. Summarize the main mechanisms of action of
   reserpine, guanethidine, and methyldopa (or
   clonidine if you wish).
2. Compare and contrast the general sites and mechanisms of action of reserpine, clonidine, and
   methyldopa with those of drugs that block adrenergic receptors (e.g., propranolol, phentolamine).
3. Explain the factors that lead to, and the characteristics of, the "rebound" phenomenon associated with sudden clonidine discontinuation.
4. Use the effects of the drugs described in this
   chapter to predict how responses to the main
   classes of adrenergic agonists (see Chapter 18)
   would be affected.

CRITICAL THINKING AND STUDY QUESTIONS

1. When you administer reserpine, guanethidine, or
   methyldopa (or any drugs in this chapter identified as being related to them), the overall level of
   sympathetic "tone" goes down. What, then, can
   you conclude about how parasympathetic tone
   will appear?

   MANY BUT NOT ALL STRUCTURES ARE
   INNERVATED BY BOTH SYMPATHETIC
   & NONSYMPATHETIC.

2. Your text notes that the effects of reserpine,
   which are mainly due to neuronal norepinephrine
   depletion, closely resemble those caused by a
   combination of alpha- and beta-adrenergic receptor blockade. Can you think of one "sympathetic"
   response that would be caused by blocking all the
   adrenergic receptors but would not be caused by
   reserpine?

   BRONCHOCONSTRICTION WOULD
   OCCUR WITH ADMINISTRATION
   OF DRUGS THAT BLOCK.

3. What are the main adverse effects of methyldopa
   that have led some to state that "frequent usage is
   difficult to understand"? Are there any situations
   in which methyldopa would actually be a preferred antihypertensive drug?

   IT IS LARGELY UNIQUE. AMOUNT
   ALL THE COMMON DRUGS.

4. A. Instructions to the patient taking clonidine
      must include an explicit warning not to stop
      taking the drug abruptly. Why? What is likely
      to happen if the patient does discontinue the
      medication suddenly?

      WITHDRAWL MAY BE FATAL
      REBOUND HYPERTENSION
      PHENOMEN, ↑ HR.

B. What other class of drugs discussed in this unit require the same warning against sudden discontinuation? How does the clinical picture differ for clonidine withdrawal compared with the withdrawal from "that other group of drugs"?

DONT STOP TAKING WITHOUT DOCTORS ORDERS. NO REBOUND FOR ALPHA RECEPTOR HOWEVER.

5. Long-term administration of either clonidine or reserpine induces supersensitivity of alpha- and beta$_1$-adrenergic receptors. When clonidine is suddenly stopped after this has occurred, there is likely to be an episode of rebound hypertension. Does this occur when reserpine therapy is stopped suddenly? Why or why not?

REBOUND OCCURS WHEN SUPERSENSITIVE ADRENERGIC RECEPTORS ARE SUDDENLY EXPOSED TO NORMAL LEVELS.

6. You may need to review material from Chapter 17 (*Adrenergic Agonists*) to answer these questions that will test your understanding of how the sympathetic nervous system and drugs that can affect it work:

    Assume we have a patient on long-term reserpine therapy and, as expected, neuronal norepinephrine levels have been rather depleted.

    What would you expect, and why, if we then administered an "ordinarily right dose" of

A. Isoproterenol, phenylephrine, or epinephrine?

RESP TO ORDINARY 'RIGHT' DOSES OF ISOPROTERENOL, PHENYLEPHRINE, NOREPINEPHRINE OR ANY OTHER DRUG THAT DIRECTLY ACTIVATES (AR.)

B. Ephedrine (ma huang)?

HARD TO PREDICT THE RESPONSE TO EPHEDRINE.

C. An amphetamine?

HAVE NO ABILITY TO ACTIVATE (AR) DIRECTLY.

CASE STUDY

Since the drugs in this short chapter are used mainly to control hypertension, we will defer a case study until Chapter 44 (Vasodilators), so you'll have time to get a better appreciation of the approaches to managing high blood pressure.

evolve To check your answers, go to http://evolve.elsevier.com/Lehne/ for Study Guide Comments from the author.

Introduction to Central Nervous System Pharmacology

OBJECTIVES

After reading and studying this chapter you should be able to:

1. Identify the main neurotransmitters of the central nervous system (CNS), and summarize some of their main physiologic effects.
2. Discuss the significance of the blood-brain barrier in the context of how it allows, or prevents, effects of drugs in general.
3. Describe how, in many cases, control of key activities in the CNS involve more than one neural pathway, each with its own neurotransmitter and set of receptors. This is generally important for understanding much of the specific information presented in later chapters in this unit.

CRITICAL THINKING AND STUDY QUESTIONS

1. How do drugs that have a pronounced (or any) effect in the brain usually get there? How do they differ, in a very general sense, from drugs that have little or no CNS effects?

   BLOOD BRAIN BARRIER IMPEDES or PREVENTS THE ENTRY OF CERTAIN DRUGS INTO THE BRAIN.

2. By what two main mechanisms can the brain's response(s) to drug be altered?

   NEUROS CAN UNDERGO ADAPTIVE CHANGES DURING PROLONGED TREATMENT OF DRUGS

3. When you get to the chapter on Parkinson's disease (Chapter 21) you'll learn that one effective approach to managing signs and symptoms of this common CNS disorder is to administer orally a drug called levodopa. Once it gets into the brain, it's metabolized to the active substance dopamine, which is a critical neurotransmitter in the brain. If we give dopamine itself, the drug is largely ineffective in managing the same disorder. Why might that be? (*Hint:* Even if we were to inject dopamine directly into a peripheral vein, it still would be largely ineffective in managing parkinsonism.)

   LEVODOPA CROSSES BLOOD BRAIN GETTING TO SITE EASILY

   DOMPAMINE DOES NOT.

4. It's been said that the way the brain controls many important functions is analogous to the way the sympathetic and parasympathetic nervous systems control the functions of many organs in the periphery. It's been said that if you block the effects one branch of the ANS, you "unmask" the effects of the other.

   What might that mean? You might want to start constructing your answer by focusing on how the ANS regulates the activities of such organs as the heart and the size of the pupil of the eye.

   (Yes, you may have trouble answering this now, but it should be a piece of cake once you work your way through this unit.)

   SYMPATHETIC

   & PARASYMPATHETIC

evolve To check your answers, go to http://evolve.elsevier.com/Lehne/ for Study Guide Comments from the author.

Drugs for Parkinson's Disease

KEY TERMS

akinesia
bradykinesia
catechol-*O*-methyltrans-
  ferase (COMT)
drug holiday
dyskinesia

extrapyramidal side
  effects
extrapyramidal system
  (of CNS)
MAO (MAO-B)
on-off phenomenon
substantia nigra

OBJECTIVES

After reading and studying this chapter you should be able to:

1. Explain the interrelationships between the CNS activities of dopamine and acetylcholine as they affect the signs and symptoms of parkinsonism and as they relate to the general biochemical approach to correcting neurotransmitter imbalances with anti-Parkinson's drugs.
2. Discuss the drug treatment for Parkinson's disease and a current consensus opinion about which agent(s) are recommended for initiating therapy in most patients with this disorder.
3. Succinctly summarize the main antiparkinsonian mechanisms of action of levodopa, carbidopa, pramipexole, amantadine, and benztropine. For each, also summarize their main adverse responses.

CRITICAL THINKING AND STUDY QUESTIONS

1. What is the fundamental underlying biochemical imbalance that seems to account for the signs and symptoms of Parkinson's disease?

2. Looking at management of Parkinson's disease with just those drugs that act on the dopamine side of the dopamine-acetylcholine imbalance provides a marvelous overview of how medications that have very different mechanisms of action can accomplish one common goal—in this case, increasing dopamine activity in the CNS. So, to appreciate that beauty, state in simple terms how each of the following drugs acts on the brain's dopaminergic system:

levodopa
pramipexole
bromocriptine
carbidopa

entacapone
selegiline
amantadine

3. How might the use of antipsychotic drugs cause a clinical syndrome that is largely indistinguishable from idiopathic Parkinson's disease?

CASE STUDY

Stan Thomas is a 57-year-old man with a 5-year history of parkinsonism. He was admitted to the medical unit at 2 PM with the major complaint of increased dyskinesias. The family provides a history of progressive memory loss and episodes of hallucinations, dramatically increased incidence of dyskinesias and tremors, frequent nausea and vomiting, and mottled discoloration of the skin. For the first 4 years since Mr. Thomas's diagnosis, he was on increasing doses of levodopa and now is receiving 2 g 4 times a day. For the last year the levodopa therapy was supplemented with amantadine (100 mg 2

55

times a day). This treatment plan was prescribed by the Thomas family's family doctor. Among other findings, Mr. Thomas's resting heart rate was 110, and he reports frequent palpitations that are confirmed on his electrocardiogram. His resting blood pressure is 95/60.

Mr. Thomas took his last dose of levodopa at noon. The physician orders Sinemet (25 mg carbidopa and 100 mg levodopa) 2 times a day.

1. What was Mr. Thomas's physician likely thinking that led to the decision to increase the levodopa dose over the last 5 years? What was hoped to be achieved with the addition of amantadine to the levodopa regimen a year ago?

REASONABLE TO ASSUME
THAT DOPAMINE RECEPTOR
STIMULATION GAINED BY BOTH
DRUGS WOULD BE ADDICTIVE OR SYNERGISTIC

2. What might be accounting for Mr. Thomas's neurologic status, the skin discoloration, and evidence of excessive cardiac stimulation; and why is the overall therapeutic plan described above almost doomed to being ineffective and bothersome?

SKIN DISCOLORATION, LIVEDO, RETICULAR,
BEGIN & REVERSABLE.

3. What are the ingredients in Sinemet? What was the likely thinking behind the hospital physician's decision to add Sinemet to the treatment plan? Based on information presented in the scenario, why does this decision appear to be potentially dangerous?

COMBINATION PRODUCT
CONTAINING LEVODOPA &
CARBIDOPA.

4. Might it be more productive for the hospital physician to prescribe selegiline (MAO-B) inhibitor instead of the Sinemet?

SHOULD BE ADMINISTERED
WITH GREAT CARE. WITH
A PATIENT WHO IS
ALREADY ON LEVODOPA.

evolve To check your answers, go to http://evolve.elsevier.com/Lehne/ for Study Guide Comments from the author.

Alzheimer's Disease

KEY TERMS

Alzheimer's disease
apolipoprotein E4
  (apoE4)
beta-amyloid

(acetyl)cholinesterase
neuritic plaque
neurofibrillary tangle
tau

OBJECTIVES

After reading and studying this chapter you should be able to:

1. Summarize the main neural pathologic changes involved in the etiology of Alzheimer's disease (e.g., formation of neuritic plaques and neurofibrillary tangles, and what they are), and the main neurotransmitter deficiency that seems to account for most of the signs and symptoms.
2. Summarize the main signs and symptoms of Alzheimer's disease and the main risk factors for developing it.
3. Identify (acetyl)cholinesterase inhibitors as the current main drug class for managing Alzheimer's disease. State the main mechanism by which these drugs seem to confer some symptom relief in Alzheimer's; summarize whether they seem to be of short- or long-term benefit, providing symptomatic relief or a true cure. Use donepezil as your example drug.
4. State the main properties of donepezil that usually make it a good first choice to treat for Alzheimer's disease. Conversely, summarize one or two key reasons that tacrine is not a preferred agent.
5. Comment on the current status of vitamin E, selegline (also see Chapter 21), and nonsteroidal anti-inflammatory drugs as agents that might relieve, delay the progression of, or "protect against" the development of Alzheimer's.

Notes: You should ask your instructor precisely what he or she expects you to know about the pathophysiology of Alzheimer's disease (AD) because that is the main new content in this text chapter. (I would consider what I've listed above for objectives 1 and 2 to be suitable.)

In terms of drug therapy (the focus of this study guide), you should emphasize the actions and uses of the cholinesterase inhibitors. You should refer to Chapter 15 (*Cholinesterase Inhibitors and Their Use in Myasthenia Gravis*) as needed to refresh your knowledge about this class of drugs. Even though that chapter focuses on the use of those drugs for myasthenia gravis (completely unrelated to Alzheimer's disease), what you learned there about their side effects, adverse responses, and toxicities apply generally to the content of what you're learning about here. Indeed, I would consider that basic knowledge from Chapter 15 fair game for testing again here. That's why the *Critical Thinking and Study Questions* below focus on that fundamental information.

CRITICAL THINKING AND STUDY QUESTIONS

1. Given the main mechanism(s) by which cholinesterase inhibitors seem to slow the progression of AD signs and symptoms, can you think of any over-the-counter drugs that can interfere with (antagonize) the desired effects of those drugs? (To answer this question, consider only pharmacologic antagonism: actions of the interactant on the same structures on which the cholinesterase inhibitors appear to act. Ignore potential interactions—such as those involving food or drugs that act in the gut—that involve altered absorption of the AD medication.)

EFFECTIVE IN AD BECAUSE THEY CAUSE A BUILDUP OF ACh WHICH ACTS ON MUSCARINIC CHOINERGIC RECP,

2. What peripheral signs and symptoms would you expect if a patient took an overdose of one of the cholinesterase inhibitors indicated for AD? To simplify things, consider that the drug is *not* tacrine (which, as you should know, can cause hepatotoxicity in addition to the typical peripheral

57

signs and symptoms). Explain how these effects occur. State simply how you would manage them if they became acute and life-threatening.

All SIGNS & SYMPTOMS of EXCESSIVE PARASYMPATHETIC ACTIVATION, PLUS EXCESSIVE SWEATING.

3. Mr. Smith, an elderly patient, has recently been diagnosed with "moderate" signs and symptoms of AD. He will begin taking a cholinesterase inhibitor. However, he also has glaucoma. A colleague states, "Gee, the drug may be a help for the AD, but it's going to worsen his eye disorder." Would you agree, and why?

NO, IT CAN BE BENIFICAL ↓ INOCULAR PRESSURE.

evolve To check your answers, go to http://evolve.elsevier.com/Lehne/ for Study Guide Comments from the author.

Drugs for Epilepsy

KEY TERMS

absence seizure
breakthrough seizure(s)
convulsion
focal seizure
gamma-aminobutyric
   acid (GABA)
generalized seizure

gingival hyperplasia
hydantoin
postictal
seizure
sodium channel
status epilepticus
tonic-clonic seizure

OBJECTIVES

After reading and studying this chapter you should be able to:

1. Differentiate between a seizure and a convulsion and between partial (focal) and generalized seizures.
2. Name and describe three cellular mechanisms (i.e., those related to ion fluxes through cells or neurotransmitter actions on cells) by which antiepileptic drugs (AEDs) act.
3. Describe the general goals of treating epilepsy and some of the problems commonly encountered in reaching them. In your consideration of the problems, you should be able to articulate social and occupational factors, not just the pharmacologic ones.
4. Discuss important considerations related to selecting an AED and then monitoring its effectiveness (or lack thereof); describe the possible side effects or adverse responses and how to deal with them.
5. State the most common reason for "therapeutic failure" of anticonvulsant drugs, and steps that might be taken to reduce the problem.
6. Summarize the likely problems that must be assessed for, and dealt with, when the decision is made to discontinue one anticonvulsant drug and switch to or start another.
7. Summarize the likely problems that must be assessed for, and dealt with, when the patient who is already receiving one anticonvulsant drug must have a second agent added to the treatment plan.

8. State why, in general, most anticonvulsants are important interactants with many other drugs, regardless of their therapeutic classification.
9. Discuss the risks and benefits of administering anticonvulsants during pregnancy (as they affect the mother and the fetus and newborn), as well as any special assessments or interventions that are indicated for the pregnant woman with epilepsy.
10. Summarize a generally accepted drug plan for intervening in status epilepticus (generalized convulsive), and state why prompt suppression of seizures is essential, but "not enough" as the only goal.

CRITICAL THINKING AND STUDY QUESTIONS

1. What is the main consideration that goes into selecting a particular AED (or drug class) for a patient with recently diagnosed epilepsy? Why might a particular drug be considered "first choice," while others might be relegated to the status of "second or third choice" and used only if the first chosen drug doesn't work? Do appreciable differences in efficacy play a big role in selecting first-, second-, (or third-) choice drugs?

THE TYPE OF SEIZURE

PARTIAL VS GENERALIZED

CONVULSIVE / NON CONVULSIVE

2. What is the most common cause, overall, for failure of AED therapy? Related to that, what seems to be the main goal in developing new AEDs? Is it because most of the drugs available now (e.g., phenytoin, phenobarbital, valproic acid, etc.) simply don't work well enough for enough patients?

NON-COMPLIANCE IS THE MOST COMMON CAUSE OF AED FAILURE.

59

3. State several pieces of information that monitoring of AED plasma levels can provide, and why it's not the only way to assess the clinical response.

1.) ASSES COMPLIANCE, RULE OUT OTHER FACTORS, CAUSE OF TOXILTY, ADJUSTING DOSES.

4. What is unusual about the dose-response relationship for phenytoin (compared with that for most other drugs)? What explains it? What are the clinical implications in terms of titrating the dose of the drug upwards in order to achieve a "better" anticonvulsant response? What are the implications in terms of how quickly the drug's effects will wane, for example, when and as the dosage is cut back if toxicity due to overdose occurs?

IT IS EASY TO GET PHENYTOIN BLOOD LEVELS INTO A RANGE THAT SATURATES & OVERWHELMS.

5. It's always a good idea to assess liver function before administering any AED long-term. Why is it particularly important to do so with valproic acid and to monitor during the course of therapy?

VALPROIC ACID, LIKE MANY ANTICONVULSANTS IS METABOLIZED EXTENSIVELY BY LIVER

6. When rapid seizure control and intravenous drug administration are needed, why is there a growing trend towards using fos-phenytoin instead of phenytoin? How do these drugs differ mechanistically or otherwise?

THEY WORK IDENTICALLY IT IS MORE PERFERED BECAUSE IT IS COMPATABLE WITH IV

7. A patient experiences status epilepticus. You know that IV therapy is essential, but with the intense tonic-clonic contractions, how do you get that IV started?

NOT AT All AN INAPPROPKIATE OR FAETIOUS QUESTION GET HELP.

8. Why is it often problematic to take a patient with epilepsy off one AED and start another? How do we do it?

MAN PROB RELATE TO PHARMACOKINET. EXCESS SIDE EFFECTS!

9. Comment on the general issues of epilepsy, epilepsy therapy, and pregnancy (or the risk of conception). "Free associate," if you will, on these questions and concepts, and state why you've come to your conclusions.

A. Physiologic changes that occur with normal pregnancy can affect actions of AEDs.

TRUE, MORE OF AN ISSUE OF GETTING DOSAGE RIGHT.

B. Because of concerns about AED therapy during pregnancy, the simple prevention of the problem is to ensure the woman is taking oral contraceptives.

ST AS SIMPLE, CONTRACEPTIVE ARE METABOLIZED & NOT AS EFFECTIVE

C. Antiepileptic drugs are teratogens, and so they should be avoided during pregnancy.

USUALLY SAFER TO MOTHER & FETUS THEN DISCONTINUING

D. If a mother must take AEDs during pregnancy, folic acid and vitamin K supplements must be given.

FOLATE SUPPLEMENTATION IMPORTANT!

E. Children born to mothers who have received AEDs during pregnancy are at greater risk of having epileptic seizures later in life.

LITTLE EVIDENCE THAT IT IS INHERITED OR THAT ANTICONVULSANT MEDS = SEZURE IN NEWBORNS.

10. A patient develops status epilepticus, characterized by generalized convulsive seizures. The physician orders a "proper" dose of IV diazepam. In a matter of a minute, the seizures stop. Is that treatment sufficient? Why or why not?

EFFECTS ARE TO SHORT TO BREAK THAT PROCESS THAT LED TO STATUS EPILEPUS.

11. You and a colleague are discussing a patient who is in a coma after head trauma. She is receiving a neuromuscular-blocking drug (and other appropriate medications) to suppress her ventilatory drive and facilitate mechanical ventilation. She is, of course, totally paralyzed from the neuromuscular blocker. The patient is also receiving IV phenytoin for seizures. Your colleague questions the use of the anticonvulsant: "The patient's in a coma and totally paralyzed... she can't have convulsions, so why give the anticonvulsant?!" Comment on this.

ARE TO PREVENT SEIZURES AS WELL. YOU CAN BE COMATOSE BE ON NEURMUSCUAR BLOCKER.

12. When many new drugs are going through clinical trials, the manufacturers compare the effectiveness of the new meds with placebos. A new drug for managing status epilepticus is being developed, but no trials comparing it with a placebo are done. Why?

STATUS EPILEPTICUSK IS FATAL UNLESS STOPPED WITH A DRUG.

13. A friend with epilepsy has read a magazine ad about a new and presumably better anticonvulsant. She's seizure-free on her current medication, but asks you, as a knowledgeable healthcare professional, whether she should ask her MD to switch her. Your thoughts?

IF THERE ARE NOT ANY PROBLEMS NO NEED TO FIX BUT SHE COULD DEF ASK HER PHYSISAN.

14. Heads-up to integrate information from other chapters in this unit: Assume a patient has epilepsy and is being treated with an oral epileptic drug. Which other meds in this unit—drugs used to manage other disorders—might pose problems with the epilepsy control? Or, stopping the administration of which drugs might cause problems too?

*DOPAMINERGIC
LOCAL ANESHTEIA
NEARLY ALL CNSSTIMULANTS*

CASE STUDY

Sara Jones, a 26-year-old woman who is 8 months pregnant, is admitted to the neuro intensive care unit with a head injury. She was an unrestrained passenger in a motor vehicle accident, and she is unconscious. On admission, she is started on an IV of D_5 1/2 NS at 50 cc/hr. Within the first 24 hours on the unit, Ms. Jones has a grand mal seizure. Standing orders on the unit allow the nurse to administer diazepam (5 mg IV). The physician is notified. She orders a loading dose of phenytoin (800 mg IV) followed by 100 mg IV doses every 6 hours; cimetidine (300 mg IV 2 times a day) is to be started to prevent acute stress ulcers; serum levels of phenytoin are to be measured the next day.

1. Explain the necessary precautions when administering phenytoin intravenously.

*CARDIOVASCULAR COLLAPSE DILUTING THE DRUG IN GLUCOSE FREE SOLUTION.
PRECIPITATE FORMING.*

2. It's common to administer histamine H_2-receptor blockers (see Chapter 72) to critically ill patients such as Mr. Jones. The purpose is to reduce secretion of gastric acid, which can prevent the development of acute stress ulcers (in the stomach)—ulcers that can suddenly bleed and cause GI hemorrhage. The physician orders cimetidine, arguably the prototype H_2 blocker. Comment on the wisdom of this order for Ms. Jones. (Sure, go ahead and look at Chapter 72.)

NO REASON TO PRESCRIBE CIMETIDINE AS THE MEANS TO PREVENT ACUTE STRESS ULCERS

3. Ms. Jones's condition is improving to the point that she can begin taking oral meds. There's a concern of recurrent generalized convulsive seizures, so the MD decides to begin oral therapy with phenytoin. A daily phenytoin dose of 200 mg isn't quite getting blood levels into a therapeutic range (10–20 mcg/ml), and the patient's EEG reveals some evidence of seizure activity. The dose is increased by 50 mg/day, to 300 mg/day, and still blood levels are a bit low; there's evidence of brief seizures. It appears that a daily dose of more than 300 mg will be required. The MD orders a dosage change to 400 mg/day—an immediate jump of 100 mg per day. Comment on this.

SMALL DOSE ↑ CAN CAUSE SIGNIFICANT ↑ IN DRUG BLOOD LEVELS AND ↑ THE RISK OF TOXICITY.

4. The physician discusses the possible use of phenobarbital for Ms. Jones. Knowing that the half-life of phenobarbital is 4 days, when could you expect plateau to be reached with this drug, once we start giving it, and if a loading-dose strategy was not used?

½ LIFE 4 DAY, WILL TAKE 2–3 WK FOR PLASMA TO REACH PLATEAU.

5. If a patient is to be switched from phenytoin to phenobarbital, what considerations need to be addressed when stopping the first agent and starting the second? Are these "things to consider" unique to a switch from a hydantoin to a barbiturate, or do they apply in a more general sense to anticonvulsant therapy? What pharmacokinetic properties of the anticonvulsants are important in terms of how we make the switch?

½ LIFES, ONSET OF ACTION, & DURATION.

6. Because Ms. Jones is pregnant, and especially because she is near term, what other special considerations and precautions would apply to the phenobarbital and/or phenytoin use?

PHENOBARBITAL CAN REDUCE LEVELS OF VITAMIN K DEPENDANT CLOTTING FACTORS, & CAUSE BLEEDING.

7. Two weeks later, Ms. Jones and her new baby daughter have improved. Ms. Jones has been relocated to the neuro "step-down" unit. She's still taking phenytoin. The nurse finds a fine rash on Ms. Jones's trunk. What might this indicate? What should be done?

SKIN RASH, WHICH CAN PROGRESS & BE DIFF TO TREAT. MUST STOP PHENYTOIN.

evolve To check your answers, go to http://evolve.elsevier.com/Lehne/ for Study Guide Comments from the author.

Drugs for Muscle Spasm and Spasticity

KEY TERMS

GABA (gamma-
   aminobutyric acid)
malignant hyperthermia

sarcoplasmic reticulum
spasticity

OBJECTIVES

After reading and studying this chapter you should
be able to:
1. Discuss some basic differences between localized
   skeletal muscle spasm and spasticity (etiology,
   manifestations, primary and adjunctive treatments).
2. Explain the basic differences, in terms of sites
   and mechanisms of action, between centrally acting muscle relaxants baclofen and dantrolene;
   and state how these different mechanisms and
   sites of action relate to the drugs' clinical uses.
3. Be sure you are familiar with the etiologies, signs
   and symptoms, and management of malignant
   hyperthermia (see Chapter 26). Likewise, be sure
   you have a good grasp of the overall pharmacology
   of the benzodiazepines as a class (Chapter 34).

CASE STUDY

*Judy Jones is a 19-year-old woman transferred from
the neuro intensive care unit to a progressive unit.
She is diagnosed as having quadriplegia from spinal
cord injury caused by a diving accident. Among
other drugs, Ms. Jones's physician has prescribed
baclofen (20 mg 4 times a day) for her.*

1. What is the main reason baclofen has been prescribed for Ms. Jones?

2. Why would baclofen, as opposed to other drugs
   discussed in this chapter (e.g., dantrolene), be
   indicated? How is the drug likely to be working?

3. What are common side effects that the nurse
   should be assessing for during Ms. Jones's treatment with baclofen?

4. After several of months of inpatient and outpatient therapy, Ms. Jones's upper extremity spasticity is confined primarily to her wrists and
   fingers, and she has been fitted with orthotics
   (splints). She has an electric wheelchair, and her
   family has purchased a van with hand controls
   that she can drive. However, the baclofen is making her so groggy that driving safely does not
   seem possible. She and her healthcare team agree
   to discontinue the baclofen. What precautions
   should be taken when this is done?

25

Local Anesthetics

KEY TERMS

amide (class of local
   anesthetic)
ester (class of local
   anesthetic)
infiltration
   (administration route)

local anesthetic, local
   anesthesia
nerve block
   (administration route)

OBJECTIVES

After reading and studying this chapter you should
be able to:

1. Describe the physiologic manner by which local
   anesthetics work.
2. Differentiate between ester and amide types of
   local anesthetics in terms of mechanism of action,
   mechanisms by which they are eliminated from
   the body, and adverse effects (particularly with
   respect to allergic reactions).
3. Describe signs and symptoms of systemic local
   anesthetic toxicity, how to recognize them, and
   how to manage them.
4. State reasons and rationales for including a vasoconstrictor (e.g., epinephrine) in a parenteral formulation of local anesthetic. Focus on the
   time-course and intensity of local anesthetic
   action, toxicity, and allergenicity as affected by
   the vasoconstrictor.

CRITICAL THINKING AND STUDY QUESTIONS

1. Why is it incorrect to assume that local anesthetics affect only pain, only sensory nerve function?

2. Assume a patient has had a documented (proven)
   allergic response to procaine. If this patient
   requires local anesthetic administration again, say
   10 years later, why is it not suitable to use tetracaine as the chosen agent? Why is it likely to be
   much safer to use lidocaine or one of the local
   anesthetic's in lidocaine's chemical class?

3. What are the key similarities and differences
   between cocaine and the more typical local anesthetics (e.g., procaine and lidocaine)?

4. Comment on the following: "Epinephrine obviously is a vasoconstrictor, clearly a drug that can
   raise blood pressure. Therefore, local anesthetics
   that contain epinephrine are contraindicated for
   patients with hypertension."
   To simplify things, assume we are talking
   about this in the context of a hypertensive patient
   who has multiple but relatively minor lacerations
   on the arms and upper body that require suturing,
   and infiltration of a local anesthetic is indicated.

CASE STUDY

*Paula Kane, 32 years old and otherwise healthy, suf-
fered traumatic amputations of four fingers and part
of the thumb on one hand during an accident at
home. There are also multiple deep lacerations of
the hand itself. She is taken to surgery to clean and*

64

close the wounds. It is obviously necessary to anesthetize the area. Bupivacaine (an amide) is selected as the drug, and it will be administered by axillary block (in the upper arm).

1. When giving her health history, Ms. Kane states that she received Novocain during her last visit to the dentist (for a tooth extraction 1 year ago) and had a "very bad reaction" to it; "I thought I was going to die." She described the reaction as hives, severe wheezing and severe tightness in her chest and throat, and light-headedness. What are your interpretations of this information?

2. What adverse effects would be of concern using any local anesthetic, but especially when doing an axillary block? Which, if any, might be modified (e.g., lessened) if the local anesthetic contained epinephrine?

3. Instead of using a regional (axillary) block, would it have been appropriate to infiltrate all the wounds with a local anesthetic containing epinephrine to "boost" the anesthetic's actions?

Five days later Ms. Kane's stumps show signs of advanced tissue death from inadequate blood flow, and there is also evidence of infection of the stumps and hand. A plastic surgeon determines that her fingers cannot be salvaged. Because Ms. Kane would be left with no fingers or thumb, she would be faced

with little meaningful function of her hand (even if it remained viable) and would have a poor cosmetic result. The surgeon recommends amputation of her hand and a portion of her forearm for subsequent fitting of a prosthesis. She has done such procedures with local anesthesia and conscious sedation (see Chapter 34) before, rather than using general anesthesia. Ms. Kane consents and returns to the operating room for the surgery.

4. Would it be appropriate to use an ester this time, provided it contains epinephrine? (As you should know by now, epinephrine is the drug of choice for managing anaphylactic reactions.)

5. Ms. Kane asks you why she had to have a local anesthetic, instead of getting a "gas" to be put to sleep (general anesthesia) during the surgery. What is your response?

6. When the local anesthetic is administered, which sensation is lost first? Which is usually last to recover? Why?

7. While Ms. Kane is recovering from her surgery, would it be appropriate to manage her pain with a local anesthetic (e.g., over the next several weeks)?

---

evolve To check your answers, go to http://evolve.elsevier.com/Lehne/ for Study Guide Comments from the author.

26

General Anesthetics

KEY TERMS

analgesia
anesthesia
balanced anesthesia
dissociative anesthesia
general
    anesthesia/anesthetic
minimum alveolar
    concentration (MAC)

malignant (as in
    malignant
    hyperthermia)
"neurolept" analgesia
volatile liquid (type of
    general anesthetic)

OBJECTIVES

After reading and studying this chapter you should be able to:

1. Discuss the concept of balanced anesthesia, that is, the overall goals of general anesthesia and the concept that no single drug has all the properties that might be considered ideal in terms of inducing surgical anesthesia.
2. Give a reasonable definition of MAC; and state how it relates to inhaled general anesthetic potency and the concentrations that must be administered to induce general anesthesia.
3. Using halothane or isoflurane as a representative inhaled general anesthetic, describe the elements of balanced anesthesia one can expect with usually effective doses of the drug given alone; those desired elements of balanced anesthesia that cannot be caused by halothane alone, and for which supplemental agents are needed; and the major toxicities with respect to the cardiovascular system.
4. Describe the uses, benefits, and limitations of nitrous oxide in general anesthesia.
5. State the roles for the following as adjuncts to general anesthesia: (a) barbiturates, especially short-acting ones (see Chapter 33); (b) benzodiazepines (see Chapter 34); opioids (see Chapter 27); and neuromuscular blockers (e.g., tubocurarine, succinylcholine (see Chapter 16). (Be sure to refer to other chapters to (re)familiarize yourself with the general actions, uses, and toxicities of these drug groups and to integrate

that information in the context of general anesthesia.)
6. Describe the basic sequence of drug administration for reversal of postanesthesia skeletal neuromuscular blockade (paralysis), the rationale for each medication that is administered, and the expected effects of each medication.
7. Describe the signs and symptoms, etiology (including the main pharmacologic causes), and management of malignant hyperthermia (see Chapter 16 and 26).

CRITICAL THINKING AND STUDY QUESTIONS

1. Why is the following statement true? "We can easily provide balanced anesthesia for our patients, but we don't have one 'balanced anesthetic' drug that's capable of doing that."

2. If we were to administer a single inhaled anesthetic (e.g., enflurane) at its MAC, and give no other adjuncts, what is the likely response in the "typical patient"? Why?

3. Is the MAC of an inhaled anesthetic an absolute, unchangeable number (you only and always must administer this drug at a concentration equal to its MAC), or can it vary? What factors might affect variations in the MAC?

4. Although halothane can be considered the prototype of the volatile liquid inhalation anesthetics, and it is still used (mainly in children), for several reasons isoflurane is often preferred, especially for adults. What are the reasons?

5. What is the main effect that nitrous oxide provides when it's used as a component of balanced anesthesia? Why can't it be used as the sole agent for producing full surgical anesthesia?

6. Some people have "sniffed" nitrous oxide for "recreational purposes." And some of them have died as a result. What's the reason for and the most likely cause of death?

7. Inhaled anesthetics that are very soluble in blood have onsets of action that are longer than those of agents that are poorly soluble in blood. This seems illogical to many people. After all, it's the blood that delivers drugs (inhaled anesthetics included) to the various organs. Wouldn't you think that the more soluble a drug was in the blood, the faster it would work? How can you explain the way things really are?

8. What area of clinical medicine (or nursing) has one of the highest (if not *the* highest) rates of substance abuse, drug diversion, and drug-induced suicide? Any guess as to why?

CASE STUDY

This is a chapter for which the topic is highly specialized (anesthesia and anesthetic agents), yet one for which the entire practice of general anesthesia depends on the knowledge and inseparable use of drugs in several categories. Therefore, there is no case study. You need to integrate knowledge from this chapter with knowledge from other chapters about, for example, neuromuscular blockers (Chapter 16); sedatives, hypnotics, and anxiety-relieving drugs (Chapter 34); analgesics (Chapter 27); and even more.

evolve To check your answers, go to http://evolve.elsevier.com/Lehne/ for Study Guide Comments from the author.

CHAPTER

27

Opioid (Narcotic) Analgesics, Opioid Antagonists, and Nonopioid Centrally Acting Analgesics

KEY TERMS

abuse (of drugs)
addiction
agonist-antagonist (type
  of opioid)
antitussive effect
endorphins
enkephalins
kappa receptor
mu receptor

narcotic
opioid
patient-controlled
  analgesia (PCA)
physical dependence
pure opioid agonist
tolerance
withdrawal syndrome

OBJECTIVES

After reading and studying this chapter you should be able to:

1. State the roles of the kappa and mu opioid receptors in analgesia, respiratory depression, and euphoria.
2. Give a precise definition(s) of **narcotic** (as applied legally to classes of drugs) and compare that with the way the typical layperson uses the term.
3. Distinguish among pure opioid agonists, agonist-antagonists, and antagonists in terms of their mechanisms of action; and place various named drugs in the appropriate category.
4. Discuss the therapeutic uses of opioid agonists, agonist-antagonists, and antagonists.
5. Discuss the adverse effects of opioids and how they are managed, both pharmacologically and with nondrug measures. The discussion should include a typical opioid agonist such as morphine, mixed opioid agonist-antagonists, and pure opioid antagonists.
6. State how meperidine differs from morphine in terms of adverse effects and proper clinical use(s).

7. Describe opioid drug-related factors that contribute to the development of physical dependence and psychologic dependence. Identify drug- and administration-related factors that affect the severity of physical dependence, as well as the severity and duration of withdrawal signs and symptoms when administration of that drug is stopped suddenly.
8. Compare and contrast acute withdrawal from an opioid (assume physical dependence has occurred) with the withdrawal signs, symptoms, and likely outcomes of unsupervised withdrawal from barbiturates, alcohol, and benzodiazepines.

CRITICAL THINKING AND STUDY QUESTIONS

1. Your text lists several pure opioid agonists in addition to the prototype, morphine. You'll see that they differ (sometimes significantly) in terms of usual doses, even when you compare them at the same administration route. Does this mean they differ in efficacy? In potency? What's the basis for your conclusions? What are the clinical implications of these differences, if there are any?

2. What is the active chemical by which heroin causes its analgesic and euphoric effects? What is responsible for codeine's main analgesic and euphoric effects?

3. How, if at all, does meperidine differ from a typical opioid (e.g., morphine, hydromorphone) in terms of (a) its use and mechanism of action as an analgesic, (b) the adverse responses it can cause when blood levels get too high, and (c) drug-drug interactions?

4. A patient arrives in the emergency department with significant ventilatory and generalized CNS depression (lethargy, reduced level of consciousness, slurred speech, blunted reflexes) that, according to the patient's friends, was unquestionably caused by "a bunch of pills" the patient swallowed. The patient is given a proper dose of naloxone, IV, but there is absolutely no change in his signs or symptoms. An additional IV dose of naloxone is given, then another. Still, no improvement in signs and symptoms and vital signs. Does this lack of response rule out an opioid as a cause of or contributor to the overdose?

5. What property(ies) of oxycodone (formulated as Oxycontin) makes this product such a popular substance of abuse and such an alleged medicolegal problem?

6. When pentazocine was approved for use, it was touted by some as the "first nonaddicting opioid." Do you have any clue about which group of individuals proved that this is untrue?

7. A patient who is known to be an ongoing, long-term IV heroin abuser was in a motor vehicle accident and is suffering significant pain from multiple limb trauma (4 severe but not com-

pound fractures), but none of the injuries is life-threatening. The paramedics have placed a peripheral IV line, and after an initial assessment the MD orders a 4-mg IV dose of morphine sulfate. After 10 minutes there is no relief of pain, nor any ventilatory depression, because (naturally) the patient is tolerant to opioids. Several additional 4-mg IV doses of morphine do nothing either, and the patient is in obviously excruciating pain. The patient has received a total of 20 mg morphine, IV, in about 20 minutes, and it appears as if nothing good (or bad) is happening.

Someone decides to give an IV injection of 40 mg hydromorphone. The patient suddenly goes into respiratory arrest. He is intubated and ventilated.

A. What property of hydromorphone probably contributed to the sudden, "big" effect?

B. The decision is made to reverse the ventilatory depression caused by the combination of the morphine and hydromorphone. Would you expect that the dose of naloxone needed to do this would be smaller than, the same as, or larger than, the "usual" naloxone dose for a patient who had not been tolerant to opioids? Why?

C. An effective dose of naloxone is given. In addition to a return of spontaneous ventilation, what else should you be prepared to deal with? Why? Which of these expected responses to naloxone would you *not* expect to see had the patient not been physically dependent on opioids? Why?

D. Reflecting on the situation you just faced, other than giving naloxone, what reasonable and safe intervention might you have used to deal with the combined morphine-hydromorphone overdose?

would it be practical and effective simply to stop the opioid abruptly and substitute a benzodiazepine or a barbiturate instead? After all, this approach is used when methadone is substituted for an opioid such as morphine or heroin.

8. You're reviewing the anesthesiologist's notes on a patient who just had a thoracotomy for cardiac surgery. You note that the patient received large IV doses of morphine. You do a quick calculation and realize the total dose is many times the average lethal dose of this drug. The patient had never received or taken an opioid before. What's going on?

12. Compare and contrast what happens to the margins of safety (or therapeutic index) for opioids and for barbiturates (or alcohol) as one continues to take higher and higher doses owing to the development of tolerance.

13. Not long ago, on a popular TV medical show, a patient with a severe tricyclic antidepressant overdose was wheeled into the ER. Upon learning the cause, the physician commented, "Why couldn't he have OD'd on a narcotic (opioid) instead?" Comment on this. (You will need to integrate your knowledge gained from studying Chapter 31, dealing with antidepressants; indeed, we ask this study question in that chapter.)

9. When propoxyphene was approved for use it was heralded as a major breakthrough in pain control. In reality, and in relative terms, how efficacious an analgesic is it? What adverse effects would you see—ones you wouldn't expect with morphine—if a patient took a very high dose of propoxyphene in an attempt to get better pain control than the proper prescribed dose provided?

14. What one thing should you remember when administering naloxone to a patient who has received an accidental overdose of an opioid such as morphine? Assume the patient is not physically dependent on opioids.

10. In order to wean physically dependent abusers of morphine or heroin, methadone is often substituted. It's been said that this is nothing more than replacing one substance of abuse with another. What does this mean? Why is this done? What is the pharmacologic or physiologic basis for this?

15. Nalmefene, a naloxone-like narcotic antagonist, has a much longer duration of action than naloxone. State one advantage and one main disadvantage of that property.

11. If the goal were to wean a person who is physically dependent on an opioid from that drug,

CASE STUDY

Lisa Wynn, 35 years old, had an abdominal hysterectomy this morning. She is ordered morphine IV via a patient-controlled analgesia (PCA) pump for her postoperative pain. The pump is set to deliver 1 mg of morphine per injection, up to a maximum of 5 mg per hour.

1. Ms. Wynn asks whether the morphine will relieve all of her pain. How would you respond?

2. She asks why she is getting PCA instead of regular injections and expresses concern that she might accidentally give her self too much. How would you explain this to allay concerns? What are some advantages of PCA?

3. What are the potential adverse effects of opioids? Can some of these side effects be desirable in some settings? How and what do you assess to help detect them?

4. It has been 8 hours since Ms. Wynn has voided postoperatively. How has the intravenous morphine contributed to her inability to void? What are your nursing interventions at this time?

5. Ms. Wynn is resting quietly now. You check to see how she is responding and find that her respiratory rate is 8/min. What would you do?

6. Ms. Wynn begins to arouse and complains of nausea. How does morphine promote nausea and vomiting? For this patient, what might be done (or given) to alleviate the sensation? When is nausea and vomiting most likely to occur in settings such as this?

7. Ms. Wynn complains of pain even though she has received the maximum amount of morphine permitted by the PCA pump. What are your thoughts about this?

8. Ms. Wynn now complains about a "respiratory allergy" from the flowers in her room. She asks you to bring her some antihistamine; your unit dose supply has diphenhydramine in it. What responses might occur with adding this drug to the morphine regimen?

9. Ms. Wynn continues to require morphine long after the usual time frame for opioids after surgery. She tells you that she cannot tolerate any pain, but the physician has decided that she must stop the morphine. You are concerned that Ms. Wynn may have been dependent on drugs before coming to the hospital and that withdrawing the morphine may lead to an abstinence syndrome. What are the initial symptoms of abstinence syndrome?

Now, consider the following scenarios.

10. After receiving a single 5-mg IV dose of morphine upon recovery from anesthesia and another identical dose 4 hours later, the house officer wishes to get Ms. Wynn off morphine and switch her to meperidine, anticipating several more days of therapy with an opioid for pain control. Would you have any concerns about the use of meperidine, and why?

11. After a day of PCA therapy with morphine and inadequate pain control from it, the resident physician orders a switch to hydromorphone. The solution is prepared at the same concentration (mg/mL) as the morphine had been prepared and is administered with the same PCA dosing limits: 1 mg hydromorphone per injection up to a total of 5 mg per hour. What do you expect might happen, and why?

12. After a day of morphine PCA (dosing noted above), the physician wishes to get Ms. Wynn on an opioid with less potential for abuse. Ms. Wynn still reports being "very uncomfortable" with pain at this time. The doctor orders that morphine be stopped and pentazocine substituted for it right away.

13. Afer a day of morphine PCA (dosing noted above), the physician wishes to get Ms. Wynn on oral morphine right away. Under what circumstances would this be a reasonable idea? How should the switch from IV to oral morphine be made, and why? What property of morphine, when administered orally, makes it unsuitable as a starting agent for immediate pain control and accounts for the lack of equivalency (in terms of analgesia) between oral and parenteral morphine doses?

evolve To check your answers, go to http://evolve.elsevier.com/Lehne/ for Study Guide Comments from the author.

Pain Management in Patients with Cancer

KEY TERMS

adjuvants (to analgesic drugs)
AHCPR (what it is, why it's important)
JCAHO (what it is, why it's important)
neurolytic (drug, effect, or procedure)
neurolytic (type of therapy)
neuropathic pain

nociceptive pain
pain affect faces scale
partial (opioid) agonist (agonist-antagonist)
patient-controlled analgesia (PCA)
phantom pain
"pure" (full) (opioid) agonist
somatic pain
visceral pain

OBJECTIVES

After reading and studying this chapter you should be able to:

1. Compare and contrast neuropathic and nociceptive pain in terms of the typical causes and the drug classes that are (or aren't) effective for managing them.
2. Describe the various tools used to assess the severity of and discomfort from a patient's pain and used to plan optimal analgesic therapy.
3. Comment on the statement that the various non-surgical interventions we use to treat cancer—cancer chemotherapy and radiation therapy—can cause pain that needs to be managed every bit as much as the pain arising from the cancer itself.
4. List and describe the main barriers or impediments to providing optimal pain control, particularly with opioids. Consider attitudes, beliefs, and even what might be described as fears involving both the healthcare providers who are responsible for prescribing and administering these drugs and the patients (and their families) who are recipients of these medications.
5. Articulate the questions you would ask of a patient to assess each of the following characteristics of a patient's pain:

- Onset and temporal pattern of pain
- Location of the pain
- Quality of the pain
- Pain intensity
- Modulating/modifying factors
- Previous treatment
- Impact on function and overall quality of life

6. Develop a prioritized list of preferred, rational, and effective drugs for a patient, given the type(s) and severities of pain. This should include both traditional analgesics and drugs identified as adjuvant (adjunctive) drug therapies.
7. Compare and contrast the benefits and limitations (or risks) of PRN pain control versus around-the-clock administration of analgesics. Don't hesitate to include in your summary the benefits of patient-controlled analgesia. Assume the patient has long-term pain that must be controlled.
8. Compare and contrast tolerance, physical dependence, and addiction as they apply to the use of opioids for pain control.
9. Summarize some general (but accurate) ways in which the elderly, very young children, and patients who are physically dependent on and abusers of opioids differ from an "otherwise healthy" young adult. Focus on problems with assessment of pain and its response to treatment, drug selection and dosing, and monitoring for adverse responses (due to either the analgesic itself or problems from other drugs the patient may be taking).
10. Tell us what the JCAHO is and why keeping the "Joint Commission" happy is good for not only your patients, but also your institution overall. If you wish, just focus on their new (2001) standards related to pain assessment and treatment, and patients' rights regarding these important issues.

Notes: A fair amount of content in the text chapter focuses on undeniably important issues, but they may be more in the domain of a medical-surgical

73

nursing course than a pharmacology course. We will focus below mainly on drug-related issues.

Do not attempt to study this chapter or answer the study questions or do the case study exercises until you have studied Chapter 27 (*Opioid [Narcotic] Analgesics*). Many of the issues raised there are more detailed but very applicable to what's presented here. However, if you are not up to speed on that content, your ability to understand, appreciate, integrate, and apply much of what's in the current chapter will be hindered considerably. In fact, you should work through the study questions and case study items from Chapter 27 and consider them an integral part of the questions and case study presented below.

The text also addresses important issues related to such other topics or drugs as cyclooxygenase inhibitors (aspirin) and acetaminophen (see Chapter 67); the effects of aspirin on platelets (see Chapters 50 and 67); cancer chemotherapeutic principles and drugs (Chapters 97–99); such adjuvant drugs as antihistamines (see Chapter 66), certain anticonvulsants (see Chapter 23) and antidepressants (see Chapter 31); bisphosphonates and their effects on bone calcium metabolism (see Chapter 70); and glucocorticoids (see Chapters 57 and 68). Chances are good that at the time you are studying the current chapter, you may not have worked through many (or any) of those other chapters.

Check with your instructor to see what, precisely, he or she expects you to "know" from those other chapters at this time. When I've asked about these drugs, below, I've usually tried to provide you with information that's sufficient to help you answer without having to be knowledgeable about all the details in those chapters.

CRITICAL THINKING AND STUDY QUESTIONS

1. A colleague says, "We ought to send Mrs. F off for an MRI scan to see how bad her pain is." Comment on this.

2. What is the most reliable method of assessing pain in a patient who is able to communicate with you? Does that method involve or depend on results of some particular clinical laboratory test? If so, which one?

3. Which drugs (or types) seem to be most effective for managing neuropathic pain?

4. It is necessary and essential to develop a long-term plan for pain management in such patients as those with cancer? What is the basic flaw, however, in following that plan rigidly?

5. Discuss the clinical approach to pain management as outlined and recommended by the AHCPR.

6. Your text notes that for many patients with mild to moderate pain, a combination of an opioid and a nonopioid (e.g., aspirin or, more commonly, acetaminophen) is useful.

   A. What is the general rationale for doing this?

   B. If we go the opioid-nonopioid combination approach, what are the general benefits of a fixed-dose combination product—one that contains both codeine and acetaminophen?

C. What is the main limitation of using fixed-dose combination products? Assume that we started therapy of mild to moderate pain with one of these, but now pain has worsened and we need to control it.

the chances that that's the approach we'd take? (This is somewhat of a bonus-question, in that it does address some issues you may not have learned about yet by reading and studying Chapters 50 and especially Chapter 67.)

D. The text notes that it's "common to combine an opioid with a nonopioid...because the combination can be more effective that either drug alone." Consider now a patient with severe visceral pain that requires morphine. Moreover, the patient has been receiving morphine, or other opioids, long enough that tolerance has developed: The morphine dose that's needed to make the patient comfortable is much higher than we'd use for a patient just starting on opioid therapy. In this situation, is it common, or necessary, or beneficial to add a nonopioid (e.g., aspirin or acetaminophen) to the regimen?

9. Your text mentions methadone (Dolophine) and levorphanol (Levo-Dromoran) in the section *Opioids to Use with Special Caution*. It states that both drugs have prolonged half-lives, *which makes dosage titration difficult*. How, specifically, does the prolonged half-life make things difficult? (This is a good review of basic pharmacokinetics, and it's important to many more drugs than these two opioids.)

7. The text notes that aspirin inhibits platelet aggregation. Indeed, even a "baby aspirin tablet" (81 mg) taken just once a day can interfere with platelet aggregation enough to cause prolonged bleeding time. (By way of comparison, a typical adult dose of aspirin for mild pain or fever is 325 mg × 2, taken every 4 hours.) Why is this important for most cancer patients who are receiving a chemotherapeutic drug for their cancer?

10. We have a patient for whom we will start opioid therapy. Our drug of choice is morphine. Our goal is to provide prompt pain control because the patient is "hurting." Why would we not start with any formulation of oral morphine? Think about not only the pharmacokinetics of morphine itself (see Chapter 27), but about some of the basic pharmacokinetic principles you learned in Chapter 4.

11. A patient with metastatic lung cancer has been taking a long-acting oral morphine sulfate preparation (MSContin), 300 mg q 3–4 hr for pain. The physician is going switch to a fentanyl patch. Identify the equianalgesic dosage for fentanyl.

8. Your text notes that there are several nonacetylated salicylates, such as choline salicylate, that don't inhibit platelet aggregation. As a result they are more suitable than, say, aspirin itself for thrombocytopenic patients. Assume we have a thrombocytopenic patient and we're contemplating using choline salicylate for managing mild pain. That sounds good to me, but what are

12. Take a trip to your favorite shopping place for OTC meds. Head to the aisle that has the sprays you might purchase for a common sore throat, and look at the "active ingredients" in several products. What ingredient, *one that's mentioned in this chapter,* do you find in many of these products? How is that agent (the drug, not the throat spray *per se*) classified, what is the purpose of giving it to some patients with long-term severe pain, and how does it work?

13. Which of the following statement(s) about pain management in the elderly is or are generally correct and supported by data? What are the clinical implications?

    (a) The elderly don't feel pain as much as younger adults. (b) They are more stoic, being able to tolerate discomfort better and easier. (c) They're more sensitive to the desired and adverse effects of opioids.

14. A colleague says, "The Joint Commission is coming for a visit next year. They're the law. If they find that we're not meeting patient and institutional goals and objectives with respect to pain, we—the nurses—will go to jail. They may even shut the hospital down." What are your thoughts on this in general and with respect to the JCAHO standards concerning pain assessment and management?

CASE STUDY

Danielle Petra, 19 years old, is on her college soccer team. She meets with the team physician and the trainer the morning after a particularly tough soccer match with a complaint of various aches and pains in one leg. She's sure it was due to an injury incurred during the game the day before, and there's no reason to suspect otherwise.

The team physician prescribes a combination of limited exercise, massage, heat and cold applications, and acetaminophen. The trainer will help with all the nondrug measures.

1. What is the probable reason that the team doctor prescribed acetaminophen instead of aspirin or another NSAID?

A week later, while practicing, Danielle falls as she's running. There was no contact—no obvious trauma that caused the fall. Her left leg is tender and swollen in the mid-femur region, and she's in terrible pain just trying to bear weight to stand or walk. Danielle is sent for an MRI of her leg. It reveals a simple fracture of the femur.

2. Is Danielle's primary pain at this time most likely neuropathic or nociceptive? Would continuation of the analgesic therapy prescribed for her pain a week ago be suitable—perhaps with simply an increase of the acetaminophen dose to cover the greater degree of pain? Why or why not? If not, what medication change might we envisage?

There's a big question about why Danielle's femur fractured during what was, for her, very routine exercise and no direct trauma. Danielle is sent for more diagnostic tests, including a biopsy of the femur. The biopsy reveals a cancer, an osteosarcoma. The first treatment plan involves initial radiation therapy, followed by a course of chemotherapy. The hope is to save not only Danielle's leg but also her life. Danielle is still in pain, but there's no reason to keep her in the hospital for more than a day. She's discharged and will be managed for now as an outpatient.

3. Would it be inappropriate at this time to switch Danielle's pain medication, knowing that she has cancer, is going to have a painful biopsy, and will be undergoing radiation and chemotherapy?

4. We are now talking about providing pain control for at least 3 weeks, and there's no certain limit to the time when analgesic drugs can be stopped. Should we now worry about our use of an opioid? If so, about what should we be concerned? Tolerance? Dependence? Addiction?

5. The clinical evidence indicates that there are no metastases of Danielle's bone cancer. A colleague suggests that we consider adding a bisphosphonate (e.g., etidronate) to her treatment plan to help control the pain. Comment on this.

The oncologist who is supervising Danielle's chemotherapy and the radiation oncologist who prescribed the radiation therapy consult after several months to do a thorough review of her progress. They consider this amount of time adequate to determine whether these therapies have been as effective as they'd like. They are not optimistic about the prognosis. Bone scans and other tests still show no metastatic disease. But the specialists agree that Danielle's leg should be amputated, in the hope of curing the cancer. Given the location of the tumor—mid-femur—they propose a hip disarticulation that will remove all of her leg.

Danielle signs the consent form, and the surgery to remove her entire leg is performed without complications.

Upon immediate postoperative recovery, Danielle is in severe pain. The surgery resident who will be in charge of her recovery for the next 5 days anticipates that she will be in severe pain for about 3 days. He orders the "proper" dose of meperidine (Demerol), given on a fixed-dose schedule, for initial pain management. His plan, he says, is to use that drug for at least those first 3 days unless Danielle says she doesn't need that degree of pain control before then.

   A. Comment on the resident's decision to use around-the-clock (ATC) dosing with an opioid, as opposed to ordering an opioid to be given PRN—as Danielle wants or feels she needs it. For now, ignore the choice of meperidine.

   B. The resident chose meperidine (Demerol) for the anticipated 3-day need for control of severe pain. Given the anticipated 3-day need for management of severe pain, what would *you* consider as another option?

7. Danielle is doing well postoperatively. She acknowledges she is in pain. According to her, however, her biggest complaint is pain and a burning/searing sensation in her lower leg and foot. Of course, she's referring to the limb that has been amputated. What is the term commonly applied to pain or other unpleasant sensations in a body part that has been amputated? What type(s) of pain is this? How might we deal with this in terms of drug therapy?

8. Danielle has made a remarkable recovery from her surgery. Her pain is controlled well with morphine administered by PCA. The prosthetics team and her surgeon would like to get her up and out of bed as soon as possible, if for no other reason than to reduce the risk of venous thrombosis that might occur from lying in bed too long. They've provided her with crutches, and the nurse is available all the time for support and assistance. Danielle gets nauseated when she stands up. What might we do about this, short term? Recall that Danielle is still taking morphine.

9. While Danielle was in the OR, once the surgery was completed but before her anesthesia was stopped and she was extubated, a prosthetic technician came in to make a plaster cast of her hip for fitting of a temporary artificial limb. Several days postoperatively the technician comes back with a temporary limb to help make some fitting adjustments for her permanent prosthesis, and to get her up on her feet, exercising and learning to walk, quickly.

Danielle is anxious. She's never looked at her amputation site. If she looks, it's likely she'll become even more anxious; there's a good chance she will become nauseated; and she may incur an acute episode of worse pain as the limb is fitted.

The MD orders an injection of "the right dose" of hydroxyzine (Vistaril) right before the prosthetist's visit. You look up the drug in a reference book and see that it's classified as an antihistamine. Is this a medication error? Why or why not?

10. After several days on morphine, Danielle's dosage requirement has increased. Is this surprising or expected? What does it reflect?

11. The MD feels it's time to take Danielle off morphine and substitute another drug for it. She's still having some pain, but her main symptom is anxiety. The doctor decides to use a very low dose of codeine, switching abruptly from the ATC morphine and adding a rather large dose of diazepam (Valium), one of the most widely used benzodiazepine anxiety-relieving drugs (see Chapter 34). Comment on problems you see.

12. While there are many things we haven't mentioned in this scenario, or our comments about it, one glaring omission stands out in my mind. I'm thinking about the JCAHO's 2001 pain management standards. Can you guess what that might be?

evolve To check your answers, go to http://evolve.elsevier.com/Lehne/ for Study Guide Comments from the author.

Drugs for Headache

KEY TERMS

aura (migraine)
calcitonin gene–related
    peptide (CGRP)
cluster headache
ergot alkaloid

ergotism
migraine headache
serotonin
serotonin syndrome
triptans

OBJECTIVES

After reading and studying this chapter you should be able to:

1. Compare and contrast common headaches, migraine headaches, and cluster headaches in terms of triggering factors, clinical presentations, and management.
2. State the common underlying neurovascular causes of migraine, including the roles of CGRP and serotonin (5-hydroxytryptamine).
2. Identify usually effective therapies for abortive and prophylactic therapy of migraine, and state which drugs are suitable for prophylaxis but not for acute intervention (abortive therapy).
3. Describe the signs, symptoms, and potential consequences of ergotism, and the main elements of managing it.

CRITICAL THINKING AND STUDY QUESTIONS

1. What is calcitonin gene–related peptide (CGRP) and what role does it seem to play in the etiology of migraine headaches? What evidence do we have to support this concept? Why and how does serotonin seem to be important in the overall pathophysiology, and in migraine management?

2. What is the main, and basically simple, reason that oral drug administration is appropriate for abortive therapy of migraines, but usually not once a full-blown migraine attack has developed?

3. What is the role of metoclopramide (Reglan) as an adjunct to treating an ongoing migraine attack? How about prochlorperazine (Compazine)? How are these drugs classified in terms of their main actions in the context of migraine headaches? A colleague says either can be used as specific and primary (the only drug) therapy for migraines. Do you agree?

4. Your text notes that ergotamine has a plasma half-life of only 2 hours (or so), but its effects may persist for as long as 24 hours. What does this suggest to you?
   (*Note:* This is not really a question specifically about ergotamine but rather an assessment of a very basic concept that helps relate to a drug's half-life and its duration of action. Can you recall another group of drugs that we pointed out that has this same relationship—short half-life, much longer lasting effects?)

79

5. The antimigraine actions of the ergot alkaloids relate, in one way or another, to promotion of cerebral vascular constriction and reduced amplitude of contraction-dilation ("pulsation") cycles. What are the *peripheral* vascular consequences of this group of drugs, and how to they relate to their main cardiovascular/vascular contraindications?

6. How might cigarette smoking pose specific problems for a patient who is taking an ergot preparation?

7. The text notes that the risk of ergotism is highest in patients with (among other things) sepsis. It also notes that sepsis contraindicates the use of an ergot alkaloid. Sepsis (septicemia) is a severe bacterial infection, so how does an infection relate to the problems with an ergot compound?

8. The text notes that there's about a 50-50 chance that patients who use sumatriptan for migraine develop "chest pressure" that is not indicative of ischemic heart disease (i.e., it is not angina pectoris as we generally apply the term). However, patients with a history or risk of coronary artery disease (CAD) may incur chest and other symptoms that truly are due to myocardial ischemia—as can be caused by coronary artery disease. In the absence of documented CAD, what risk factors place patients who use sumatriptan at risk of this myocardial ischemic episode?

9. What in the world do ergot alkaloids have to do with the Salem (Massachusetts) Witchcraft Trials in the late 1600s? Or with thousands of deaths in Europe in about AD 857 and again in the 11th century from a condition called Holy Fire or, later, St. Anthony's Fire? I mean, back then we never knew of anything called migraine headache, ergot alkaloids, and all that jazz! (OK. This is nontestable stuff [unless your prof likes to write "extra credit" questions, as I do], but perhaps fodder for an interesting show of your knowledge of both pharmacology and history.)

10. Hop on an Internet search engine such as Google and search for articles on Chinese restaurant syndrome. Explain how this phenomenon may be important to people who suffer recurrent migraine headaches.

11. Take a trip to the OTC pain-reliever aisle of your favorite pharmacy or supermarket. Compare the ingredients in, and per-dose cost of, Excedrin Migraine and regular Excedrin. What do you find?

CASE STUDY

Jane Smith, 29 years old, presents at your clinic with the chief complaint of severe, frequent headaches that begin mid-morning and grow progressively worse throughout the day. She admits to occasional nausea and vomiting associated with the headaches. She is frequently asked to work double shifts, and so her sleep cycle is irregular at best. Her headaches are pulsatile and usually unilateral. All laboratory findings are within normal limits. Mrs. Smith has been married for 4 years and she and her husband are planning to begin having children.

1. Mrs. Smith reports that her headaches are more frequent and much worse when she is menstruating. Is this a typical finding?

2. Mrs. Smith is asked to try to correlate the onset of her headaches with her diet. She says the following tend to cause really bad headaches: prepared (canned or dry) soups and broths, hot dogs, cold cuts (especially salami and bologna), flavored potato or corn chips (e.g., barbeque-flavored chips), and Chinese foods. What do you make of this information? What ingredient that's common to these foods may be the migraine trigger?

3. Mrs. Smith tells you that she's tried OTC pain relievers, and after going through the list of things she's tried, you find that plain acetaminophen doesn't work at all. Is that surprising?

4. What are some prescription drug options that might be ordered for this patient for long-term prophylaxis of migraine, and what factors would dictate whether one would be particularly suitable (or unsuitable)? (To answer this question fully, you may need to review or read ahead in the chapters cited in our response to get more complete on alternative drugs.)

5. In reviewing Mrs. Smith's OTC meds further, you learn that ibuprofen and aspirin (or aspirin-containing combination products) seem to give her some headache relief. However, they also tend to cause wheezing and, increasingly, hives. She says that the wheezing and breathing difficulty are getting to be worse than the headache relief the meds provide. What should you be thinking and planning in the way of further evaluation?

6. Let's assume that Mrs. Smith has documented asthma. What drugs certainly or probably should *not* be prescribed for her, given this

information? Think of both OTC and prescription drugs, whether they would be used for prophylaxis or abortive migraine therapy. Give us some of your reasons for your comments and your thoughts on what prophylactic drug might be worth a try.

The physician, comfortable with the diagnosis of migraine, orders sumatriptan 6 mg, SC, dispensed as a self-injector (e.g., Imitrex STATdose pen).

7. How often should sumatriptan be administered for aborting a given migraine attack, and what is the maximum recommended dose per 24 hours?

8. What other medical conditions should be assessed for and ruled out before sending the patient off with a prescription for a sumatriptan self-injector?

9. The physician then orders ergotamine tartrate, 3 mg, with the goal of starting the patient on longer-term oral therapy right away. What are your thoughts about this order?

10. What lifestyle and dietary changes would you review with this patient before discharge? We've addressed some of them in earlier questions. What else needs to be considered?

11. Mrs. Smith learns about the drug therapy and is taught all the important lifestyle modifications that will help with the frequency and severity of migraine attacks. She says, "Now that I'm going to be taking effective drugs, can I do more or less what I want and like with my diet, sleep, and so on?" How would you respond?

12. Let's assume that Mrs. Smith was placed on ergotamine rather than a triptan. If she were to develop an infection that required antibiotic therapy, are there any particular antibiotics (or antibiotic classes) that should be avoided? Ignore the issues of antibiotic allergies or resistance and think specifically of interactions with antimigraine drugs.

13. Mrs. Smith starts to experience signs of depression after trying to deal with her migraines, and having to use triptan injections, for many months. She visits another doctor, who does not get a complete history and so writes a prescription for one of the selective serotonin reuptake inhibitor antidepressants (SSRIs such as fluoxetine [Prozac]. What, if any concerns, are there with this?

14. We mentioned that Mrs. Smith and her husband are planning to start a family. How does this relate to our selection of prophylactic and abortive therapies—and the need to implement lifestyle and dietary changes as well?

evolve To check your answers, go to http://evolve.elsevier.com/Lehne/ for Study Guide Comments from the author.

Antipsychotic Agents and Their Use in Schizophrenia

KEY TERMS

akathisia
atypical antipsychotic
   drug
butyrophenone (drug
   class)
conventional
   antipsychotic drug
depot preparation (of
   drug)
dystonia
extrapyramidal (system
   or side effects)

high-potency
   antipsychotic
low-potency
   antipsychotic
neuroleptic malignant
   syndrome
phenothiazine (drug
   class)
seizure threshold
tardive dyskinesia

OBJECTIVES

After reading and studying this chapter you should be able to:

1. Describe the principal indications for antipsychotic drugs.
2. Compare and contrast chlorpromazine and haloperidol with respect to their mechanisms and onsets of antipsychotic action, uses, and the relative incidence of central nervous system and peripheral autonomic side effects.
3. Explain why antipsychotic drugs may cause side effects or adverse responses that mimic many signs and symptoms of Parkinson's disease. (Related to this, you should be able to explain why excessive doses of dopaminergic drugs used for parkinsonism may trigger some signs and symptoms of schizophrenia.)
4. Summarize the main signs and symptoms of extrapyramidal side effects caused by antipsychotic drugs and acceptable therapeutic approaches to minimize or reverse them.
5. Associate the neuroleptic malignant syndrome as a relatively rare but serious adverse reaction to antipsychotic drugs; describe its signs and symptoms and time of onset after starting

antipsychotic drug therapy; state interventions that should be implemented if/when neuroleptic malignant syndrome is suspected or confirmed.
6. Highlight the key differences between and similarities of antipsychotics that are called high-potency and those called low-potency.
7. State why clozapine, which is considered a prototype of the atypical antipsychotics, is not a first-line drug for managing schizophrenia, but does seem to be preferred to phenothiazines for managing levodopa-induced psychosis. Discuss special monitoring that must be implemented and special instructions that should be given to the patient who is receiving clozapine, regardless of the use.

CASE STUDY

John Newman is a 52-year-old man admitted to the hospital for symptoms of schizophrenia. He has been hospitalized previously and when discharged was taking thioridazine (Mellaril), 600 mg/day, as the initial antipsychotic drug therapy. His wife reports that he had done well until he stopped taking his medication 3 days ago. On admission Mr. Newman complained of a headache, insomnia, gastric distress, and sweating. During the admission procedure Mr. Newman appeared to be responding to voices. He cried out, "Please help me. They are trying to kill me. They put poison in my food; the medicine is poison too. Please don't make me take it."

The attending physician who sees Mr. Newman upon admission prescribes chlorpromazine (Thorazine), 50 mg IM stat, followed by 150 mg qid by mouth for maintenance therapy.

1. Comment on the selection of thioridazine as the initial antipsychotic drug. Is this a reasonable starting drug? Why or why not?

2. Briefly describe the reason Mr. Newman may experience orthostatic hypotension.

3. A new nurse on the unit complains to you that she has noticed a rash on her hands since she has been working with Mr. Newman. She comments, "Maybe I caught something from him." What could you tell her that might allay her fears?

4. When Mr. Newman's chlorpromazine is increased to 800 mg a day to control his symptoms, he complains of twitching, tremulous fingers. What does this likely represent? What plan of action might come next?

5. It has become obvious that Mr. Newman's antipsychotic therapy is causing extrapyramidal side effects, equivalent to drug-induced parkinsonism. Dopaminergic drugs (e.g., levodopa) are indicated for relieving parkinsonian signs and symptoms. Would it be appropriate for Mr. Newman? Why or why not?

6. You are giving report to a colleague who will be taking care of Mr. Newman on the next shift. He comments that Mr. Newman should have received haloperidol for the initial management of his acute psychosis "because it's a high-potency antipsychotic, and so it controls symptoms better than chlorpromazine." Comment on that, and briefly describe the alleged differences between low- and high-potency antipsychotic agents.

7. If Mr. Newman had received haloperidol (Haldol) instead of chlorpromazine for his acute therapy, what adverse side effects would he be most likely to experience?

8. What would a plan of action be if Mr. Newman displayed these adverse side effects?

9. While Mr. Newman is taking chlorpromazine, and as the dosage is being adjusted, it's necessary to check his blood pressure and heart rate in the supine, sitting, and standing positions. Why?

10. After a couple of weeks on chlorpromazine, Mr. Newman reports that he is having trouble focusing his eyes in order to read. What action of chlorpromazine may account for this effect, and what other related effects should you be assessing for?

11. Assume that after a reasonable course of therapy with chlorpromazine, Mr. Newman's schizophrenia signs and symptoms do not improve sufficiently. The physician plans a switch to clozapine. What special concerns should use of clozapine raise, and why was it not selected as the initial therapy (instead of a phenothiazine)?

evolve   To check your answers, go to http://evolve.elsevier.com/Lehne/ for Study Guide Comments from the author.

Antidepressants

KEY TERMS

electroconvulsive
  therapy (ECT)
MAO inhibitor
monoamine ("biogenic
  amine")

SSRI
tricyclic (and tetracyclic)
  antidepressant

OBJECTIVES

After reading and studying this chapter you should
be able to:

1. Describe the main clinical features (signs and
   symptoms) of depression, the various main types
   and etiologies of this general term, and the types
   of subjective or objective responses that you can
   use to state with reasonable certainty that any
   antidepressant that might be prescribed is "working" as we'd wish.
2. Compare and contrast the mechanisms of action
   and main adverse effects of tricyclic antidepressants (TCAs), SSRIs, and MAO inhibitors. State
   the role(s) of each class in a step-wise approach
   to managing depression pharmacologically, that
   is, which is/are generally first-line, which is/are
   generally used only as a last resort, and why.
3. Explain the general mechanism by which MAO
   inhibitors and mixed- and indirect-acting sympathomimetics (e.g., ephedrine and tyramine) interact, the expected outcomes of such interactions,
   and ways to reduce the chance that such adverse
   effects occur.
4. Describe general precautions that are necessary
   when switching a patient from a TCA to an
   MAO, and explain the rationale(s) behind the precautions.

CRITICAL THINKING AND STUDY QUESTIONS

1. You know from your text that all the antidepressants do "something" to monoamines in the brain.
   What are those monoamines?

2. Which class of drugs is generally preferred for
   starting drug therapy of depression? Explain this
   in terms of time to symptom relief, overall efficacy, and side effect or adverse response profiles.
   What else should be considered in terms of drug
   selection suitability for a particular patient?

3. Describe the autonomic side effects profile for
   the tricyclics, and identify some common conditions that would weigh against using these drugs
   (as opposed to other antidepressants).

4. A patient with refractory depression is being
   treated with an MAO inhibitor. She develops
   cholecystitis and excruciatingly painful bile duct
   spasm. Ordinarily an opioid is indicated for short-
   term pain relief before gallbladder surgery.
   Which analgesic is generally preferred for spasm
   of the gallbladder or bile duct, and would it be
   suitable for this patient? Why?

5. Not long ago, on a popular TV medical show, a
   patient with a severe TCA overdose was wheeled
   into the ER. Upon learning the cause, the physi-

85

cian commented, "Why couldn't he have OD'd on a narcotic (opioid) instead?" Comment on this (you will need to integrate your knowledge gained from studying Chapter 27).

6. In your text, or in a reference book or on the Web, look up the generic name, dose, and indications for the brand-name product Sarafem. Do the same for the proprietary drug Prozac. Are these different drugs? Are they prescribed, for their indications, in different dosages? What does this tell you about how some drugs are marketed and about how some drug manufacturers can find not only new uses for "old" drugs, but also legitimate ways to keep a revenue stream by patenting new uses for those old drugs medications? (See also item 3, right below.)

7. Apropos question 6, what are "unlabeled uses" for a drug? Any idea how many unlabeled uses there are for fluoxetine, the prototype SSRI?

CASE STUDY

Tom Sledd, a 35-year-old high school teacher, comes to the community mental health center because of feelings of depression for the past 2 weeks. He complains of crying spells, has been unable to sleep throughout the night, is unable to go to work, and has no desire to eat. He denies suicidal intentions. Amitriptyline hydrochloride (Elavil) 50 mg tid is prescribed for Mr. Sledd.

1. Briefly explain the mechanism of action of TCAs such as amitriptyline in reducing the symptoms of depression.

2. Why is Mr. Sledd taking the antidepressant in divided doses, since antidepressants have a long half-life?

3. Why should the acutely depressed patient ordinarily be given no more than a one-week supply of an antidepressant at a time?

4. The day after his initial visit, Mr. Sledd tells you that he does not feel any better. He wants to know how long after initiation of drug therapy he can expect to experience a decrease in the severity of his symptoms. What do you tell him?

5. Why are TCAs or SSRIs used instead of a monoamine oxidase (MAO) inhibitor to start antidepressant therapy for the majority of patients?

6. Why was an SSRI not prescribed for Mr. Sledd instead of a TCA?

Now assume that Mr. Sledd is 50 years old, has been married happily for 25 years, and has three children (aged 16 through 20). Mr. Sledd has held a job in a major corporation for 20 years, and has been promoted up through the ranks. There are no obvious job-related concerns.

Mr. Sledd has essential hypertension, diabetes mellitus (type 2), and hyperlipidemia (primary hypercholesterolemia). He is taking usually appropriate doses of metformin, an ACE inhibitor, and atorvastatin (Lipitor). All the drug (and other) therapies are working well; there are no notable adverse effect, interactions, or the like. At a 6-month visit to his primary care MD, Mr. Sledd says that he feels fine physically, but is a little "overwhelmed by all the stuff" that's going on in his life, and he probably is a little depressed. He repeats this, and his lab tests are still fine, at a doctor's visit 6 months later. Mr. Sledd emphatically denies any thoughts of suicide. He's just "not as happy" as he'd like to be.

The MD asks Mr. Sledd whether he (Mr. Sledd) thinks he might benefit from an antidepressant. Mr. Sledd has subtly hinted that he'd like to "take something for the way I feel, emotionally."

The MD is thinking of prescribing an SSRI, and not thinking of referring Mr. Sledd to a psychotherapist for adjunctive therapy (psychotherapy). The MD will pick a particular SSRI, and allow several months to elapse before re-evaluating the need for therapy with this antidepressant.

7. Do you think this is a reasonable approach? Why or why not? What are the pros and cons of this doctor's decision to treat with an SSRI?

8. Six months after the MD started Mr. Sledd on an SSRI, Mr. Sledd has another routine checkup with his doctor. The doctor asks Mr. Sledd whether he's "feeling as well (mentally) as he'd like," and whether Mr. Sledd feels he's experiencing any adverse effects from the SSRI or the combination of it with his other meds. Mr. Sledd isn't sure he's feeling as well as he could. The MD orders no blood tests for the SSRI, but decides to try increasing Mr. Sledd's daily SSRI dose by 50%. His goal is to allow a month or so of therapy with the increased dose, and let Mr. Sledd report back about how well this therapy change is working. What are your thoughts?

evolve To check your answers, go to http://evolve.elsevier.com/Lehne/ for Study Guide Comments from the author.

Drugs for Bipolar Disorder

KEY TERMS

bipolar illness
diabetes insipidus

polyuria

OBJECTIVES

After reading and studying this chapter you should be able to:

1. Identify the typical manifestations and clinical course of bipolar disorder and the drugs used to manage them.
2. Describe the best way to determine therapeutic lithium levels.
3. Describe why and how body sodium balance is important in maintaining steady blood lithium levels and responses to the drug, and identify drug-related and diet-related aspects that affect those lithium levels and effects.
4. State the main elements of patient assessment and patient education with respect to detecting the development of both beneficial and excessive lithium effects.

CRITICAL THINKING AND STUDY QUESTIONS

1. Which drugs are considered perhaps the most common cause of excessive or toxic effects of lithium or at least a main problem in maintaining steady lithium levels and effects?

2. A patient with bipolar illness presents in the psychiatric section of the emergency room with an obvious episode of profound mania. The physician checks serum lithium levels and finds that they are below the therapeutic range. She orders a stat dose of oral lithium and discharges the patient with a prescription for a daily lithium dose that is approximately twice the previous maintenance dose. Comment on this approach.

3. A patient with a long history of bipolar illness, with one element of the therapy including lithium, develops an adrenal cortical tumor. How might it affect the patient's response to the lithium? What might you predict if the patient developed liver dysfunction, say, from excessive long-term alcohol consumption or hepatitis?

4. Another opportunity to look ahead to the cardiovascular unit and the chapter on diuretics: You will find that there are four main classes of drug for initiating therapy of essential hypertension: diuretics, angiotensin-converting enzyme (ACE) inhibitors, beta-adrenergic blockers, and calcium channel blockers. You already know that diuretics may complicate control of serum lithium levels. What about the other classes of antihypertensive?

CASE STUDY

Doris Roberts, a 35-year-old woman, is brought to the hospital because she has become increasingly hyperexcitable over the past 5 days, and now she is "in a rage," according to her husband. She has talked on the phone almost continuously because, *she says, she's trying to start a business. She's called friends and relatives all over the country, at all hours of the night, to tell them her news. She went on a spending spree to buy new clothes and equipment for her business and accumulated almost $10,000 worth of debt before she was caught writing bad checks. Her husband was called when she tried to purchase a car and the bank reported that she had insufficient funds to cover the check. And her husband says, when she's not "like that" she has bouts of crying and just seems to want to be "left alone."*

On admission, Mrs. Roberts moves about restlessly, waving her arms in a threatening manner while loudly berating her husband and hospital staff. She demands to be released from "this jail" and curses the nurse who interviewed her. The physician prescribes lithium carbonate 300 mg qid.

1. Given the patient's current condition (and behavior), comment on the likely immediate benefits of administering lithium.

2. Discuss reasons for poor adherence to a medication regimen in patients such as Mrs. Roberts.

3. Why is it important for patients who take lithium to maintain an adequate and consistent (from day to day) intake of sodium (salt)?

4. What are the main signs and symptoms of lithium toxicity?

5. Mrs. Roberts tells you she is supposed to be taking a drug for her blood pressure. What information must you obtain about this in order to provide safest care?

6. What information is essential for Mrs. Roberts to know about taking lithium?

7. What adjuvant medication may be used in the treatment of bipolar disorders?

8. Mrs. Roberts's family wants to know whether the lithium will "cure" her depression or whether the antidepressant will do the same for the manic phase of her illness. They also want to know whether therapy will be "for the rest of her life." Your thoughts?

evolve To check your answers, go to http://evolve.elsevier.com/Lehne/ for Study Guide Comments from the author.

Sedative-Hypnotic Drugs

KEY TERMS

anterograde amnesia
barbiturate
benzodiazepine
hypnotic (drug or effect)
induction (of liver
   microsomal enzymes)

oxybarbiturate
porphyria
REM sleep
sleep latency
thiobarbiturate

OBJECTIVES

After reading and studying this chapter you should be able to:

1. State why benzodiazepines are almost always preferred to a barbiturate, whether the clinical goal is managing insomnia or anxiety (see Chapter 33 and 34. Summarize the key advantages of benzodiazepines for managing these common conditions.
2. Identify the drug used for diagnosis and treatment of benzodiazepine overdosage; explain its basic mechanism of action; and state what you might reasonably conclude if a patient who is obtunded from a multiple drug overdose does (or does not) respond to this diagnostic/treatment agent (given at usually effective doses).
3. Describe the important considerations when using benzodiazepines (or zolpidem or zaleplon) for insomnia, for example, nondrug adjunctive measures, and generally accepted time limits on the duration of drug therapy.
4. Compare and contrast the "withdrawal syndrome" associated with abrupt discontinuation of benzodiazepines (whether used for anxiety or insomnia) with that of barbiturates. (As you work your way through other chapters in this unit, you should be able to do the same for abrupt discontinuation of opioids and of alcohol.)
5. Summarize the main points about "sleep fitness"—things people can do to help them go to sleep, stay asleep, and sleep restfully, without the need for medications.

Note that you'll find additional information about several drugs discussed in this chapter in other chapters, particularly Chapters 31 (*Antidepressants*) and 34 (*Management of Anxiety Disorders*). Be sure to integrate the information.

CRITICAL THINKING AND STUDY QUESTIONS

1. With barbiturates, there is a good relationship between onset and duration of action: Slow-acting agents such as phenobarbital tend to have long durations of action. In contrast, fast-acting agents (thiobarbiturates such as thiopental) have brief durations. For the benzodiazepine class, overall, does such a relationship between onset and duration exist? Why or why not?

2. Since virtually all the benzodiazepines can cause similar effects and with roughly equivalent intensities if the "right" dose is given, why are some preferred for managing anxiety and others are indicated mainly for helping someone fall or stay asleep?

3. A patient who is receiving triazolam, a short-acting benzodiazepine hypnotic, decides to self-medicate with diphenhydramine to relieve signs and symptoms of a seasonal allergy (hay fever). What is your major concern (if any) with this combination, and what advice would you give to a patient who reports this intent to you?

4. In order to sleep, some people consume some alcohol. Others take melatonin, which is sold OTC as a nutritional supplement, not as a sleep aid. However, the majority of OTC sleep-aid medications contain another drug as the "active ingredient." What is it? How is it classified? What other properties does this drug have—what other effects can it cause—that would necessitate a thorough health history before recommending that a patient take the medication?

5. Compare benzodiazepines and barbiturate hypnotics with respect to the following properties. (In many cases, you can use relative terms such as "high" or "low" for your answers.)

   Potential for abuse

   Potential for leading to physical dependence

   Frequency of interactions with other drugs-due to induction of hepatic drug-metabolizing enzymes

   Relative safety (i.e., difference between toxic and therapeutic doses with acute administration)

   Development of tolerance

   Relative safety with continued administration (i.e., what happens to the margin of safety?)

   Maximum ability to depress CNS function (assume oral dosing)

   Maximum respiratory depressant activity (oral dosing)

6. An MD who claims to be a sleep specialist has two main classes of patients: those who have trouble falling asleep and those who fall asleep easily but awaken soon after they fall asleep. For the former he prescribes a short-acting barbiturate. For the latter group he prescribes barbiturates that have a slow onset of action but a relatively long duration of action, thereby increasing the chance that the patient won't awaken prematurely. Does this make sense to you? Consider pharmacokinetics and overall concepts about the barbiturates.

7. Although drug therapy of insomnia typically should last for a relatively brief time, many patients have been taking prescribed hypnotics for months or years in a row. What factors may contribute to this?

8. A patient schedules an appointment with her physician complaining that she is unable to sleep at night because of significant lower back pain. Which, if any, of the hypnotic drugs or drug classes discussed in this chapter would be suitable for managing the pain that is causing the sleeplessness? Why?

9. A patient presents in the emergency department with significant CNS depression (lethargy, reduced level of consciousness, slurred speech, blunted reflexes) that, according to the patient's friends, was unquestionably caused by "a bunch of pills" the patient swallowed. The patient is given a proper dose of flumazenil, but there is absolutely no change in his signs or symptoms. Does this lack of response rule out a benzodiazepine as a cause of or contributor to the overdose?

10. Are there any hypnotic or sedative drugs with which alcohol does not interact, making it relatively safe for the patient to have a few "adult beverages" right before he or she takes the medication?

11. As part of the recommendations for "sleep fitness" the text advises not to read or watch TV while in bed trying to fall asleep. Why might you disagree with this?

CASE STUDY

A patient has insomnia. He has trouble falling asleep, but once it's "lights out," he sleeps pretty well and feels refreshed each morning.

He gets a prescription to take a benzodiazepine hypnotic at 8:30 PM to help him fall asleep. His usual bed time is 9:30 (That's what happens when prime-time TV is terrible, or you just get older.)

1. He calls back a week later saying that he's been taking the medication as instructed, but he feels terribly groggy through most of the next morning. You check and see that this drug causes a peak CNS depressant effect in 60 minutes. Its plasma half-life is about 2 hours.

   If the patient is taking the proper dose in the evening, at the recommended time, he should have very little of the administered drug left in his system next morning. What, then, might explain the "hangover?"

2. Given the hangover problem, would it be advisable to instruct the patient to take the medication much earlier than usual so the residual effects of the drug are gone by next morning?

3. Upon learning of the hangover problem, the MD switches the prescription to zolpidem (Ambien). It causes peak CNS-depressant effects in about 2 hours; it's quickly metabolized to inactive compounds, and the overall incidence of residual daytime effects such as hangover is only about 1%–2%.

The problem here is that the patient didn't get explicit instructions. The MD meant to have the patient stop taking the benzodiazepine and then start the zolpidem. The patient thinks he's supposed to be taking both now, an hour or so before bed time.

What do you expect will happen? Note that the zolpidem isn't a benzodiazepine.

4. You're in the ED and will be assigned to this patient. You are made aware of the "drug cocktail" the patient took and are "guaranteed" he took nothing else. You know that there is a specific benzodiazepine antagonist, flumazenil (Romazicon). You know that it only works to antagonize benzodiazepine effects. Should you *not* give it since the patient has taken two other CNS-depressant drugs?

5. The patient survives and is discharged the next afternoon. Does the incident he experienced mean he should no longer be prescribed either the benzodiazepine hypnotic or the zolpidem?

evolve To check your answers, go to http://evolve.elsevier.com/Lehne/ for Study Guide Comments from the author.

Management of Anxiety Disorders

KEY TERMS

anxiolytic (drug or
    effect)
generalized anxiety
    disorder
obsessive-compulsive
    disorder

posttraumatic stress
    disorder
social anxiety disorder
social phobia

Most of the drugs presented in this clinically oriented chapter have many uses and are described in more detail in other chapters in this unit. Be sure to consult that information and integrate it in the context of the management of the various anxiety disorders presented here. Be especially sure to integrate material in this chapter with those in the previous chapter (*Sedative-Hypnotic Drugs*). There you'll find more information about the benzodiazepines, which as a class are also important drugs for anxiety.

OBJECTIVES

After reading and studying this chapter you should be able to:

1. Summarize the consensus about the recommended duration of insomnia therapy with hypnotics.
2. Compare and contrast the effects of buspirone (BuSpar) and a typical benzodiazepine (e.g., alprazolam) that might be prescribed for generalized anxiety disorder. Focus on the tendency to cause generalized CNS depression; interactions with other CNS depressants (e.g., alcohol, benzodiazepines, and barbiturates); pharmacokinetics, particularly with respect to onsets of action; and suitability for managing such other disorders as epilepsy and skeletal muscle spasm.

CRITICAL THINKING AND STUDY QUESTIONS

1. Since benzodiazepines—a large class of drugs—are often used to manage both insomnia and anxiety relief, what property(ies) of the individual drugs are usually considered when choosing one member of the class for a particular indication? A classmate says they differ in terms of mechanisms of action and potency, and that's the basis on which we choose one over another.

2. A patient has both daytime anxiety and difficulty falling asleep. The MD decides to prescribe just one drug: a benzodiazepine indicated for managing anxiety. Do you think this physician is ignoring the patient's other complaint, the sleeping problem? Why or why not?

3. What properties of buspirone (BuSpar), other than chemical structure, "set it apart" from benzodiazepines?

4. Your text notes that ketoconazole (a member of the azole antifungal group), erythromycin (a macrolide antibiotic), and grapefruit juice can increase buspirone's blood levels and effects? What's this all about? What should pop into your mind almost automatically when you see comments like the one we just made?

93

CASE STUDY

Al Torney is a 21-year-old college student who comes to the campus health center. He carried a 2.8 GPA until the first semester in his junior year. Now at the end of his first semester of his third year, he's failed courses in English, U.S. government, and ethics. He used to be very active, taking time away from his studies to run about 10 miles a day (he doesn't even "break a sweat") and participate in a host of intramural activities in the evenings and on weekends.

Mr. Torney expresses extreme worries about upcoming exams but also about "things in general." He says he's tense and worried. He describes himself as quite restless all the time. He can't concentrate on studying as well as he did. Sometimes he sleeps OK, but often he has trouble at night. He may fall asleep easily but wake up in the middle of the morning; at other times he just lies in bed and worries. He feels his heart pound and has chest tightness. He's dizzy, has trouble catching his breath, and says both hands get "awfully sweaty." Mr. Torney denies any thoughts of suicide or worthlessness. He wants to be able to focus, just not worry all the time.

His physical exam is largely normal and aside from the bout with mononucleosis he's been very healthy. However, his resting heart rate is 95 and he's checked his pulse during some of his "spells"; and it's been as high as about 120.

All these symptoms are unusual for him. "I've never felt like this before," he says. They began several months ago. We've ruled out infectious disease and medications as contributors to his signs and symptoms.

1. What's the most likely initial diagnosis?

Mr. Torney is placed on alprazolam (Xanax 0.25 mg tid) with instructions to return to the health center in 2 weeks.

2. How is alprazolam classified, and how, in general, does the group of drugs to which it belongs exert their main CNS effects?

3. How might we increase the likelihood that Mr. Torney will be more compliant in taking his prescribed medication? Encouragement and

providing strategies to stay compliant are not likely to be too effective.

4. Since sleepiness may be a problem for Mr. Torney (it may hinder his ability to stay awake and alert to study), what other anxiety-relieving drug might be considered instead of alprazolam or a benzodiazepine with a similar profile?

5. Since there seems to be a strong "sympathetic" component to Mr. Torney's signs and symptoms, is there yet another class of drugs that might be given a try, at least for a short time?

6. Mr. Torney wants to continue the "tradition" of hitting the bar with his buddies on Thursday nights, but he does want to have a couple of beers when he and the guys grill out on the weekends. He says he doesn't drink much alcohol, but you still are concerned that he may not abstain completely while he's on medication. In what direction might this direct your choice of medication, and why?

7. If Mr. Torney is placed on a low dose of alprazolam and promises to drink only small amounts of alcohol, should there be any concern about an adverse interaction?

8. Fast-forward. Mr. Torney has taken recommended dosages of his alprazolam daily for several months to manage his anxiety. We know this doesn't seem to reflect proper (short-term) use of an anxiety-relieving medication, but it's

happened anyway. What might you expect if Mr. Torney were to stop taking his medication abruptly? What does this *physiologic response* indicate?

9. Mr. Torney drops by to pick up a prescription for yet another month's supply of his alprazolam. You notice he appears a little groggy, and you ask if he's been drinking. He denies it, but says he's had some allergies lately and has been taking a nonprescription allergy medication. What is that most likely to be, and why would it cause the drowsiness?

10. Assume that one evening Mr. Torney gets a little down-in-the-dumps and takes 15 days' worth of alprazolam all at once. His friend hauls him off to the emergency department, but his buddy doesn't really know what, precisely, his friend took. What is the drug of choice to help diagnose and treat acute toxicity of benzodiazepines? How does it work? Of what other groups of CNS-active drugs will it reduce or block the effects?

11. Mr. Torney finishes his meeting with you by mentioning again his 2.8 GPA and recent failures of his English, government, and ethics courses. He asks for your advice: "What am I gonna do after college?" What might you recommend?

evolve To check your answers, go to http://evolve.elsevier.com/Lehne/ for Study Guide Comments from the author.

Central Nervous System Stimulants and Their Use in Attention-Deficit/Hyperactivity Disorder

KEY TERMS

ADHD
amphetamine
indirect-acting sympathomimetic

methylxanthine
narcolepsy

OBJECTIVES

After reading and studying this chapter you should be able to:

1. Discuss the CNS and peripheral autonomic effects of the amphetamines and the general mechanism by which they occur.
2. Describe the most common adverse and toxic effects of amphetamines and their management. Include the issues of tolerance, physical dependence, and abuse in your discussion.
3. Describe the various generally accepted drug treatments for attention-deficit/hyperactivity disorder.
4. Explain why CNS stimulants such as amphetamines and methylphenidate are beneficial for managing manifestations of hyperactivity disorder.

Note: Amphetamines cause significant autonomic (adrenergic) effects. Be sure to review relevant content from Chapters 12 (*Basic Principles of Neuropharmacology*), 13 (*Physiology of the Peripheral Nervous System*), and 17 (*Adrenergic Agonists*) so you can apply that information to the new information presented here.

CRITICAL THINKING AND STUDY QUESTIONS

1. Most drugs, and all neurotransmitters, work by acting as agonists on specific cell receptors.

Norepinephrine and dopamine are good examples. Why, then, is it correct to say that amphetamines (or methylphenidate) do *not* act as typical agonists, even though they cause obvious pharmacologic effects?

2. A morbidly obese adult patient who is taking recommended doses of amphetamines long-term develops episodes of "heartburn" (reflux of gastric acid into the lower esophagus) and decides to self-medicate with sodium bicarbonate (baking soda), an antacid that also alkalinizes the urine. Sodium bicarbonate is taken daily for several days in an attempt to alleviate the stomach discomfort. What is the likely outcome of this?

3. It is relatively common for schoolteachers (particularly in elementary school grades) to diagnose ADHD in some of their students and to recommend that the child's parents or guardians place him or her on methylphenidate. Comment on this.

CASE STUDY

A 19-year-old man is brought to the emergency department. He is hallucinating and exhibiting combative and confused behavior consistent with acute psychosis. His pupils are dilated but not fixed. A neurologic assessment reveals no evidence of stroke. Blood pressure is 220/116; the pulse is 130 and irregular. An electrocardiogram reveals dysrhythmias (sinus tachycardia with occasional premature ventricular contractions) and other changes indicative of myocardial ischemia (the underlying cause of angina pectoris).

A friend who accompanied him to the hospital states that he "swallowed some pills," but he does not know what they were. No other drugs, including alcohol, were consumed. The underlying cause of the overdose was amphetamines, but at the time you and your team do not know that.

1. What drug would be most appropriate for managing the acute psychosis, given the fact that at the time the underlying cause is not known?

2. Why are the patient's pupils dilated?

3. Concerned about the patient's blood pressure, the physician orders the "right" dose of phentolamine, an alpha-adrenergic blocker. What effects might you expect this drug to cause?

4. Assume that instead of administering the alpha blocker the physician turns his attention to the tachycardia and dysrhythmias. He orders propranolol, a beta-adrenergic blocker, reasoning that it will slow heart rate, has antidysrhythmic actions, and is also used as an antihypertensive. What effects would you expect from this drug?

5. Given your answers to questions 3 and 4, above, what one drug would be more suitable for managing the adverse cardiovascular effects of the amphetamine overdose?

evolve To check your answers, go to http://evolve.elsevier.com/Lehne/ for Study Guide Comments from the author.

Drug Abuse I: Basic Considerations

KEY TERMS

addiction
Comprehensive Drug
    Abuse Prevention and
    Control Act of 1970
DEA drug schedules
dependence (physical,
    psychologic, and
    cross-dependence)
DSM-IV
drug abuse
physical dependence

psychologic dependence
tolerance (and cross-
    tolerance)
reinforcing property (of
    drugs)
"reward circuit" (in
    brain)
withdrawal syndrome

OBJECTIVES

After reading and studying this chapter you should be able to:

1. State why drug abuse can be considered "culturally defined." Discuss medical and social norms that might be applied to say that a pattern of drug use or misuse and whether the use or misuse of a particular drug (or class of drugs) constitutes drug abuse.
2. Discuss psychologic and drug related factors that contribute, in a broad sense, to substance abuse.
3. Describe several of the common mechanisms by which tolerance to a drug's effects can develop, and state whether tolerance development depends on properties of the drug or on processes inherent in the body.
4. Differentiate between physical and psychologic dependence.
5. Describe the alleged roles or purposes of the Controlled Substances Act.
6. State the prescribing requirements and restrictions on DEA Schedule II, III/IV, and V medications.

Note: Meeting many of these learning objectives and commenting on the critical thinking items will be easier (and almost certainly more meaningful) after you have studied the previous chapters in this unit.

CRITICAL THINKING AND STUDY QUESTIONS

1. Is tolerance to a drug's effect(s) a phenomenon that applies only to drugs with a potential for abuse or to those that act only or mainly in the CNS?

2. Since all drugs cause more than one effect, will tolerance to one or several effects of a particular drug necessarily be accompanied by tolerance to all the rest? Does tolerance to all of a drug's effects necessarily occur to comparable degrees? Give examples to support your answer.

3. Is tolerance to a drug's effects necessarily a bad (or unwanted) thing? Give examples to support your answer.

4. Is the assignment of a drug to one of the DEA schedules permanent? If not, what is the main factor in the decision to change the assigned schedule, and therefore change restrictions on the prescribing, possession, and use of these agents?

5. What is the main criterion used to state correctly that someone has become physically dependent on a drug?

6. Check policies, guidelines, and laws that apply to and in your agency and state regarding substance abuse and misuse by healthcare providers. (*Note:* No comments are given about this on the website; this is information you need to find on your own.)

evolve To check your answers, go to http://evolve.elsevier.com/Lehne/ for Study Guide Comments from the author.

Drug Abuse II: Alcohol

KEY TERMS

acetaldehyde syndrome
aversion therapy (with
  disulfiram)
cirrhosis (hepatic)
delirium tremens
fetal alcohol syndrome

Korsakoff's psychosis
Wernicke's
  encephalopathy

OBJECTIVES

After reading and studying this chapter you should be able to:

1. Differentiate between beneficial and detrimental effects of alcohol. (You need to acknowledge, as do we, that there are conflicting reports about the benefits of alcohol and the simultaneous risks.)
2. Discuss the metabolism of ethanol with respect to the following: the roles of alcohol and aldehyde dehydrogenases, the rates of alcohol metabolism as a function of blood alcohol levels, and the general mechanism(s) by which acute high-dose and chronic "moderate" alcohol consumption affect elimination of many other drugs that undergo hepatic metabolism.
3. Identify the major non-hepatic route of elimination of alcohol and its medicolegal implications.
4. Identify several drugs—and nondrug measures—that have some hope of stopping or reducing the problems of chronic alcohol intake.
5. Compare and contrast the typical signs, symptoms, and outcomes of acute "unsupervised" withdrawal from alcohol with those of acute withdrawal from barbiturates (see Chapter 33 and 37) and from opioids (see Chapter 27).
6. Comment on the frequent use of aspirin to manage some of the common signs and symptoms of alcohol-induced "hangover." Describe whether (and which and why) other over-the-counter analgesics might be preferred for managing hangovers.

CRITICAL THINKING AND STUDY QUESTIONS

1. Why do we get "high" (have our "inhibitions released") when we consume small amounts of alcohol? It is, after all, a CNS depressant... isn't it?

2. Why do breathalyzer tests, such as those law enforcement officers may administer to a suspected drunk driver, "work"? After all, doesn't the degree of impairment depend on brain levels of alcohol, which are estimated best by measuring the blood alcohol concentration?

3. A fellow down the hall in the dorm brags about how much alcohol he can consume and how infrequently he gets a hangover from it. He says that after drinking lots of alcohol sometimes he takes aspirin before bedtime. At other times he'll use acetaminophen instead. Comment on whether these hangover remedies are a good idea, and explain the reasons for your answers.

100

4. What happens to the margin of safety of alcohol as one becomes tolerant to the subjective responses to this drug? You should remember that the margin of safety is a comparison of the lethal dose and an effective dose.

5. A patient with a condition totally unrelated to alcohol intake receives a prescription. Instructions that come with the drug, however, say "Don't take with alcohol." What are the main reasons for this warning?

6. What problems may be encountered when a woman consumes alcohol during her pregnancy?

7. A judge hearing a drunk-driving case mandates that the defendant, found guilty of his infraction, undergo mandatory disulfiram (Antabuse) therapy in addition to receiving other sanctions. Comment on this.

evolve To check your answers, go to http://evolve.elsevier.com/Lehne/ for Study Guide Comments from the author.

Drug Abuse III: Major Drugs of Abuse (Other than Alcohol)

KEY TERMS

abuse (of a drug)

hallucinogen (type of drug)

maintenance therapy (as with methadone)

misuse (of a drug)

nicotine replacement therapy

opioid

psychedelic (drug or effect)

psychostimulant

psychotomimetic

suppressive therapy (as with methadone)

tetrahydrocannibinol (THC)

OBJECTIVES

After reading and studying this chapter you should be able to:

1. Summarize the main points raised in Chapter 36 regarding the general issues of substance abuse, and apply that knowledge to what is presented in this chapter.
2. Recognize that the five main pharmacologic groups of frequently abused substances (in no particular order and excluding those labeled miscellaneous in the text) are (a) opioids, (b) generalized CNS depressants that act through mechanisms that don't involve opioid receptors, (c) psychostimulants, (d) psychedelics and psychotomimetics, and (e) anabolic steroids.
3. State whether there are any specific antidotes (e.g., receptor antagonists) for the substances of abuse (or pharmacologic groups) noted in objective 2. Identify those groups and their antagonists.
4. Compare and contrast the patterns of abuse for the drugs or drug groups listed in objective 2 and summarize their main behavioral (CNS) and systemic effects.
5. Describe the signs, symptoms, and treatment for acute or long-term use or overdose of the drugs or drug groups listed in objective 2.

6. Describe the key signs and symptoms of opioid withdrawal, its clinical management, the likely clinical outcome of unsupervised or untreated opioid withdrawal, and similarities and differences of "severe" withdrawal from opioids and severe withdrawal that from alcohol.
7. Discuss the issues of tolerance and cross-tolerance to drugs, focusing on the opioids and barbiturates.
8. Cite at least two examples for which signs and symptoms of abuse (or overuse) of a particular substance (or drug class) cause radically different acute effects that are dose-dependent. (**Hint:** Low-dose alcohol consumption causes signs and symptoms that reflect, but are not actually due to, CNS stimulation, whereas higher doses cause obvious signs and symptoms of CNS depression. In addressing this you might want to focus on such drugs as phencyclidine, PCP).

Note: The introduction to this chapter in the text states that many of the substances or drug classes that are important in the context of substance abuse have been discussed in previous chapters, and so the discussion of the basic pharmacology and abuse-related issues in the text *will be brief.* We will do the same here in terms of brevity and focus. Be sure to review the information from other chapters and integrate it with what is presented here.

CRITICAL THINKING AND STUDY QUESTIONS

1. What, to your way of thinking, differentiates misuse of a drug from abuse of one? Give some examples.

102

2. Consider two individuals, one who is a long-time abuser of opioids and another who is a long-term abuser of alcohol. Both have developed significant physical dependence to the substance. Both undergo acute, unsupervised withdrawal. What are the likely outcomes from the withdrawal syndromes characteristic to each class of drugs?

3. The text notes several classes of often-abused substances (drugs or drug classes). With which drug or groups of drugs do the patterns of barbiturate abuse, toxicity, and withdrawal share the most similarities?

4. What might be the reason barbiturate abuse has declined dramatically over the last 15 or so years?

5. Physician Robert Mendelsohn once said, "We are prone to thinking of drug abuse in terms of... illicit drugs such as heroin, cocaine, and marijuana. It may surprise you to learn that a greater problem exists with millions...dependent on legal prescription drugs." What do you think is the point of this quote? What are your overall thoughts, personally or professionally?

evolve To check your answers, go to http://evolve.elsevier.com/Lehne/ for Study Guide Comments from the author.

Diuretics

KEY TERMS

aldosterone
diuretic (drug or effect)
glomerular filtration rate
 (GFR)
hyperuricemia
hypokalemia
hyponatremia
loop diuretic (high-
 ceiling diuretic)

osmotic diuretic
ototoxicity
potassium-wasting
 (-sparing) diuretic
thiazide
tubular reabsorption
tubular secretion

OBJECTIVES

After reading and studying this chapter you should
be able to:

1. State the common mechanism(s) by which all
   diuretics increase urine production.
2. Classify the following as potassium-sparing or
   potassium-wasting diuretics: thiazides, loop
   diuretics, spironolactone, and triamterene; and
   state why knowing the effects of diuretics on
   renal potassium excretion is clinically important.
3. State factors that should be considered when
   selecting a diuretic. Consider efficacy of the various agents, dose-response relationships, and the
   potential for adverse effects in patients with other
   disorders. For which pathologies are the various
   diuretics (see objective 2) suitable?
4. Describe the adverse effects and contraindications of (or precautions for) the diuretics (or
   diuretic classes) listed in objective 2.
5. State expected effects of thiazides and loop
   diuretics on blood levels of glucose, lipids (e.g.,
   various cholesterol fractions and triglycerides),
   uric acid, calcium, and magnesium; identify
   the pre-existing conditions that might require
   extra caution if using these diuretics is anticipated.
6. After reading this chapter and Chapter 46, dealing with digoxin, state how changes of serum
   potassium levels affect the effects of the digoxin,
   and what the likely impact of hypokalemia or
   hyperkalemia would be on therapy with the cardiac glycoside.

7. Be able to state whether combinations of named
   diuretics are rational or not, and give a reason
   why. For example, is it reasonable and rational to
   administer two thiazides, or two loop diuretics, to
   the same patient?
8. Compare and contrast the mechanisms of action,
   clinical uses, and typical adverse effects of mannitol with those of a thiazide or loop diuretic.

Given the main uses of diuretics, it's important to
integrate content from this chapter with others, particular those dealing with hypertension (Chapter 45)
and heart failure (Chapter 46). Also several questions
in Chapter 40 of this study guide deal with agents that
affecting the volume and ion content of body fluids,
which are directly relevant to the actions, uses, and
problems with some of the diuretics.

CRITICAL THINKING AND STUDY QUESTIONS

1. Thiazides induce diuresis mainly through an
   action in the distal tubules and they exert relatively "modest" effects on urine output.
   Furosemide acts in the loop of Henle and can
   cause copious urine production. How and why
   do these different sites of action account for the
   differences in the peak responses to these drugs?

2. What properties give furosemide a therapeutic
   advantage over the related loop diuretics
   (ethacrynic acid, bumetanide, and torsemide)?
   Do any of the loop diuretics have a disadvantage
   over the others?

3. Parenteral furosemide can move so much fluid from the circulatory system into the urine, and do it so quickly, that it can cause significant and prompt reductions of blood pressure. A patient presents with a hypertensive crisis caused by an overdose of cocaine, which has vasoconstrictor activity. Comment on whether it would be suitable to administer furosemide to manage the excessive blood pressure.

4. Your text notes that the optimal adult daily dosage for hydrochlorothiazide is 12.5 mg to 25 mg. A patient with edema fails to derive sufficient benefit from 25 mg/day, nor from a trial of 50 mg/day. Serum potassium levels are normal due to adjunctive use of oral potassium supplement. All other things being equal, which change in the therapeutic plan is most likely to be effective: (1) increase the hydrochlorothiazide dose to 100 mg/day, (2) switch from hydrochlorothiazide to polythiazide, which is more potent (optimal dosages are only 2 mg to 4 mg/day), or (3) switch to furosemide or another loop diuretic?

5. A main indication for using furosemide is also a condition in which an osmotic diuretic (i.e., mannitol) should be used with great caution, if at all. What is that condition, and why is the statement true?

6. Without a doubt, loop diuretics are more efficacious than thiazides at increasing renal sodium excretion and urine volume. However, the risk of causing hyponatremia is much greater with a thiazide. Indeed, loop diuretics can be administered to treat hyponatremia. Explain this paradox.

7. A patient with chronic edema due to heart failure is taking digoxin, a loop diuretic, and oral potassium supplements. He experiences an acute flare-up of rheumatoid arthritis, for which he is prescribed indomethacin, which is a very efficacious inhibitor of prostaglandin synthesis. What response(s) would you expect from this medication addition?

8. A patient with a newly diagnosed adrenal cortical tumor is scheduled for surgery to remove the gland. In the meantime, he is experiencing significant fluid retention and serum electrolyte imbalances, all of which are contributing to significant edema and hypertension.

   What main serum ion imbalances would you expect? Given the pathophysiology, which diuretic would be most appropriate to provide symptomatic relief until the tumor can be removed? Which diuretics would be contraindicated because they might aggravate one or more of the serum ion imbalances caused by the tumor?

9. A patient presents in the emergency department with signs and symptoms resulting from significant overuse of a loop diuretic. With respect to the following, what would you expect to find, what might the consequences be, and what interventions might be suitable? Explain how you came to each conclusion.

   Blood pressure and heart rate
   Serum sodium, potassium, and chloride levels
   Blood pH
   Hematocrit
   To keep things simple, assume the patient is taking no other drugs that might interact or pose other problems.

10. A patient presents in the emergency department with symptomatic hypokalemia (occasional cardiac dysrhythmias, a variety of neuromuscular and neurologic dysfunctions, muscle weakness, and ileus) from excessive doses of a potassium-wasting diuretic. The physician orders oral potassium supplements and triamterene in an attempt to get serum potassium levels up. Comment on this approach.

CASE STUDY

John Sanders, 65 years old, has a history of mild type 2 diabetes, for which dietary modification alone seems to provide reasonable blood glucose control without the need for antidiabetic drugs. He reports developing "mild" heart failure, manifested mainly by mild fluid retention and ankle edema, for which his physician prescribes a typical dose of hydrochlorothiazide (50 mg each morning). Blood pressure, measured at rest on three occasions, is 130/88. Heart rate at rest is 80 and regular. There are no other significant findings.

Three weeks later Mr. Sanders calls to report that his ankles are much less swollen and puffy, but he has been feeling weaker. He has checked his blood pressure: It's 128/84, which is not uncommon (and is quite good) for a man his age. He reports a significant increase in urine output (volume and frequency), and he is "always thirsty." However, the main reason for his call is to report that he is in excruciating pain: One of his great toes is red and swollen; it hurts "just to look at it; I can't even put on my sock without it hurting so bad."

1. What might explain Mr. Sanders's feeling of weakness?

2. Could any drug-related effect(s), in addition to the expected diuresis, account for Mr. Sanders's polyuria (increased urinary volume and frequency) and polydypsia (insatiable thirst leading to frequent drinking)?

3. What is the most likely explanation for Mr. Sanders's swollen, painful toe? Could it have been drug-induced? If so, how?

4. Could any of the above problems have been avoided if Mr. Sanders were placed on furosemide instead of the thiazide when diuretic therapy was started originally?

Mr. Sanders is evaluated again. His serum potassium level is 3.5 mEq/mL (low end of normal). He is placed on oral medications for type 2 diabetes to control his blood glucose levels; and he receives proper therapy for an acute gout attack and long-term control of serum uric acid levels. The physician needs to address the hypokalemia.

5. Would it be rational for the physician to prescribe both triamterene and oral potassium supplements, to be taken daily, in an attempt to get fast and good control of Mr. Sanders's serum potassium levels?

6. When might it be more appropriate for the doctor to order spironolactone instead of the triamterene?

After 6 months of therapy with hydrochlorothiazide and triamterene Mr. Sanders seems to be doing well in terms of keeping his CHF and blood pressure in check. His diabetes and hyperuricemia medications are controlling his blood glucose and uric acid levels.

7. The physician decides to stop the hydrochlorothiazide and triamterene and place Mr. Sanders on Dyazide instead? What are the advantages, if any, of doing this?

8. A year later Mr. Sanders's signs and symptoms of CHF have returned and are assessed by various measures as being worse than when therapy started. Comment on the decision to double the dose of Dyazide.

9. Instead of doubling the dose of the Dyazide, the physician decides to go back to therapy with two different diuretics. The triamterene will continue at the same dose; the hydrochlorothiazide will be switched to a therapeutically equivalent dose of a more potent thiazide diuretic. Is this reasonable? Might there be a more efficacious alternative?

evolve To check your answers, go to http://evolve.elsevier.com/Lehne/ for Study Guide Comments from the author.

Agents Affecting the Volume and Ion Content of Body Fluids

KEY TERMS

metabolic acidosis and
    alkalosis
"normal" saline
osmolality (or
    osmolarity)
percentage (as applied to
    the concentration of a
    solution)

respiratory acidosis and
    alkalosis
volume contraction
    (isotonic, hypertonic,
    hypotonic)

OBJECTIVES

After reading and studying this chapter you should be able to:

1. Identify and describe the common etiologies of and treatments for isotonic, hypertonic, and hypotonic volume contraction.
2. Identify and describe the common etiologies of and treatments for respiratory and metabolic acidosis and for respiratory and metabolic alkalosis.
3. Identify the main hormone responsible for regulating renal potassium excretion (or retention), and state that hormone's simultaneous effects on renal handling of sodium and water.
4. Describe the link between serum insulin and potassium levels, explaining why hyperinsulinism leads to hypokalemia.
5. Identify the main potassium salt that is preferred (in most situations) for preventing or managing hypokalemia, and state why it is generally the preferred salt.

There's much good information in this chapter that relates directly to content in other chapters in this unit and elsewhere. Be sure to integrate the content here about such issues as hypertonic/hypotonic volume contraction/expansion with material dealing with diuretics (see Chapter 39).

CRITICAL THINKING AND STUDY QUESTIONS

1. Your text notes that for hypertonic volume contraction we can infuse 5% dextrose intravenously. It is rapidly metabolized to carbon dioxide and water, and so it is described as the "osmotic equivalent of water."

    How many grams of dextrose (D-glucose) are there in a 5% solution?

    What is the osmolality (osmolarity) of a 5% glucose-in-water solution? (The molecular weight of glucose is 180.) What's the osmolality of pure water?

    How might that statement about osmotic equivalency be misleading? If they were truly osmotically equivalent, as infused, could we not simply infuse or inject plain sterile water instead of the 5% glucose?

2. Tom and Dick are identical twins. Both are 6 feet tall, weigh 70 kg, and until just now were completely healthy and taking no medications. Within a 24-hour span, Tom loses 6 liters of fluid via a combination of the GI, urinary, and skin (sweating) routes. Lab tests reveal he has developed isotonic volume contraction.

    Dick loses the same amount of fluid via the same combination of routes, also over 24 hours. He develops hypertonic volume contraction.

    What simple explanation could account for these different outcomes?

3. A student looks in a comprehensive reference book and sees numbers that correctly show that urine potassium concentration is much lower when an effective loop diuretic is given than it is in normal urine. He then states, "That's impossible; you've told us that loop diuretics are potassium-wasting." Clear up the confusion for this young lad.

4. When hypokalemia occurs in response to a potassium-wasting diuretic and the goal is to prescribe an oral potassium supplement to replace the extra amount lost in response to the diuretic, how do we determine the dose of the potassium supplement?

5. To answer the above question it's helpful to collect a urine sample when the response to the diuretic has stabilized. Since the intensity of a drug's response is related to the blood concentration of the drug (more or less), how can you estimate when the diuretic's blood level has stabilized?

6. You learned in the previous chapter that two main groups of diuretics are the thiazides and the loop diuretics (e.g., furosemide). Both meet the traditional definition of *diuretic:* They increase urine volume (cause fluid loss via the urine) by increasing renal sodium excretion.

   Loop diuretics are far more efficacious than thiazides (at maximum recommended doses). The former can increase urine production by about eight times the "normal," compared with a peak of about three times for a thiazide.

   However, the thiazides are much more likely to cause hyponatremia, often called *dilutional hyponatremia,* which is not unlike what this chapter refers to as a *hypotonic state.* Indeed, loop diuretics are sometimes used to help *treat* hyponatremia. How can it be that the *more efficacious* diuretic is *less likely* to cause hyponatremia?

7. A person who lives on the Maine seacoast (altitude 0) goes on a photo expedition to Mt. Elbert, in the Sawatch Range of Colorado (the highest point in the state, altitude 14,433 feet). What blood acid-base changes would you expect, and how would it occur as this camera bug tries to adapt to this oxygen-poor environment?

   What drug or drug class might be administered to this photographer to help normalize blood acid-base balance? Constantly rebreathing into a paper bag or carrying around a tank of 95% oxygen plus 5% carbon dioxide just isn't practical.

CASE STUDY

Bob James has recently developed congestive heart failure. Because of this, his lungs have rales one-third of the way up from the base on each visit to the doctor. For several months he has been taking 20 mg of furosemide to eliminate the excess fluid, but it apparently is not working.

1. What laboratory values are important to assess in Mr. James?

2. The doctor orders that Mr. James receive potassium chloride 40 mEq IV push for his very low potassium level of 2.5 mEq/L. What is your response to this?

Mr. James has stabilized after a day in the hospital. In planning for discharge, the doctor decides to increase the oral furosemide dose to 40 mg bid and to add oral potassium chloride, 20 mEq bid.

3. Mr. James now knows he needs to keep his potassium up. He asks you what foods that he might like would be high in potassium. What are your thoughts? Given the patient's history, what other nutrient information about these potassium-rich foods is important to know? Who is probably the best person to give such dietary advice?

4. Oral potassium supplements are available in various dosage forms: tablets meant to be swallowed, tablets meant to be dissolved in some liquid or liquid beverage and then drunk, and liquids that can be added to a beverage and drunk. Which is preferred for initial therapy? What is the major hindrance to compliance with these preferred dosage forms?

5. Mr. James says, "I know salt isn't good for my heart and blood pressure. I've heard about salt substitutes. Are they OK for me? " How would you respond? What type of salt substitute would you recommend? What types are there?

6. In planning for his discharge, it is important for Mr. James to recognize some differences between hypokalemia and hyperkalemia. How will you help him remember these differences and what he needs to do at the first sign of either of these conditions?

evolve To check your answers, go to http://evolve.elsevier.com/Lehne/ for Study Guide Comments from the author.

Review of Hemodynamics

KEY TERMS

afterload
baroreceptor reflex
cardiac output
contractility (ventricular)
ejection fraction (of the
  ventricle)
natriuresis
natriuretic peptide(s)
peripheral resistance

postural hypotension
preload
renin-angiotensin-
  aldosterone system
Starling's law of the
  heart
stroke volume
venous capacitance
venous pressure (central)

OBJECTIVES

After reading and studying this chapter you should
be able to:

1. Summarize the main physiologic roles of the
   arterial and the venous "sides" of the circulatory
   system, particularly as they affect blood pressure
   and venous return to the heart.
2. Describe the processes that contribute to venous
   return.
3. Write the equation by which you calculate cardiac output, and state the main physiologic and
   pathophysiologic factors that can affect (increase
   or decrease) each of the two elements that determine cardiac output.
4. State the main neural and hormonal controls over
   blood pressure. What endogenous chemicals
   (neurotransmitters, etc.) help regulate arterial
   blood pressure?
5. Compare and contrast the roles and mechanisms of
   the renin-angiotensin-aldosterone system, the kidneys (both aldosterone-dependent and aldosterone-
   independent mechanisms), and the autonomic
   nervous system, with respect to regulating hemodynamics (i.e., blood pressure, blood flow, and
   cardiac contractility).
6. Explain why and how increases of arterial pressure can affect overall hemodynamics and ultimately lead to congestive heart failure.

Be advised: You will need to integrate the information in this chapter with information found throughout most of the rest of the unit.

CRITICAL THINKING AND STUDY QUESTIONS

1. What must peak left ventricular systolic pressure
   be in order for the ventricle to eject blood into the
   systemic circulation?

2. Starling's law states that as the length of myocardial cell fibers increases, the force developed by
   those cells increase. This can be translated into
   the whole ventricle: As left ventricular volume
   increases (greater LV filling from increases of
   end-diastolic volume and pressure), the strength
   of blood ejection increases (all other factors being
   equal). Is Starling's law without limit? Can one
   keep on stretching the myocytes, or the ventricles, and have contractile force keep going up?
   Why or why not?

3. Describe the three main systems that regulate
   blood pressure, and explain in simple terms (you
   will learn more about the details in later chapters)
   basically "how they work."

4. Is the baroreceptor reflex a bidirectional pathway? That is, do changes of heart rate *reflexly*
   affect blood pressure, just as changes of blood
   pressure reflexly affect heart rate?

5. Someone argues with you that activation of the baroreceptor reflex by a sudden fall of BP does *not* change *only* heart rate. Are they correct? Why or why not?

6. Can the heart function with no autonomic nerve (sympathetic and parasympathetic) control at all? Cite a real and quite common clinical example that proves your contention.

7. A patient is having a bout of paroxysmal supraventricular tachycardia, characterized by an inordinately high ventricular rate that's due to a very rapid atrial rate. The physician massages the patient's neck and heart rate normalizes; no drug was given. What's going on?

8. What is the most important determinant of coronary artery blood flow? What "drives" blood through the coronaries? When during the cardiac cycle does coronary blood flow occur?

evolve To check your answers, go to http://evolve.elsevier.com/Lehne/ for Study Guide Comments from the author.

chapter 42

Drugs Acting on the Renin-Angiotensin-Aldosterone System

KEY TERMS

angiocdema
angiotensin-converting
    enzyme (ACE)
angiotensin II (A II)
bradykinin and
    bradykininase

dysgeusia
juxtaglomerular
    apparatus (of kidney)
kinase II
nephropathy
renin

OBJECTIVES

After reading and studying this chapter you should be able to:

1. Describe the main components of the renin-angiotensin system (RAS) and how the overall system is regulated physiologically.
2. State the main effects of aldosterone on renal handling of sodium, potassium, and water. Identify the main physiologic stimulus for aldosterone release, and describe what increased aldosterone release is likely to do to hemodynamics (blood volume, pressure, cardiac function) and blood electrolyte composition.
3. Name the classes of drugs (and a prototype for each) that can affect blood pressure by altering the RAS or targets of its activity, and state how they cause those effects.
4. Describe the effects of angiotensin-converting enzyme (ACE) inhibitors on blood pressure and on renal regulation of sodium, potassium, and water excretion.
5. Compare and contrast the actions of angiotensin II–receptor blockers (antagonists/receptor blockers such as losartan) with those of an ACE inhibitor.
6. State the two main contraindications for administration of ACE inhibitors and angiotensin-receptor blockers (ARBs).

Important note on terminology: As indicated in your text, angiotensin-converting enzyme, bradykininase, and kinase II are essentially the same

enzymes. ACE is by far the oldest and most widely recognized term. Specific names are generally used to rcfcr to specific substrates for these enzymes. **ACE** is used when the substrate is angiotensin, which gets converted to angiotensin II by that enzyme. **Kinase II** has been introduced recently as the enzyme that inactivates bradykinin, but the term **bradykininase** has been in use longer, and it's arguably more informative since it tells you what the precise substrate actually is.

CRITICAL THINKING AND STUDY QUESTIONS

1. State the three main mechanisms by which ACE inhibitors lower blood pressure. Which two of them occur with such drugs as losartan, and how is losartan classified? (Stated differently, which effect of ACE inhibitors are lacking in such drugs as losartan?) Are the mechanistic differences between ACE inhibitors and losartan (and relatives) clinically significantly different?

2. As you learned in Chapter 39 (*Diuretics*), the diuretics commonly used (alone or in combination with ACE inhibitors or ARBs) for edema or hypertension have the following properties: (1) they all increase renal sodium excretion; and (2) thiazides and loop diuretics also increase renal potassium loss (potassium-wasting), while such agents as triamterene reduce renal potassium loss (potassium-sparing).

113

A. What are the theoretical advantages of using any of the above diuretics in combination with an ACE inhibitor or ARB, whether for hypertension or edema?

B. Despite the theoretical advantages addressed in question 2(A), which class of diuretics should not be used with ACE inhibitors or ARBs, and why?

C. When an ACE inhibitor or ARB is added to a diuretic regimen (or the converse is done, adding a diuretic to the ACE inhibitor or ARB),

3. Explain, in simple terms, why ACE inhibitors are considered highly beneficial for most patients with "mild or moderate" renal dysfunction (as from diabetes mellitus, and assuming no other specific contraindications), but bad (if not clearly dangerous) for patients with severely compromised renal function caused by significant renal artery stenosis. Your answer needs to include some indication of your knowledge of systemic blood pressure and pressures in the glomerular vasculature (glomerular filtration pressure) and how they're affected by angiotensin II and by ACE inhibitors.

4. What gender-related factor is an absolute contraindication to the use of an ACE inhibitor? What is the concern of ignoring the contraindication? Do ARBs differ from ACE inhibitors in this respect?

5. What is the main pharmacokinetic factor that often affects the decision to choose one ACE inhibitor over the several alternatives?

6. A small but important number of patients who receive ACE inhibitors experience cough that is so bothersome that they can't take the drug any longer. What accounts for this? Would you expect the incidence or severity of cough to be less with an ARB (e.g., losartan), and why?

7. What seems to be the main advantage of eplerenone (Inspra), a very new drug, over its older "alternative?" What is that alternative, and how do these drugs exert their main antihypertensive actions?

CASE STUDY

Tom Lee, who has a history of heart failure (currently NYHA Class 2), was admitted to the medical unit with complaints of a 10-pound weight gain, swollen ankles, and increasing shortness of breath over the past week. Although furosemide (a loop diuretic was partially effective in alleviating the signs and symptoms until now, the physician feels it is necessary to add an ACE inhibitor. Mr. Lee is starts taking captopril (12.5 mg PO, tid). His blood pressure is currently 150/94. Significant history includes an anterior wall myocardial infarction 12 months ago; he has also been told that he has renal artery stenosis involving the right kidney.

1. Describe the pharmacologic effects of captopril.

2. Knowing what you do about captopril's absorption, when would you recommend Mr. Lee take his medication?

3. Identify factors that trigger the release of renin and the subsequent activation of the renin-angiotensin system. These would include general triggering factors (in any person) as well as ones that might apply specifically to Mr. Lee, given his history.

4. What are the two most important physiologic actions of angiotensin II?

5. What are the main indications for ACE inhibitors?

6. What must you be concerned about shortly after Mr. Lee takes his first dose of captopril? Recall that he is already taking a diuretic. Related to this, what general precautions should be taken to reduce the risk or severity of this "most concerning" potential problem?

7. Comment on the advisability of adding triamterene (see Chapter 39) to the furosemide or switching from furosemide to triamterene while maintaining ACE inhibitor (or ARB) therapy. Assume that the reason for considering these options is that the current dosage of furosemide isn't "enough."

8. Is Mr. Lee's unilateral renal arteriolar stenosis of concern with respect to using captopril or any other ACE inhibitor?

9. All other things being equal, would prescribing an ARB such as losartan be a reasonable alternative to prescribing an ACE inhibitor?

10. If Mr. Lee were diabetic, would that have any impact on the decision to use an ACE inhibitor? Would the type of diabetes—type 1 or type 2 ("insulin-dependent" or "non–insulin-dependent," respectively)—make a difference?

11. If the patient were a 28-year-old married woman with essential hypertension, would an ACE inhibitor or an ARB be a reasonable treatment? Why or why not?

evolve To check your answers, go to http://evolve.elsevier.com/Lehne/ for Study Guide Comments from the author.

Calcium Channel Blockers

KEY TERMS

calcium channel
dihydropyridine (class of
   calcium channel
   blocker)

nondihydropyridines
   (classes of calcium
   channel blockers)

OBJECTIVES

After reading and studying this chapter you should be able to:

1. Give a brief description of the calcium channel; describe the relationships between intracellular and extracellular calcium concentrations as they affect smooth and cardiac muscle contractile function.

2. Describe the functional "linkage" between beta-adrenergic receptors and calcium channels in the heart.

3. Compare and contrast the sites of action of nifedipine (as the prototype dihydropyridine type of calcium channel blocker, or CCB) with those of diltiazem (or verapamil, which is largely equivalent to diltiazem). Explain how the differences between the dihydropyridines and verapamil (or diltiazem) affect their clinical uses and the most common side effects.

4. Identify other drugs, noted and described in this unit, that should not be administered with CCBs owing to the risk of excessive depression of cardiac contractility, rate, and electrical activity. Specify whether these precautions apply to dihydropyridine type of CCBs, just to verapamil or diltiazem, or to all CCBs. Explain why.

Notes: For material specific to this chapter, focus your studying on nifedipine as the main dihydropyridine, and consider verapamil and diltiazem to be "equivalent" to one another as the main nondihydropyridine agents. Be sure to integrate content in this chapter with relevant material in other *Cardiovascular Unit* chapters, particularly drugs for hypertension (see Chapter 45), angina (see Chapter 49), and dysrhythmias (see Chapter 47).

You should be able to recognize the common term *dihydropyridine* (as a class of CCBs), know that nifedipine is in that class (as are several other drugs) and what the cardiac and vascular spectrum of activity is. As far as verapamil and diltiazem go, it's far more important to know that they *aren't* dihydropyridines and how they act differently from dihydropyridines than it is to know that verapamil is a phenylalkylamine and that diltiazem is a benzothiazepine. It's beyond rare to hear a clinical healthcare professional use the terms *phenylalkylamine* or *benzothiazepine,* know what they mean, or that the nondihydropyridine CCBs are in one of these classes.

CRITICAL THINKING AND STUDY QUESTIONS

1. Consider the notion that there is a "functional linkage" between beta-adrenergic receptors and calcium channels. Does this mean that calcium channels and beta-adrenergic receptors are the same thing? That all the effects of administering a CCB are equivalent to those of administering a beta-adrenergic blocker?

2. In the United States roughly 10 different calcium channel blockers are approved for use, and nearly twice that number of different formulations (oral meds with different durations of action, products intended for intravenous use, etc.). And, of course, there are two main classes of calcium channel blockers: the dihydropyridines (nifedipine and most others) and the nondihydropyridines (e.g., and verapamil, diltiazem).

   Can you make any sweeping generalizations about the approved uses for these various drugs, formulations, or groups? For example, could you correctly state that "all dihydropyridines are approved for angina, but not for hypertension," or that "all the long-acting/slow-release dosage forms are indicated for hypertension but not for angina"? It certainly would be helpful to your learning if you could make such general comments as those.

3. You and a colleague are arguing over the effects of nifedipine on the heart. One of you says the drug has no effect on that organ. The other states that it causes cardiac stimulation. Who's right?

4. Assume a patient will be taking several drugs, one of which is a calcium channel blocker. What three characteristics or properties should automatically come to mind in terms of excessive or otherwise unwanted or adverse effects of such medication combinations? What questions should you ask—and answer, or at least assess for—in such settings?

5. A patient has extensive atherosclerotic lesions of several coronary arteries, which are contributing to various signs and symptoms of regional cardiac ischemia. One colleague argues nifedipine would be an ideal treatment for this patient because the drug will dilate the coronary arteries. Another argues that the opposite would be true; the nifedipine might actually worsen things, perhaps to the point of inducing acute myocardial ischemia or a myocardial infarction. Who is "right," and why?

6. Some CCBs require coadministration of a beta-adrenergic blocker, yet some formulations of the very same drug might not. With other CCBs, it's usually necessary to *avoid* giving a beta blocker. To which CCBs (or CCB groups) are we referring, and what are the main reasons that a beta

blocker might be needed.... or might need to be avoided? Explain this apparent paradox.

7. A patient with angina receives a prescription for an extended-release dosage form of nifedipine. The instructions specifically advise to swallow the medication whole, and not to crush, break, chew, or bite the product. Why is this, and what might happen if the patient ignores this warning? While we're at it, why, in general, do manufacturers make extended-release (or other slow-release or long-acting) dosage forms as alternatives to ones that are pharmacologically identical but have different pharmacokinetic profiles?

8. Prescriptions for verapamil, nifedipine, and certain other calcium channel blockers should carry a warning on the label along the lines "Don't take with grapefruit juice." A colleague tells you that that's because grapefruit juice is rich in calcium, and it will counteract the effects of these calcium channel blockers. Comment on the accuracy of her statement; explain why she might be wrong and give the correct reason or explanation.

CASE STUDY

Check the case studies for Chapter 45 (Drugs for Hypertension) and Chapter 49 (Drugs for Angina Pectoris). Case-based material dealing with calcium channel blockers is integrated in them.

Cindy Dunn, 67 years old, has a history that includes long-standing coronary artery disease with angioplasty (4 years ago) and coronary artery bypass surgery (2 years ago), peripheral vascular disease in her right leg, essential hypertension, and chronic obstructive pulmonary disease (e.g., emphysema). Despite the many and significant risks, Mrs. Dunn continues to smoke about half a pack of cigarettes a day. She takes a "baby aspirin" (81 mg) occasionally for prophylaxis of myocardial infarction. She was given a prescription for a "statin" (lipid-lowering drug; see Chapter 48) but hasn't been at all compliant with it for the last 2 years. She takes sublingual nitroglycerin "as needed" when exertion causes signs or symptoms of angina pectoris.

She visits your clinic for a routine exam that she's put off time and again for the last 18 months. Her blood pressure, in the supine position (and documented again after 30 minutes rest) is 160/96 mm Hg. Resting heart rate is 110.

The physician writes a prescription for immediate-release nifedipine, saying that it'll probably help both Mrs. Dunn's angina and her high blood pressure.

1. To what chemical class of calcium channel blockers does nifedipine belong, and what does that mean in terms of its direct effects on the peripheral vasculature (blood pressure) and the heart?

2. Do you agree with the notion that nifedipine might help both the angina and the hypertension? Formulate your answer to address the general issue of beneficial effects of this drug for these conditions and for issues pertinent to Mrs. Dunn.

3. A colleague comments on the prescription for nifedipine for Mrs. Dunn. She says, "Hmmm, Mrs. Dunn has COPD, doesn't she? I'll bet you Mrs. Dunn is going to start wheezing or developing full-blown bronchospasm as soon as she takes the nifedipine!" Do you agree with your colleague's assessment and predictions? Why or why not?

4. Two weeks after starting the rapid-acting nifedipine Mrs. Dunn comes back with complaints of palpitations, a flushed face, increased frequency and severity of angina, a weight gain of 15 pounds, and swollen ankles.

What is likely to account for these findings? Her blood pressure is back to where it was before she started the nifedipine, yet you know that after 1 week on the nifedipine her blood pressure had been coming down nicely. Your colleague states it's because Mrs. Dunn hasn't been taking her medications. What do you think?

5. Soon after one of her oral nifedipine doses, Mrs. Dunn becomes exceptionally light-headed. She feels her heart "pounding in (her) chest," which is now becoming tight and heavy—all indications of angina and maybe an imminent MI. In this situation, is Mrs. Dunn's sublingual nitroglycerin going to be helpful? Would you have any concerns?

6. Upon seeing Mrs. Dunn again, the physician reconsiders the initial decision to start Mrs. Dunn on rapid-acting nifedipine. One option now is adding metoprolol ("cardioselective" beta blocker) to the rapid-acting nifedipine regimen. What are your thoughts on this?

7. What probable advantages would there have been from starting therapy with diltiazem or verapamil (in extended-release formulations), instead of the nifedipine or another dihydropyridine?

Vasodilators

KEY TERMS

afterload

capacitance vessels

lupus-like syndrome

nitrovasodilator

nitric oxide

preload

resistance vessels

vasodilator (drug)

OBJECTIVES

After reading and studying this chapter you should be able to:

1. Identify the main ways that we can pharmacologically cause vasodilation; state the drugs (or drug classes) that have vasodilator action and describe how they cause blood vessels (e.g., arterioles) to dilate.
2. State what "unloading" the left ventricle means and why it can be beneficial in a patient with hypertension and/or heart failure.
3. Identify the pathologic conditions for which vasodilation and its consequences are beneficial; describe how excessive vasodilation can cause adverse effects that can actually worsen many of the conditions for which vasodilators are given.
4. State the expected compensatory cardiac and renal responses that occur when a drug that does nothing but dilate arterioles is given, and identify adjunctive drugs that might be used to control those responses.
5. Describe the metabolism of nitroprusside in the context of (a) the metabolite that is responsible for the vasodilation and (b) the metabolite that is responsible for the drug's potentially fatal toxicity. State precautions that need to be taken with respect to administering nitroprusside as safely as possible and monitoring for its desired and adverse effects.
6. Describe clinical settings in which diazoxide might be indicated (parenteral administration) and the likely adverse responses to it (cardiovascular and otherwise).

Be sure to integrate content in this chapter, which largely deals with drugs used to lower blood pressure, with content from other chapters (e.g., other antihypertensive drugs, see Chapter 45; drugs for heart failure, see Chapter 46).

CRITICAL THINKING AND STUDY QUESTIONS

1. Some agencies automatically add sterile sodium thiosulfate to their nitroprusside solutions right before the drug is administered. Why?

2. Given the effectiveness of nitroprusside, why and when would anyone want to use parenteral diazoxide for managing a hypertensive crisis?

3. A patient with severe hypertension has been receiving nitroprusside to control blood pressure, but it's clear that cyanide toxicity is developing. The drug has to be stopped. What, then, can be done to control the blood pressure?

4. Some vasodilators cause significant orthostatic hypotension, others do not. What action mainly determines whether orthostatic hypotension will occur or be severe? (*Hint:* To answer this question, consider the normal physiologic responses that prevent us from developing orthostatic hypotension; then consider the drugs that interfere with that.)

119

5. Vasodilators of just about any type often cause compensatory reflex tachycardia and edema. What are the mechanisms by which these unwanted effects occur? What adjunctive drugs may need to be prescribed to counteract them? (Assume no contraindications to the use of those adjuncts.)

A week after beginning the hydralazine, Mr. Allen's blood pressure is back to where it was before he began taking the drug. He has gained about 7 pounds (3 kg) over that time and developed some swelling in his ankles, too. But he insists that he has been eating healthy foods, and not at all in excessive quantities; he swears he's been taking his medications as ordered. Assume that's true.

2. What might explain the return of the hypertension, the weight gain, and the ankle swelling?

CASE STUDY

George Allen, a 50-year-old man who is 5' 10" tall and weighs 90 kg, has both stage II essential hypertension and congestive heart failure. They are seriously compromising his quality of life. He has difficulty walking up one flight of stairs without experiencing significant fatigue and dyspnea. These problems persist despite daily use of usually effective doses of furosemide (loop diuretic; see Chapter 39) and captopril (ACE inhibitor; see Chapter 45).

Mr. Allen's physician discontinues the diuretic and ACE inhibitor and prescribes oral hydralazine, 10 mg taken 4 times a day, with the plan to reevaluate in a week and probably titrate the dose up to 20 mg 4 times a day.

Before Mr. Allen leaves the physician's office, you teach him how to measure his blood pressure, and you are satisfied that he can do it accurately. Mr. Allen will keep a log of his blood pressure and pulse rate, measuring both just before each hydralazine dose. He'll also weigh himself daily and keep a log of his daily activities and symptom onset and severity.

Mr. Allen reports that after taking the hydralazine for 2 days his blood pressure is "coming down nicely," (BP = 106/60) but his resting heart rate now hovers around 100 and it spikes to about 120–130 when he stands. He feels light-headed about an hour after taking his medication, and he's getting "some chest discomfort... it feels 'tight,' as if someone's standing on my chest."

1. What properties of hydralazine may contribute to Mr. Allen's relative increase in heart rate, the light-headedness, and the chest discomfort? The drug is, after all, simply an arteriolar dilator.

3. What other drug(s) might be added to control the unwanted cardiovascular and renal responses to the hydralazine? Why?

4. Would it be reasonable for the physician to add nifedipine or another type of dihydropyridine calcium channel blocker to the regimen?

5. Would it be reasonable for the physician to add both verapamil and a beta blocker to Mr. Allen's treatment plan in order to get really good control over the tachycardia?

6. Mr. Allen is now taking "usual" doses of hydralazine, metoprolol (a cardioselective beta blocker), and furosemide. He lost the extra weight he gained while taking just the hydralazine, and his blood pressure and heart rate are approaching target levels set by the physician. Mr. Allen calls to report that he's feeling achy,

and he has a fever. What needs to be investigated and which drug or drug combination that is part of his current therapy might be the culprit?

7. Comment on whether it would have been better to start Mr. Allen on hydralazine to manage his hypertension and heart failure at the outset. Why start with the ACE inhibitor, for example?

evolve To check your answers, go to http://evolve.elsevier.com/Lehne/ for Study Guide Comments from the author.

Drugs for Hypertension

KEY TERMS

afterload reduction
comorbid condition(s)
eclampsia, preeclampsia
hypertension (primary,
    secondary, essential)
"JNC VI"

monotherapy
step-down therapy
papilledema
pheochromocytoma
white coat hypertension

OBJECTIVES

After reading and studying this chapter you should be able to:

1. State how the following contribute to the regulation of blood pressure, and name the classes of antihypertensive drugs that target one or more of these processes or structures when they are given to lower an elevated blood pressure:
    Heart (via the contractile force developed by the left ventricle)
    Peripheral vasculature
    Parasympathetic nervous system
    Sympathetic nervous system
    Renin-angiotensin-aldosterone system (including the kidneys themselves)
2. State the criterion (criteria) used to classify hypertension as "essential hypertension."
3. State the factors that, in addition to blood pressure *per se,* are used to classify the severity of hypertension according to the "Joint National Commission–VI."
4. Explain how many (most) of the pathophysiologic processes that occur during long-term hypertension simultaneously contribute to the development of heart failure.
5. State the major factors that go into determining which antihypertensive drug (or drug combination) would be most suitable for a patient with a stated severity of essential hypertension; in addition state how specified comorbidities (e.g., heart failure, diabetes, asthma, etc.) would affect the drug choice, that is, weighing in favor of or against a particular class of drugs.

6. Given a list of pre-existing comorbidities, state whether named antihypertensive drugs (or drug groups) would or would not be appropriate, and give reasons for your answers.
7. State the gains to be expected, in terms of blood pressure control, by progressively increasing the dosage of one antihypertensive drug vs. adding drugs in other classes to the initial agent.
8. State the benefits to be gained, in terms of blood pressure control, by switching from one drug in a particular class to another agent in the same class (e.g., switching from one beta blocker to another).
9. List and describe several nondrug (e.g., lifestyle) factors that should be encouraged to manage essential hypertension, regardless of the drug(s) used.
10. Describe general goals for safe management of a hypertensive emergency, and name drugs that would be suitable for such a situation.
11. Discuss the etiology of hypertension during pregnancy; include a discussion of preeclampsia and eclampsia, as well as the roles of antihypertensive drugs and magnesium sulfate. State the "definitive cure" for hypertension in eclampsia.

As noted in the text, the contents of this chapter include many drugs and disorders that are discussed in more detail in other chapters. Be sure to review that information and integrate it as needed with the new information presented here.

There are many other chapters in this unit that describe drugs used to manage hypertension. Be sure to consult them and integrate that material. The study questions (and the case study) presented here supplements information you should find elsewhere.

CRITICAL THINKING AND STUDY QUESTIONS

1. How can too great a daily intake of salt (sodium chloride) raise blood pressure? If one drastically *reduces* his or her daily salt intake, what compensatory responses that might actually tend to

122

increase blood pressure occur? What might be the greatest risk if a patient is taking a thiazide and drastically reduces daily salt intake?

2. You're listening to a nurse practitioner with years of clinical experience give a continuing ed presentation entitled "Initiating Antihypertensive Drug Therapy in Ambulatory Patients. She states, "It's a no-brainer to pick and prescribe an antihypertensive drug; what's more difficult is selecting the *right one* for the patient." What might she mean by this, and why is it important?

3. We have three "average" hypertensive patients. Mr. A is taking a recommended dose of hydrochlorothiazide. Mr. B is taking a beta blocker. Mr. C is taking captopril. None of these patients is experiencing adverse responses to his medication, but none is experiencing adequate lowering of blood pressure either. We are sure that the maximum recommended dosages of each are being given, that there are no problems with eliminating (excreting and metabolizing) the drugs, and no interacting drugs are being taken.

   What would you expect, in the way of better blood pressure lowering, if we switched Mr. A to another thiazide, Mr. B to another beta blocker, and Mr. C from captopril to a different ACE inhibitor?

4. State the three main mechanisms by which ACE inhibitors lower blood pressure. Which two of them occur with such drugs as losartan, and how is losartan classified? (Stated differently, which effect of ACE inhibitors do such drugs as losartan lack?) Are the mechanistic differences between ACE inhibitors and losartan (and relatives) clinically significantly different?

5. Many ambulatory patients with essential hypertension are taking alpha$_1$ blockers such as prazosin. Why would that alpha blocker be used rather than a nonselective alpha$_1$ or alpha$_2$ blocker such as phentolamine?

6. What concern might you have about using a diuretic as an antihypertensive drug for a pregnant woman? (We are not talking about a woman with preeclampsia or eclampsia, but rather more modest elevations of pressure.)

7. A patient with hypertension is placed on prazosin and hydrochlorothiazide. The patient asks, "Why do I have to take two medications for my blood pressure?" What is the rationale for this?

8. It's pretty obvious (we hope) that administering a nonselective beta-adrenergic blocker such as propranolol to a hypertensive patient with asthma is a bad idea—a dandy way to cause significant bronchospasm, maybe even kill the patient.

   A. Instead of propranolol, would a cardioselective beta blocker be preferred for this asthma patient?

   B. Comment on potential concerns about using a diuretic as an antihypertensive medication for a person with asthma.

9. A colleague who is discussing a pregnant woman with eclampsia states that the woman should get magnesium sulfate to lower her blood pressure. Comment on this.

To simplify things, assume we are talking about this in the context of a hypertensive patient who has multiple but relatively minor lacerations on the arms and upper body that require suturing, and infiltration of a local anesthetic is indicated.

10. Joe Smith has stage III hypertension and the physician decides to prescribe oral hydralazine. In a couple of days his BP is falling nicely towards the lower target BP. After another 5 days Mr. Smith calls the MD's office. He is complaining of "fluttering" in his chest.

    A. What probably accounted for the chest flutters?

    B. When Mr. Smith visits the office to check on his palpitations, what would you expect to find in the way of his body weight and blood pressure? Why? What meds might need to be added to control the cardiac responses, the weight gain, and the blood pressure?

13. What properties of nitroprusside make it such a good drug for managing hypertensive emergencies or for providing controlled hypotension during surgery? Which of those properties, and others, make this such a potentially dangerous drug at the same time? Given the properties you have identified, what precautions must be taken and what prerequisites must be met if this drug is to be administered?

14. Take a trip to your local retail pharmacy or the OTC medicine aisles of your favorite supermarket. Look for several rather new products that are advertised as relieving nasal congestion, but labeled "For people with high blood pressure." (These may have such initials as HBP—high blood pressure—on the label.) What is the active ingredient in those products? While the medication in them may be OK for people who shouldn't take an adrenergic agonist (e.g., people with hypertension), it may not be good for people with other common disorders. What is the decongestant ingredient in those products? For whom might this ingredient pose risks, and why?

11. A patient has essential hypertension. She develops a cold and a profuse and bothersome runny nose. She'd like to take an OTC decongestant for a couple of days, and the ones that contain an adrenergic agonist certainly work well. Should she avoid such products "no matter what"?

12. Comment on the following: "Epinephrine obviously is a vasoconstrictor, clearly a drug that can raise blood pressure. Therefore, local anesthetics that contain epinephrine are contraindicated for patients with hypertension."

CASE STUDY

Joe English is a 50-year-old man with a 12-year history of hypertension and coronary artery disease. He was taking atorvastatin (see Chapter 48) to keep his serum cholesterol levels in check. His hypertension had been managed with oral clonidine (how is it classified, how does it lower blood pressure?), which kept his blood pressure around 130/86 mm Hg for 4 years. However, he discontinued the clonidine abruptly 2 days ago because he ran out of his pills and decided to wait a while to go to town to get a refill.

1. What would you expect from this sudden discontinuation of the clonidine?

When Mr. English arrives at the physician's office his blood pressure is 220/140 and his heart rate is 110. Respiratory rate is 24/min. There is some papilledema, but pupil function and other reflexes appear intact. He is alert and oriented, and there's no evidence of target organ damage (brain, kidneys, etc.). The paramedics are called and he is transported and admitted to your small, rural hospital.

2. What drug might the MD administer in the office to get a quick start on safely lowering blood pressure before the paramedics arrive?

3. How might Mr. English present differently if he had been on long-term metoprolol (cardioselective beta-adrenergic blocker) therapy instead of the clonidine, and had discontinued that drug abruptly?

4. What other classes of oral antihypertensives are associated with a "rebound" phenomenon characterized by significant and quickly developing rises of heart rate and/or blood pressure?

Prompt drug therapy is indicated, but you cannot quickly locate a physician to order the proper IV drug(s). A colleague suggests pricking open a capsule of nifedipine (rapid-acting dosage form of this dihydropyridine calcium channel blocker; see Chapter 43) and squirting the contents under Mr.

English's tongue. "I know lots of doctors and nurses who say this works well," he says, "and we have some in the medication drawer on the unit."

5. What would you expect if you followed this plan?

Mr. English received the sublingual nifedipine. He is now hypotensive (BP 70/40) and tachycardic (R = 120) and is becoming unresponsive. The physician arrives, assesses the situation, and orders the ordinarily right dose of intravenous phenylephrine.

6. What is the rationale for administering the phenylephrine?

7. If the physician orders the "usual recommended" dose of phenylephrine, what response(s) would you expect, and why?

8. The physician orders a rapid IV infusion of a large volume of fluid, instead of a vasoconstrictor drug, to raise Mr. English's acutely lowered blood pressure. What fluid (e.g., 0.9% NaCl or something else) would be appropriate? Why?

Let's back up and reassess treating Mr. English's acute hypertensive episode from the start. Remember that the goal is to lower blood pressure safely and not do greater harm to other medical conditions he may have (or cause new problems). Comment on the suitability of the following drugs, given by themselves parenterally, in this scenario.

A. Furosemide

B. Chlorothiazide (the only thiazide diuretic available in an injectable formulation)

F. Propranolol

G. Metoprolol

C. Enalaprilat, the injectable dosage form of enalapril, which is an angiotensin-converting enzyme inhibitor.

H. Labetalol

D. Diazoxide

E. An alpha-adrenergic blocker such as phento-lamine

evolve To check your answers, go to http://evolve.elsevier.com/Lehne/ for Study Guide Comments from the author.

Drugs for Heart Failure

KEY TERMS

afterload
cardiac glycoside
digitalization (digitalize)
dyspnea
ectopic focus/foci (of
    cardiac electrical
    activity)
heart failure (and
    congestive HF)
ino(vaso)dilator

inotropic (drug or effect)
Na^+, K^+-ATPase
orthopnea
preload
sarcomere
sodium pump
Starling's law of the
    heart
vagotonic (effect of
    digoxin)

OBJECTIVES

After reading and studying this chapter you should be able to:

1. Summarize the essence of Starling's law of the heart as it relates to the length of the heart cells' contractile proteins (sarcomeres), and translate that into factors that relate ventricular end-diastolic volume (or central venous pressure) with the amount of contractile force the entire left ventricle develops during systole. State how those relationships are altered as heart failure develops.

2. Describe the characteristic signs and symptoms of heart failure, including those that would qualify for being called "congestive."

3. Summarize the characteristics or measures that are used to "assign" a patient with heart failure to the four American College of Cardiology/ American Heart Association stages and those that make up the New York Heart Association classes.

4. Discuss the goals for the treatment of chronic and acute heart failure.

5. Recognize and be able to describe the roles, benefits, and limitations of the following drugs (or drug groups) in the setting of long-term management of heart failure:
   - Angiotensin-converting enzyme inhibitors (and angiotensin-receptor blockers)
   - Diuretics
   - Spironolactone
   - Beta-adrenergic blockers
   - Digoxin

6. Describe what *afterload* and *afterload reduction;* explain why afterload reduction is of benefit in the management of heart failure.

7. State the main direct and indirect cardiac contractile and electrophysiologic effects of digoxin, and describe the relationship between serum potassium levels on them. You might want to focus on digoxin's effects on atrial and ventricular automaticity and electrical impulse conduction rates through the AV node; they are the most important clinically.

8. Explain how digoxin's desired effects lead to beneficial systemic hemodynamic and metabolic/endocrine effects, when the drug is "working properly," to provide the desired clinical outcomes.

9. Explain why digoxin is a mixed blessing for management of chronic heart failure, particularly with respect to problems related to the frequency and severity of toxicity.

10. Describe why the use of such diuretics as furosemide as an adjunct to digoxin can be considered a double-edged sword—beneficial on one hand, but also one that can increase the risk of digoxin toxicity.

11. State the cardiac and other (noncardiac/extracardiac) signs and symptoms that are consistent with digoxin toxicity—those that would lead you to suspect intoxication of the drug even before you have electrocardiographic and blood test results. State the first thing that should be done—or given as an instruction to the patient— when digoxin toxicity is suspected.

Note: Many of the drugs discussed in this chapter are described in more detail in other chapters. Be sure you review that material and integrate it into this discussion on heart failure and its pharmacologic management. In addition, be sure you've studied and understood the material in Chapter 41 (*Review of Hemodynamics*).

CRITICAL THINKING AND STUDY QUESTIONS

1. It's often said that "the heart fails backwards." Assume a patient has severe, long-standing systemic (arterial) hypertension, which of course has immediate impact on the structure "right in back" of it: the left ventricle. Trace the "backwards spread" of failure (just follow the normal pathway for blood from the venous to the arterial side and through the heart chambers, but do it backwards). Describe how Starling's law attempts to compensate for the initial insult. (*Hint*: Remember that a pressure gradient [pressure difference] is responsible for moving blood from one compartment to another, or through a vessel, and that increased pressure during diastole increases resting stretch of the affected heart chamber.)

2. When the heart fails, the contractile proteins lengthen (stretch). According to Starling's law, that will cause a compensatory increase in contractile force development. What causes this "stretch"? Is it an active or a passive process?

3. How does digoxin "shift" a Starling curve that describes a failing heart towards a curve that more closely reflects what a normal heart does?

4. Cardiac output, which is reduced in most cases of heart failure, is determined by the following formula: CO = Heart Rate × Stroke Volume. From a therapeutic viewpoint, which do we almost always try to change (HR or SV)? Why, and how?

5. Cells in the failing heart hypertrophy and "remodel." Are these beneficial over the long run? What are the consequences? Which drugs that are typically used for managing heart failure—inotropes, diuretics, or others—seem to exert desired effects on this remodeling/hypertrophy process? How?

6. Most of the discussion in this chapter is centered on heart failure characterized by low cardiac output: "low-output failure." Is there such a thing as "high-output cardiac failure"? Can you think of a couple of examples in which that might occur, at least initially?

7. When usual therapeutic doses of digoxin are given for heart failure, what is the main expected effect on heart rate—the one arising indirectly from its beneficial hemodynamic effects? How and why does that effect occur?

8. What is the main *direct* electrophysiologic (and electrocardiographic) change that occurs with administration of digoxin, even at therapeutic blood levels and with normal serum electrolyte levels? The magnitude of this change roughly parallels the digoxin blood level.

9. Although digoxin toxicity can cause just about any type of dysrhythmia you can imagine, two electrocardiographic changes are most common. What are they, and why do they occur?

10. A patient presents with acute heart failure. Blood pressure is quite low. A colleague says, "Give some phenylephrine.... That'll help!" How is phenylephrine classified? Would it be the "right" drug to give in this setting? Why or why not?

11. Another patient arrives with acute heart failure and very low blood pressure. There's no trauma, no evidence of blood loss. Yet another colleague says, "Infuse some saline.... That'll get his blood pressure up!" Comment on this approach.

12. Ponder this hypothetical situation. You're in a small hospital that is suddenly swamped with many patients with acute heart failure. There's no dopamine available, and all the dobutamine has been used up too. You have a patient who requires an IV positive inotropic agent. Of course, you want to avoid giving an agent that will cause peripheral vasoconstriction. What combination of adrenergic drugs could you administer that would, in essence, provide exactly the same, and only the same, effects as dobutamine? How did you arrive at that answer?

CASE STUDY

Todd Black, a 68-year-old hypertensive patient, was being treated for congestive heart failure and had been taking digoxin (0.25 mg daily) for the last 3 years. Assessment placed him in NYHA Functional Classification II over that time, during which he has gained approximately 20 kg. Over the last year, he reports, he has been "getting real tired real easy" when he goes out for walks or shopping, and so he's basically stayed home to watch TV or read the papers, but can easily do things for himself around the house or when he goes out.

At the time you see him in the physician's office, blood pressure now is 170/110, heart rate is 110 and

regular, and respiratory rate is 22. He weighs 95 kg and is 175 cm tall. His ankles are puffy, his jugular veins distended, and his belly protruding and "full." He can't lie flat on the bed to sleep; he sleeps in a semireclining position with three pillows under his head.

1. What criteria are used to "place" a given patient into an NYHA functional classification, and what does being in Class II mean?

2. Given the little bit of history noted above, give your thoughts on the medical approach to Mr. Black's heart failure over the last 1 to 3 years.

3. What might you reasonably conclude are contributing pathophysiologic factors to Mr. Black's BP and heart rate, his weight gain, and his easy fatigability?

4. What is the term used to describe Mr. Black's need to sleep semireclining, with pillows propped under his head? What physiologic/pathophysiologic problem(s) account(s) for this?

5. In a sample of Mr. Black's blood, would you expect serum sodium and potassium concentrations to be high, normal, or low? Why?

6. Why are serum potassium levels of particular importance for patients receiving digoxin? What is the relationship between K levels and digoxin's actions?

7. Why might a beta-adrenergic blocker (e.g., propranolol) seem, at first glance, to be a good add-on to Mr. Black's digoxin therapy? In thinking about it more, do you think administering a beta blocker at this time would be wise?

8. How do metoprolol and carvedilol differ from propranolol, which could be considered the prototype of beta-adrenergic blockers? What are the theoretical advantages of using one of those alternatives?

9. Would starting Mr. Black on an oral ACE inhibitor and hydrochlorothiazide sending him home in an hour or two with instructions to come back in 2 weeks be a good option?

10. Would it be better simply to double Mr. Black's digoxin dose?

Mr. Black is admitted to the hospital. He receives parenteral doses of furosemide, carvedilol, and electrolytes, such that his cardiac output is brought closer to normal and serum electrolytes are all

within normal limits. The digoxin is not stopped because blood levels are in the therapeutic range.

11. Of the above drugs, which was most likely to have helped Mr. Black's symptoms the quickest?

Mr. Black is discharged on captopril, metoprolol, furosemide, and digoxin. Verapamil is also prescribed to control Mr. Black's blood pressure. Each is prescribed at the "usual" recommended dose.

12. With this combination of drugs, are you concerned that the furosemide might cause hypokalemia, thereby increasing the risk of digoxin toxicity? Why or why not?

13. Based on the information provided, do you think it is necessary to prescribe verapamil in addition to the other meds for the purpose of managing Mr. Black's hypertension?

14. What other concern(s) might you have about the combination of captopril, metoprolol, furosemide, digoxin, and verapamil?

15. If you thought it was necessary to eliminate one of those drugs from the overall medication plan (it probably is necessary), which would it be, and why?

16. If you could get Mr. Black's regimen down to a "bare minimum" of drugs, which would you choose? Why? Assume that the underlying problem with Mr. Black's heart failure is left ventricular dysfunction (i.e., reduced stroke volume) and that there are no specific contraindications to the drug(s) you choose. If there were congestive symptoms due to volume overload, which drug would you add to the therapeutic plan?

17. Long-term, what does digoxin therapy for heart failure really accomplish? What important outcome is not associated with digoxin therapy?

evolve To check your answers, go to http://evolve.elsevier.com/Lehne/ for Study Guide Comments from the author.

Antidysrhythmic Drugs

KEY TERMS

automaticity (of
   cardiac tissues)
blood dyscrasia
cinchona alkaloid
cinchonism
heart block
Holter monitor
prodysrhythmic
   effect (of drugs)

reentrant activation (of heart)
RF catheter ablation
supraventricular dysrhythmia
torsades de pointes
Vaughan Williams
   (classification)
ventricular dysrhythmia
Wolff-Parkinson-White
   syndrome

OBJECTIVES

After reading and studying this chapter you should
be able to:

1. State the normal electrophysiologic roles of the
   following specialized portions of the heart: sinoatrial node, atrial myocardium, atrioventricular
   node, and His-Purkinje system.
2. State what each of the following parts of a normal
   EKG represent in terms of contractile or electrophysiologic activities of the heart: P wave, QRS
   complex, T wave, PR interval, and ST segment.
3. Explain the pathophysiology involved in the
   development of dysrhythmias, focusing on the
   main electrophysiologic properties of heart cells
   and tissues: automaticity, conduction velocity,
   and refractoriness.
4. Define the terms *first-degree, second-degree,* and
   third-degree heart block. Describe how you can
   tell by inspecting the EKG that these are occurring. Identify the drugs that can cause heart
   block; include in your list not only antidysrhythmic drugs, but other drugs discussed in Unit VII
   (there are several important ones).
5. Describe how the type of dysrhythmia affects the
   selection of drugs used to manage it.
6. Recognize the Vaughan Williams classification as
   one that is used for antidysrhythmic drugs, and
   state the general principles that determine
   whether a drug "fits" in a particular category of it.
   State whether this classification scheme is clinically useful to the extent that it predicts adverse

responses, side effects, or even clinical uses
caused by every member of a given class.
7. Summarize current trends and opinions about
   pharmacologic management of dysrhythmias (as
   opposed to nondrug interventions like catheter
   ablation or to no treatment) based on the
   anatomic origin, severity, and acuity of the
   rhythm disorder.
8. Describe the side effects or adverse responses
   that can be caused by virtually any antidysrhythmic drug, and those that are unique to quinidine,
   amiodarone, procainamide, and disopyramide.

Many other drugs used for dysrhythmias are discussed in more detail in other chapters because they
have other clinical uses. These include beta-adrenergic blockers and calcium channel blockers.
Therefore, focus here on the short list of drugs,
above, (used only for controlling dysrhythmias).

CRITICAL THINKING AND STUDY QUESTIONS

1. What are the predominant ion movements during
   phase 1 of the cardiac cell action potential? Phase
   2? Phase 3? Which antidysrhythmic drugs exert
   their main electrophysiologic effects on each of
   these parts of the action potential?

2. In addition to controlling dysrhythmias, what do
   antidysrhythmic drugs have the potential to do in
   terms of cardiac electric effects? Are "all antidysrhythmic drugs created equal" in this respect?

3. What part of the EKG gives you information that the electrical impulse conduction rate through the AV node is being slowed? What part of the EKG gives you information about conduction rate through the ventricles?

4. Instructions for some drugs (beta blockers are a good example) carry the warning, "Do not administer to patients with second-degree or greater heart block." What is heart block, and what are the different degrees of it?

5. Compare and contrast the main clinical uses and most common side effects (particularly those "outside the heart") of quinidine, procainamide, and disopyramide, which are all in the same Vaughan Williams class. (It's OK to peek in your text.) Given the information you've summarized about these three drugs, what can you conclude about this classification system?

6. A patient who is taking digoxin and furosemide for heart failure presents in clinic for scheduled blood work and an EKG. His pulse is irregular and slow (50), and the EKG reveals second-degree heart block and frequent premature atrial contractions. A possible cause is digoxin intoxication, whether from a frank overdose or from hypokalemia. Since this patient's dysrhythmia primarily is supraventricular and quinidine is mainly used for supraventricular dysrhythmias, what are your thoughts about using this drug for this patient? Would a beta-adrenergic blocker or a calcium channel blocker (specifically diltiazem or verapamil) be a reasonable, or better, alternative to quinidine? Explain your reasoning.

7. You're reading about a drug in a reference book and see information that states that the drug may prolong the QT interval on the EKG. What should this mean to you? What dysrhythmias might such a drug cause in susceptible patients? What are its characteristics? Do you have any idea about how many drugs have this QT-prolonging property, and what drug classes they belong to?

8. Identify the antidysrhythmic drug(s) that...
   - may cause a clinical syndrome indicative of or resembling hypothyroidism.
   - may cause many of the signs and symptoms of systemic lupus erythematosus.
   - probably ought to be avoided, if possible, by patients who are at risk from antimuscarinic (atropine-like) effects.

9. An apparently healthy man of 35 years is having dinner at a restaurant. After eating a few bites of food, he becomes dizzy and faints. He reports that his heart was racing and he was becoming light-headed right before he passed out. He has never experienced such a response before. He is brought to the ED; all vitals are normal, as is the EKG (normal sinus rhythm), but it's probable he suffered some sort of arrhythmia. After spending 24 hours in the hospital to rule out a myocardial infarction (results are negative for MI), he's discharged with instructions to visit his personal physician. His personal MD orders a Holter monitor to record his EKG continuously for 24 hours. Comment on the likelihood that this monitoring technique will show anything meaningful.

CASE STUDY

Vic Brown, an overweight 75-year-old retiree, underwent open-heart surgery 5 days ago. His history includes stage II hypertension, renal insufficiency, a 2-pack-per-day smoking habit, and a stroke 5 years ago.

The physical therapists were in to help Mr. Brown transfer to a chair. Following transfer to a recliner, Mr. Brown complained that his "heart felt like it was racing." About that time, the nurse walked in to check because the cardiac monitor revealed a heart rate of 160, which the nurse called supraventricular tachycardia (SVT). The nurse asked Mr. Brown to bear down to simulate a Valsalva maneuver.

After obtaining a full set of vital signs, the nurse placed a call to the doctor. Fifteen minutes later, the doctor returned the call and ordered stat doses of digoxin and adenosine. This regimen was unsuccessful, so the doctor ordered a 1-mg test dose of verapamil, followed by another 4 mg if tolerated.

The physician arrived on the unit, examined the EKG, and questioned whether the rhythm might be ventricular tachycardia (VTACH), not supraventricular. By this time, Mr. Brown was feeling weak with a blood pressure of 66/46. A bolus of lidocaine (100 mg) was administered, followed by a 2 mg/min continuous drip. Fifteen minutes later, Mr. Brown remained in VTACH. Cardioversion was attempted but was unsuccessful. Finally, 5 hours later, Mr. Brown converted to a normal sinus rhythm with a stable blood pressure. Over the next few days he was started on oral therapy with quinidine, digoxin, and long-acting procainamide.

1. Explain the differences between supraventricular and ventricular tachycardias. Is an atrial dysrhythmia necessarily the same thing as a supraventricular dysrhythmia?

2. What was the purpose of having Mr. Brown perform a Valsalva maneuver? Was that an appropriate intervention, given Mr. Brown's history? Might there have been another nondrug option for trying to convert the dysrhythmia?

3. Mr. Brown's doctor originally prescribed digoxin and adenosine to control the dysrhythmia? What was he thinking in terms of how these drugs might work?

4. Since the adenosine-digoxin combination did not normalize Mr. Brown's ventricular response, what can you conclude about the origin of his dysrhythmia?

5. Aside from monitoring Mr. Brown's EKG and blood pressure, what else should the nurse be assessing to detect adverse effects of the lidocaine that was subsequently administered?

6. Based on the information presented in the scenario, comment on the rationale for ultimately controlling Mr. Brown's dysrhythmia with a combination of quinidine, digoxin, and long-acting procainamide.

7. If the MD chose to treat Mr. Brown with both digoxin and quinidine, what would you expect this combination of drugs to do to the patient's AV nodal function and to ventricular contractility? What pharmacokinetic interaction would you expect when giving these two drugs together and what might need to be done to manage it?

Prophylaxis of Coronary Heart Disease: Drugs That Lower LDL Cholesterol Levels

KEY TERMS

atherogenesis
atherosclerosis
bile acid sequestrant
coronary artery (heart)
   disease (CAD; CHD)
cholelithiasis

fibrates (class of drugs)
HMG-CoA reductase
myoglobinuria
myositis
rhabdomyolysis
statins (class of drugs)

OBJECTIVES

After reading and studying this chapter you should be able to:

1. Describe the general physiologic and biochemical processes of lipoprotein synthesis and regulation of serum lipoprotein levels.
2. Name the drug class that is generally the first choice to treat hypercholesterolemia, and summarize its fundamental mechanism of action.
3. Describe the signs and symptoms of rhabdomyolysis; identify the main class of drugs associated with it, its clinical consequences, and factors (drugs and other) that increase the risk of this syndrome.
4. Compare and contrast the lipid-lowering mechanisms of action, clinical indications, and side effects, for the following: (a) the statins, (b) fibric acid derivatives, (c) niacin, and (d) bile acid sequestrants.
5. Develop a teaching plan that will maximize therapeutic benefits from dyslipidemia therapy for patients taking one or several lipid-lowering drugs, and describe adjustments when interactants (that you should specify as being clinically important) are prescribed.

CRITICAL THINKING AND STUDY QUESTIONS

1. According to some studies, there are millions of people who have dyslipidemias and are, therefore, at a greater risk of some long-term and potentially deadly cardiovascular disease. They would benefit from lipid-lowering drugs (in addition to exercise, diet, etc.). Why aren't these millions getting treatment?

2. The enzyme HMG-CoA, the "rate-limiting step" in cholesterol synthesis, is the target of the statins' activity. Can you describe, in your own words, what *rate-limiting step* means? Use an analogy totally unrelated to pharmacology or biochemistry, if you wish.

3. What is the pathophysiology involved in rhabdomyolysis and the most dangerous consequence of it?

4. What is arguably the most important factor that increases the risk of rhabdomyolysis in a patient taking a statin? Assume he or she has normal liver and kidney functions to begin with.

5. One of your patients, who has recently diagnosed hypercholesterolemia has just had his atorvastatin prescription filled. He calls to say, "The label on the pill bottle says 'Don't take with grapefruit juice.' What's up?" So, what *is* up?

6. Hop on the Web and find out when cerivastatin was approved for use in the United States and when it was pulled from the market (and why). What does this information suggest to you about the drug approval process in recent times? Go back to Chapter 3 and review the importance of phase 4 in the drug development and drug approval and monitoring period (postmarketing drug surveillance). What lessons are there to learn from the cerivastatin situation? Do they apply to the remaining and still-approved agents that are classified like cerivastatin?

1. What would you tell her about cholesterol levels and their relationship to disease processes?

2. Identify the major lipoproteins and their functions.

3. What nondrug therapies help lower total cholesterol and increase HDL cholesterol? Why is this important?

4. Why are these effective nondrug therapies often *not* effective?

5. After several weeks on her statin, Mrs. Walters calls to tell you she's feeling "achy." "It may be the flu," she says. What advice would you give to Mrs. Walters, and why?

CASE STUDY

Edith Waters is a 52-year-old Caucasian woman who had a thorough physical exam last week. Her family history is, she thinks, negative for hypertension, coronary artery disease, myocardial infarction, and stroke. Her consumption of fats comes mainly from a high daily intake of fast foods. Mrs. Waters's physician called her with the following lab work results: cholesterol 285 mg/dL, HDL 33 mg/dL, and LDL 129. Because of the elevated cholesterol and a low HDL, Mrs. Waters is considered to be at an increased risk for coronary artery disease. The doctor has placed Mrs. Waters on a restricted diet in an attempt to lower serum cholesterol and mentioned that if this does not correct the problem, he may need to place her on medication. She asks you about her newly diagnosed problem.

Mrs. Walters gets her aches and pains checked by the physician. The apparent cause turns out to be some overexertion and muscle stress caused by a camping trip and lots of hiking. (She is, after all, trying to exercise more to help alter her lipid profiles favorably.) She continues her statin therapy. Her total cholesterol levels have come down somewhat, but not nearly as much as the MD would like. Her triglyceride levels are falling nicely too. However, her LDL cholesterol is still way too high. The physician decides to add cholestyramine to the statin regimen.

6. How is cholestyramine classified in terms of its lipid-lowering action? How does it work?

7. What are Mrs. Walters's "complaints" most likely to be, especially soon after the cholestyramine therapy starts?

8. Through expected actions of the cholestyramine, Mrs. Walters may experience some nutritional problems. What are they, specifically, and why do they occur? What might be recommended to combat them if they become clinically significant?

9. A colleague says, "You know, the cholestyramine may help Mrs. Walters, but it may counteract some of the good effects of the statin." To what is she referring, and is she correct? If so, what instructions need to be given to Mrs. Walters?

10. What might we expect, if anything, in the way of interactions if the patient takes either of her lipid-lowering drugs at the same time she takes her warfarin?

11. If Mrs. Walters were placed on niacin to lower cholesterol levels, why might she want to take aspirin before each dose? Is there another approach, which still involves the use of niacin, that might eliminate or at least reduce the problem for which aspirin prophylaxis might otherwise be needed?

12. Since aspirin can alleviate some of the problems due to niacin, what do you think is involved in causing the signs and symptoms in the first place? (*Note:* To answer this you may need to skip ahead to Chapter 67.)

13. Why would gemfibrozil not be a good choice for Mrs. Walters as a lipid-lowering drug, at least at this stage of her therapy?

Now we have a new piece of information: Mrs. Walters has had atrial fibrillation and she's taking warfarin daily for prophylaxis of thromboembolism as the result of the dysrhythmia.

evolve To check your answers, go to http://evolve.elsevier.com/Lehne/ for Study Guide Comments from the author.

Drugs for Angina Pectoris

KEY TERMS

angioplasty (PTCA)
chronic-stable angina
ischemia
nitric oxide
percutaneous
  transluminal coronary

Prinzmetal's angina
transdermal delivery
  system (for drug)
unstable angina
vasospastic angina

OBJECTIVES

After reading and studying this chapter you should be able to:

1. Summarize the main factors that affect myocardial oxygen demand and oxygen supply, and their relationships to angina pectoris.
2. Describe, compare, and contrast chronic-stable angina, vasospastic (Prinzmetal's) angina, and unstable angina in terms of etiology and clinical presentation and drug therapy for each.
3. Describe the mechanisms of action and therapeutic and adverse effects of organic nitrates (e.g., nitroglycerin), calcium channel blockers (verapamil, diltiazem, nifedipine), and beta-adrenergic blockers in terms of angina therapy with nitroglycerin.
4. State whether the drugs listed in objective 3 can be used interchangeably in angina management. If not, why not? Include in your discussion comparisons of the various groups of beta blockers (e.g., nonselective vs. cardioselective) and calcium channel blockers (e.g., verapamil or diltiazem vs. nifedipine or another dihydropyridine).
5. Summarize the pros and cons of using long-acting oral or topical (transdermal) nitroglycerin or nitroglycerin-like drugs for angina prophylaxis and acute intervention compared with intermittent use of sublingual nitroglycerin.
6. Identify the group or class of antianginal drugs with which sildenafil interacts; state the mechanism and likely consequences of it.

CRITICAL THINKING AND STUDY QUESTIONS

1. A colleague argues that angina is caused by anoxia. Why is this statement false? What is anoxia? What is the real problem in the etiology of angina and the correct term used to describe that underlying condition?

2. The same colleague states that depressing cardiac contractility with a drug is bad for a patient with angina because it lowers the "pressure pulse" created by the heart when it contracts (during systole). Why is this incorrect?

3. For years nitroglycerin was said to exert its antianginal effects by selectively and specifically dilating the coronary arteries, thereby delivering more oxygenated blood to ischemic regions of the heart. Give two pieces of evidence to show that this is not correct.

4. You have read in several places that the cardiac effects of beta-adrenergic blockers (use propranolol as a prototype) and calcium channel blockers like verapamil and diltiazem are "the same"

138

because activation of beta$_1$ receptors is linked to opening of calcium channels. Block beta$_1$ receptors and calcium channels don't open. Is the converse true? Block calcium channels and expect reduction in beta-receptor activation?

5. Given the line of reasoning given in question 4 comment on whether beta blockers and calcium channel blockers are "similar enough" that one could use either for managing angina. (**Hint:** Is there a particular etiology of angina in which one type of drug would be beneficial, the other not?)

6. Rapid-acting oral forms of verapamil or diltiazem are often beneficial in angina. How do they work? What about a rapid-acting form of nifedipine, the other prototypic calcium channel blocker?

CASE STUDY

John Carter is a 75-year-old man admitted to the hospital with substernal "burning" that was not relieved by 3 sublingual nitroglycerin (NTG) tablets taken 5 minutes apart. In the emergency room he was given a nitroglycerin IV drip (33 mcg/hour) that relieved his discomfort. Mr. Carter has been admitted to the coronary care unit. He has no changes in his EKG and is without discomfort. The physicians believe he is having classic angina and not a myocardial infarction (MI).

The physician orders blood tests for marker enzymes (AST, ALT, troponin, and creatine kinase isozymes) that might indicate MI; the results are negative for MI. There have been no changes in Mr. Carter's EKG. The physician orders that Mr. Carter be weaned from the NTG drip and that NTG transdermal patches (10 mg/24 hours) be started. Mr. Carter is also started on long-acting diltiazem

(Cardizem-CD; 30 mg once daily), which will be his antianginal drug therapy once he is discharged.

As the nurse assigned to this patient, you have to decide how to wean him from the NTG drip, start the patches, and assign the time for the diltiazem to meet the needs of the patient. It is 11:00 AM when you receive the order for these medications. Mr. Carter also tells you he has a severe headache.

1. Briefly describe when you would apply the NTG transdermal patch and how this schedule relates to weaning the NTG drip, knowing that Mr. Carter has the headache.

2. Mr. Carter asks why, when he took his three NTG sublingual tablets before he was admitted to the hospital, the medication "did not work." Based on what you should know about NTG sublingual tablets, explain why Mr. Carter experienced no relief.

3. Mr. Carter is told to wear the NTG patch for only 12 hours at a time. He asks why he shouldn't wear it all the time (around the clock). What is the reason?

4. Would it be appropriate for the physician to add a beta blocker to the nitroglycerin-to-diltiazem regimen later if Mr. Carter continues to have angina?

5. Mr. Carter was discharged on long-acting diltiazem to control his angina. Why is that medication plan insufficient?

6. The physician now prescribes sublingual nitroglycerin tablets in addition to the long-acting calcium channel blocker. Remembering that during the previous angina attack three tablets didn't provide relief, Mr. Carter states that next time he'll be sure to take more than three tablets. What should you advise him about this, and why?

7. Several weeks after starting on the long-acting diltiazem, Mr. Carter complains of constipation. Is this unusual or worrisome? How would you respond if Mr. Carter stated that he's heading off to the drug store to purchase some "strong laxatives" to combat the problem?

evolve To check your answers, go to http://evolve.elsevier.com/Lehne/ for Study Guide Comments from the author.

Anticoagulant, Antiplatelet, and Thrombolytic Drugs

KEY TERMS

anticoagulant (drug or effect)

antiplatelet (drug or effect)

antithrombin

activated partial thromboplastin time (APTT)

cyclooxygenase(s)

deep venous thrombosis (DVT)

disseminated intravascular coagulation (DIC)

embolus (pl., emboli)

extrinsic pathway of coagulation

fibrinolysis

glycoprotein IIb/IIIa

international normalized ratio (INR)

intrinsic pathway of coagulation

percutaneous angioplasty (PCI/PCA)

prostacyclin

prothrombin time (PT)

stroke (ischemic, thrombotic, hemorrhagic)

thrombocytopenia (incl. heparin-induced)

thrombolytic (drug or effect)

thromboxane A$_2$

thrombus (pl., thrombi)

tissue plasminogen activator

OBJECTIVES

After reading and studying this chapter you should be able to:

1. Give an overview of the pathways involved in hemostasis, including platelet plug formation and reinforcement of platelet plugs, and mechanisms by which the body protects against widespread coagulation.

2. Explain the differences among anticoagulant, antiplatelet, and thrombolytic drugs in terms of what they do (what coagulation processes they affect) and what their main clinical uses are. Likewise, state the main difference between a thrombus and an embolus.

3. Describe the usual etiologies of arterial vs. venous thrombosis and how prophylactic or interventional drug therapies for these two situations are similar or different.

4. Give a short summary of how and where heparins exert their desired anticoagulant effects; and describe mechanisms and risks of paradoxical increases in thrombotic events associated with heparin-induced thrombocytopenia.

5. Compare and contrast unfractionated heparins and low-molecular-weight (LMW) heparins in terms of mechanisms of action, pharmacokinetics, dosing (schedules), suitability for outpatient therapy, and monitoring of response(s).

6. Summarize the key points that describe the differences between warfarin and heparin: mechanisms, onsets, and sites of action; and monitoring (see the section *Contrasts Between Warfarin and Heparin in the text*).

7. Compare and contrast the actions and uses of aspirin with those of warfarin and heparin, and state the typical "targets" for the lab test that is used to monitor the response to each.

8. Summarize instructions you would give to an outpatient who is taking warfarin about the use of aspirin for relief of common headache, pain, or fever; explain situations and conditions when it is acceptable to take both warfarin and aspirin and situations in which doing so can be dangerous.

9. Summarize general precautions and guidelines (including drug selection and monitoring) that apply when anticoagulation is indicated for a pregnant woman. In particular, what adjustment to the dosage of warfarin should be made?

10. Describe what the glycoprotein IIb/IIIa receptor is and what the clinical significance of blocking that receptor is.

11. State whether and how streptokinase, alteplase, and tenecteplase differ in terms of mechanism(s) of action, pharmacokinetics (time-course of action), and relative safety. In your discussion, consider the need to repeat administration.

12. State the main adverse response that is shared by anticoagulants, antiplatelet, and thrombolytic drugs.

141

CRITICAL THINKING AND STUDY QUESTIONS

1. Compare and contrast unfractionated heparin and LMW heparins in terms of (a) composition; (b) mechanism of action; (c) administration routes and dosage determinations; (d) bioavailability and implications thereof, including duration of action; (e) need for monitoring during therapy and the clinical test(s) used to monitor; and (f) consequences and management of excessive effects.

2. Excessively low platelet counts (thrombocytopenia) typically are associated with excessive bleeding or frank hemorrhage. Why, then, is it essential to monitor platelet counts and assess for thrombocytopenia and also assess for evidence of intravascular clotting (thrombosis) during heparin therapy? After all, heparin is classified as an *anti*coagulant, and its main site of action is not on platelets.

3. Is the etiology of atrial thrombi that form during atrial fibrillation more similar to that by which arterial thrombi or venous thrombi form? Which class(es) of drug(s) discussed in this chapter is/are indicated for managing these thrombi, and why are they indicated at all since we can rather easily stop the fibrillation electrically or with suitable antidysrhythmic drugs?

4. Some patients are prescribed both warfarin and aspirin. Others are given such instructions as, "Don't take aspirin if you have a headache, fever, or mild joint pain" (if you're taking warfarin). Why the apparent inconsistency in these diverse opinions? What problems might arise from giving aspirin to a patient taking warfarin, and how do they occur?

5. Apropos the above, is acetaminophen (e.g., Tylenol, the major OTC "nonaspirin" product for headache, fever, and pain) a "safer" alternative to aspirin for warfarin-treated patients? Why or why not?

6. What is the INR? Identify the drug for which this measurement is used for following the clinical response and state why is it preferred to reporting the prothrombin time?

7. What pharmacokinetic properties of warfarin make it susceptible to interactions with a variety of other drugs, and what are some common examples of those interactants?

8. Any idea about the approximate percentage of strokes that can occur in patients with persistent atrial fibrillation (AF) could be prevented by anticoagulant (e.g., warfarin) therapy? Any idea of the percentage of patients discharged from the hospital with AF who are actually taking prescribed warfarin? Can you think of some physician-centered and patient-centered reasons why far fewer AF patients are placed on anticoagulants than perhaps should be?

9. Why are patients who have hypertension generally not good candidates for anticoagulant therapy, particularly in the ambulatory/outpatient setting?

10. Explain this apparent paradox: For patients at risk of stroke (e.g., a patient with long-standing AF), too little anticoagulation (or none at all) increases the risk of stroke. For otherwise identical patients, too much anticoagulant does the same. While we know that too much of any drug can be just as bad as too little, there's something rather unique about stroke—in particular, its pathophysiology. What is that? (Assume that there are no contraindications, such as hypertension, that apply to the use of anticoagulants.)

11. A patient visiting your rural town is brought in to the emergency department with chest discomfort and enzyme alterations and EKG changes indicative of myocardial infarction. Nothing about this man's history is known other than a comment from his wife that he's had a heart attack before and received "some drug to open up the arteries in his heart."

    The MD believes the present problems are due to multiple thrombotic occlusions of several branches of the left main coronary artery. An IV streptokinase infusion is started, and after 1 hour there's no evidence of any clinical improvement that would indicate that the clots are dissolving. The drug was diluted properly, the usually correct dose was given, and there's no doubt that the IV line was patent. What's the most likely explanation for the *lack of response* to the streptokinase?

12. For prophylaxis of thrombosis and reduction in the risk of heart attack, low-dose aspirin (e.g., 81 mg/day) seems sufficient. How, biochemically, does it work? Would very high doses of aspirin "work better"? Why? For the purpose of answering this question, ignore potential adverse effects of aspirin on, for example, the gut. Focus on clotting pathways.

13. There's growing evidence that a combination of dipyridamole and aspirin (marketed as Aggrenox) can significantly reduce the inci-

dence of ischemic stroke or transient ischemic attacks (TIAs) in patients with a history of these events, compared with results obtained with aspirin or dipyridamole alone. Your patient, who has had recurrent TIAs, is placed on a regimen of *dipyridamole alone*. The MD says it has excellent antiplatelet effects all by itself. Comment on this.

CASE STUDY

Susan Kelly is 35 years old and weighs 100 kg. She works at a job that requires her to sit near a conveyor belt in a factory during her 8-hour shift, 5 days a week. She smokes cigarettes occasionally, has "about three" beers a night, and has been on oral contraceptives (estrogen-progestin combination products) for the last 12 years. Outside work she has a largely sedentary lifestyle and rarely participates in any physical activities of even a modest nature.

Mrs. Kelly presents in the emergency department with discomfort in her left thigh that she describes as being much worse when she walks. Her left leg is swollen, warm, and rather red looking. "It just came on," she said. "I wasn't doing any exercise or anything."

1. Based only on this information, what is the most likely diagnosis?

2. What hemodynamic factor usually contributes to this disorder? Which aspects of Mrs. Kelly's history were likely to have contributed to its development?

3. What is the most worrisome complication of venous thrombosis?

Mrs. Kelly is admitted to your hospital for treatment. The physician orders a heparin drip prepared as 20,000 units of unfractionated heparin in 1000 ml of D₅W (to be infused at 800 U/hr), a heparin bolus of 5000 units IV, and bed rest. The appropriate blood test to assess the effects of the heparin and to guide dosage adjustments is to be done in 6 hours.

4. Explain why heparin was ordered. A colleague says it's to dissolve the clots in Mrs. Kelly's leg.

5. What blood test is mainly used to monitor the effects of unfractionated heparin? What is a typical "target" for this value in such patients as Mrs. Kelly?

6. When should blood samples for monitoring the clinical response to unfractionated heparin be taken when the drug is given by intermittent IV injection, by continuous IV infusion, and by subcutaneous injection?

7. Among other blood tests for monitoring the course of Mrs. Kelly's therapy, the physician orders periodic platelet counts. Since heparins don't have direct antiplatelet effects, why is this done?

8. There's always a chance for excessive anticoagulation with heparin. What is the most serious concern? What antidote should be administered if it occurs? How does it work? And finally, would this antidote be effective for managing excessive effects of other drugs that affect some other aspect of clotting, such as aspirin, warfarin, and a thrombolytic?

After a couple of days on heparin, Mrs. Kelly's doctor wants to start her on warfarin (5 mg per day).

9. Since Mrs. Kelly will be switched to warfarin, why wasn't that used (instead of the heparin) from the start?

10. Explain the statement, "Warfarin certainly affects the blood (in terms of clotting), but the blood isn't its site of action." If you had a laboratory in which you could test the effects of various drugs on the blood, how might you prove that the blood isn't warfarin's site of action?

11. When a patient's anticoagulation therapy is started with unfractionated heparin and the time comes to switch to warfarin, can the heparin be stopped at the same time the warfarin is started? Why or why not?

12. What test is used to monitor the clinical response to warfarin? What are typical "targets" for alterations of this measurement?

13. Mrs. Kelly's warfarin has been started. Blood tests to monitor her response to heparin were done 4 hours after each heparin dose. What will the 4-hour test to assess the response to the first warfarin dose show, and why?

14. What is the usually recommended medication for an overdose of warfarin? In general terms, how does it work?

15. Is it possible for a patient to consume so much vitamin K–rich food, long enough, that their response to warfarin is virtually nothing?

16. Mrs. Kelly, in her zeal to "become more healthy," wants to start a daily exercise regimen, eat the "right" foods, and start taking multivitamins. We've addressed problems arising from excessive vitamin K intake. Are there any other vitamin-related concerns we should have while she is taking warfarin?

evolve To check your answers, go to http://evolve.elsevier.com/Lehne/ for Study Guide Comments from the author.

Management of Myocardial Infarction

OBJECTIVES

After reading and studying this chapter you should be able to:

1. Describe the pathophysiology related to myocardial infarction (MI).
2. Discuss methods for reperfusion.
3. Describe the adverse effects of reperfusion therapy.
4. Explain adjunctive drug therapy including anticoagulants.
5. Discuss treatment methods for patients experiencing an acute MI.

CASE STUDY

Les Guy is a 47-year-old male admitted to the emergency room with severe chest pain that radiated into his left arm and started about 2 hours ago. He experienced some sweating, weakness, and nausea. His EKG shows elevated ST segments in the inferior leads, and his creatine kinase and MB isoenzyme are slightly elevated. Streptokinase was administered in the emergency room, and he was transported to the coronary care unit. His admission orders included heparin 5000 unit bolus and a heparin drip at 1000 units per hour, ASA 160 mg PO stat, nitroglycerin drip at 10 mcg per hour and increase as needed to control pain, maintain blood pressure (BP) greater than 110 systolic, and metoprolol 50 mg 2 times a day.

1. Describe what occurs to cause MI.

2. Identify the clinical presentation of a patient experiencing an MI.

3. Briefly describe the classification and action of streptokinase and its purpose for use in acute MI.

4. Why are heparin and aspirin administered? When should they be started?

5. What is the difference between an anticoagulant drug (heparin) and a thrombolytic drug (streptokinase)?

6. Describe why metoprolol is used in MI.

7. What would be some contraindications for beta blockers in acute MI?

9. Identify the drug therapy to treat the complications of an MI.

8. Identify the most common complications of an MI.

Drugs for Deficiency Anemias

KEY TERMS

anemia
cobalamins (and
    cyanocobalamin)
erythropoiesis
ferritin
hypochromic (re: red
    cells)
intrinsic factor
iron deficiency anemia

macrocytic anemia
megaloblastic anemia
microcytic anemia
pernicious anemia
pteroylglutamic acid
Schilling test
transferrin

OBJECTIVES

After reading and studying this chapter you should be able to:

1. Summarize the roles of erythropoietin, iron, vitamin B_{12}, and folic acid in erythropoiesis (red blood cell production).
2. State the main factor that determines daily iron requirements, and how the body "adjusts" iron uptake from dietary sources to ensure adequate levels yet prevent iron overload.
3. List several foods or food groups that are naturally rich sources of iron.
4. State three common conditions that lead to iron deficiencies, and state whether it is usually reduced iron delivery or increased iron demand that contributes to the imbalance.
5. Describe the physiologically essential relationships among vitamin B_{12} and folic acid and the major physiologic roles of "active folate"; the main physiologic roles of each; and the signs and symptoms of deficiency.
6. Describe the consequences of vitamin B_{12} deficiency on neural function, erythrocyte count and appearance (as in a blood smear), coagulation, and immune system function; summarize the signs and symptoms a patient with pernicious anemia is likely to have; and discuss therapy for mild, moderate, and severe cases of the disorder. Consider that the hypothetical patient is an adult.
7. Summarize the likely fetal consequences of folate deficiency in the pregnant mother and the general

guidelines about folate supplementation in women, especially during pregnancy. State the trimester(s) in which adequate maternal folate intake is particularly critical.

Be sure to check Chapter 105 for information about deferoxamine and its use to manage iron poisoning.

CRITICAL THINKING AND STUDY QUESTIONS

1. On average, the RDA for iron is about 10 times the body's actual physiologic requirement for this mineral. Why?

2. A patient with macrocytic anemia of unknown cause is prescribed very large doses (>1 mg/day) of folic acid on a long-term basis. Eventually, blood counts return to normal. Why, then, should you have concerns about this approach?

CASE STUDY

Marge North, 58 years old, presents with severe pallor and has glossitis (smooth, beefy, red tongue), fatigue, and weight loss. The physician suspects anemia caused by deficiency of either vitamin B_{12} (pernicious anemia) or folic acid.

148

1. What substance usually is deficient as the root cause of pernicious anemia, and how does that deficiency affect nutrient absorption?

Vitamin B$_{12}$ deficiency is confirmed. Mrs. North is told she has pernicious anemia and will need to receive B$_{12}$ supplements.

2. How is vitamin B$_{12}$ essential to the development of red blood cells?

4. Mrs. North says she has a friend with the same problem and he had to get frequent injections that were very painful. Is there anything you can tell her to allay her concerns?

3. Mrs. North says that she "eats healthy," with lots of fresh green vegetables and grains in her diet. She asks whether eating more of those foods or different kinds of foods will cure her problem. How would you respond to this?

5. Ms. North asks what is likely to happen if she doesn't take her meds. "Give me the worst-case scenario," she says. Your response?

A. What is the most likely finding that the pathology lab would detect in looking at a smear of her blood under the microscope? Would that finding alone differentiate between anemia due to B$_{12}$ deficiency (pernicious anemia) and that due to folate deficiency?

6. Mrs. North is also prescribed an additional drug. What do you think it might be, and why?

7. Mrs. North wants to know why she doesn't have to take iron pills right now. What is your response?

B. Mrs. North is told she will be given a Schilling test to help diagnose the cause of her anemia. Explain what that is and what other findings would lead to a relative certain diagnosis of B$_{12}$ deficiency?

evolve To check your answers, go to http://evolve.elsevier.com/Lehne/ for Study Guide Comments from the author.

Hematopoietic and Thrombopoietic Growth Factors

KEY TERMS

colony-stimulating factors
cytokine(s)
erythropoietin
hematopoiesis

interleukins
red cell aplasia
thrombocyte
thrombopoiesis

OBJECTIVES

After reading and studying this chapter, you should be able to:

1. Discuss the need for epoetin alfa.
2. Describe the treatment modality for risk of infection by elevating neutrophil counts.
3. Describe the adverse effects of filgrastim.
4. Discuss medication used after failure of a bone marrow transplant.

CRITICAL THINKING AND STUDY QUESTIONS

Bobby Carter, a 5-year-old with acute lymphoblastic leukemia, has had a bone marrow transplant. Sargramostim (Leukine) 250 μg/m^2 is ordered.

1. Identify the rationale for this therapy.

2. You would monitor this patient for which adverse side effects?

CASE STUDY

Chuck Mann is a 45-year-old patient who has had chronic renal failure for 20 years. He has been maintained at home leading a relatively normal life. Mr. Mann weighs 67 kg. Recently he has become more anemic, and the diagnosis is a lack of erythrocyte production. He is prescribed epoetin alfa (erythropoietin) to help maintain his erythrocyte count.

1. What does erythropoietin do?

2. Why give Mr. Mann epoetin alfa?

3. How would you administer epoetin alfa to Mr. Mann?

4. As the nurse monitoring Mr. Mann long-term for his chronic renal failure, what do you need to assess as a result of his taking epoetin alfa?

5. The physician has ordered for maintenance therapy: 12.5 units per kg 2 times per week for Mr. Mann. How many units will you give him in one dose?

6. Identify at least two other clinical situations when hematopoietic growth factors would be used.

Drugs for Diabetes Mellitus

KEY TERMS

alpha-glucosidase (and its inhibitors)
biguanide
diabetic ketoacidosis (DKA)
euglycemia
"glitazones"
glycosylated hemoglobin HbA$_{1c}$
hyperinsulinism
insulin resistance
ketosis (and ketone bodies)
lactic acidosis
lente (semilente, ultralente) insulins
neutral protamine Hagedorn (NPH)

recombinant DNA (technology, as for making synthetic or semisynthetic "human" insulins)
sliding scale (for insulin dosing)
sulfonylurea
suspension (pharmaceutic formulation)
thiazolidinedione
type 1 diabetes mellitus
type 2 diabetes mellitus
unit (of insulin)

OBJECTIVES

After reading and studying this chapter you should be able to:

1. Discuss the physiologic effects of insulin on carbohydrate, lipid, and protein metabolism, and identify the body cells and tissues that are most dependent on insulin for providing glucose as the main metabolic "fuel."
2. Differentiate between the two major types of diabetes mellitus based on etiology, demographics, and treatment.
3. State three classic signs or symptoms of diabetes mellitus; identify the main pathophysiologic risks from long-term, poorly controlled diabetes mellitus.
4. Describe the values and limitations of monitoring diabetes mellitus therapy based on urine testing and blood testing for glucose and ketones.
5. State what HBA$_{1c}$ is, what it reflects (in terms of blood chemistry), and why it is an important adjunct to static (total) blood glucose levels in monitoring the response of diabetes to therapy.

6. State the main goals of therapy for all patients with diabetes in terms of both symptom control and quantitative targets for fasting blood glucose levels and for HBA$_{1c}$.
7. Differentiate among the different types of insulin for therapeutic use in terms of their mechanisms of action, pharmacokinetics (onsets, duration), and administration routes. Identify the pharmaceutical formulations that can be given intravenously and those that cannot, and explain which pharmaceutic property governs whether IV administration is safe or not.
8. Discuss insulin resistance in terms of what it means, factors that contribute to it, and things that can be done to reduce the problem.
9. Identify the main groups of drugs that can interfere with diabetes therapy (of any type), whether by directly altering blood glucose levels or by interacting with the current antidiabetic drug(s).
10. Identify the main groups of oral antidiabetic drugs (and a prototype of each); compare and contrast their main mechanisms of action and their main adverse responses; and describe the drug-drug interactions (including mechanisms and likely outcomes of them) specific to the oral agents.
11. Describe appropriate interventions for acute or chronic hypoglycemia.
12. Describe the potential maternal and fetal consequences of poorly controlled blood glucose levels during pregnancy; assuming you have a pregnant woman who is being treated for diabetes (type 1 or 2), describe drug therapy changes that usually are indicated until parturition.
13. Summarize the general cause, signs, symptoms, and clinical outcomes of diabetic ketoacidosis. What alterations in carbohydrate and fat (lipid) metabolism occur to contribute to the biochemical and clinical problems?

CRITICAL THINKING AND STUDY QUESTIONS

1. State why it is false to assume that all patients with "non–insulin-dependent" diabetes mellitus (NIDDM) never need insulin. In your answer,

152

consider why using the term *NIDDM* can be misleading in terms of what might be needed (or expected by the patient), drug therapy-wise.

2. What accounts for the polyuria that is a common feature of "severe" hyperglycemia? How does it relate to the etiology of diabetic polydypsia? What diuretic (that you should have learned about in Chapter 39) works in a manner similar to that by which the hyperglycemia of diabetes leads to polyuria?

3. A urine sample from a patient with diabetes mellitus is negative for glucose. What can you conclude about his or her blood glucose level at the time the urine sample was donated? Does the *type* of diabetes this patient has affect what you can deduce from the absence of urine glucose? Include in your comments how you would explain to the diabetes patient why urine testing for glucose will not be part of the daily monitoring routine.

4. What is neutral protamine Hagedorn, a component of NPH insulin? What does this protein do to the mechanisms of action, pharmacokinetics, and route of administration for this insulin?

5. Related to question 4, how do lente, semilente, and ultralente insulins differ in terms of onset and duration of action, mechanism of action, and safe administration route(s)? What cation is a component of these insulins, and why is it there?

6. What's the basic rationale to explain why many persons with insulin-dependent diabetes administer a mixture of insulins, say, regular insulin injection and semilente insulin?

7. How do animal-derived (e.g., beef or pork) insulins differ in terms of mechanism of action and adverse responses from the synthetic or semisynthetic insulins? Since animal-derived insulins are comparatively cheap, and the cost of drugs is an important consideration, what's the advantage of the newer expensive insulins made by recombinant DNA technology?

8. Until "not all that long ago," insulins were available in many "strengths" (units/mL)—not just the U-100 and U-500 insulins we have now. Can you state one or more reasons why now we only have two strengths?

9. What serum ion imbalance would you expect in a patient who has received an inadvertent overdose of insulin? Why.

10. A patient has type 2 diabetes and is a candidate for oral antidiabetic drug therapy. Despite all reasonable attempts to get him to do "eat healthier," he sips coffee throughout the day and doesn't eat or drink anything else except at dinnertime—one meal a day. Which would be most appropriate for this patient—metformin, a sulfonylurea (e.g., glipizide), or a glitazone (e.g., pioglitazone or rosiglitazone)—as the main drug therapy? Assume there are no contraindications to either drug. Compare and contrast the effects of metformin and of a sulfonylurea (or glitazone) on regulating blood glucose levels and the risks of an excessive lowering of blood glucose (hypoglycemia).

11. What is the major adverse effect of metformin (one that is not shared by any other antidiabetic drug), and what are the major factors that increase the risk of it?

12. A patient who is taking an oral antidiabetic drug consumes a couple of glasses of wine at a party and soon begins sweating and complaining of headache, light-headedness, and chest tightness. What drug or drug class is the likely cause of these signs and symptoms of a likely interaction with alcohol, and how do they occur?

13. Beta-adrenergic blockers are considered important drugs for patients who have had a myocardial infarction and who have mild symptoms of heart failure (provided there are no other contraindications). Assume a 55-year-old patient with this history was now diagnosed with type 2 diabetes and placed on oral hypoglycemic drug therapy. What should be done about the beta blocker? What are the concerns about beta blockers in this patient or any patient with diabetes mellitus?

14. A patient presents in the emergency department with severe hypoglycemia (60 mg/dL) from excessive effects of an antidiabetic medication, and generalized convulsions of unknown etiology. The physician orders the proper dose of phenytoin (anticonvulsant; see Chapter 23) to be diluted in 5% dextrose-water and given IV. What is wrong with this medication order?

15. A patient with diabetes of 5 years duration is being treated with oral medications for the disorder. There is good evidence that organ and nerve damage from poor diabetes control is increasing, but the patient insists that he has been taking his medications faithfully and checking his blood glucose each day, with fasting (morning) readings of "about 100 mg/dL." Indeed, when he comes to the clinic a finger stick reveals a blood glucose level of 110 mg/dL—close enough to the patient's stated levels. However, there is reason to suspect that the patient is not complying with medication, diet, and exercise recommendations.

    What blood test might be useful to help determine whether the patient has actually been compliant, at least for the last 2 to 3 months? Why? How often should it be done as an add-on to periodic (or even daily) measurements of total blood glucose?

16. A general approach for diabetic patients who develop hypoglycemia is to eat or drink something that contains sugar (sucrose), which is broken down to glucose that helps restore blood glucose levels when it's absorbed. This works regardless of the antidiabetic drug being used—except for one. Identify that drug or drug class, and explain why oral sucrose administration is not likely to be of help when hypoglycemia occurs during treatment with it.

17. Which diuretic can be administered to quickly and effectively increase the renal excretion of excess blood glucose—an effect that certainly would be desirable if a patient's blood glucose levels become dangerously high?

18. To monitor (if not facilitate) the "success" of diabetes therapy (regardless of the type, severity, or treatment modalities), it's important to monitor blood glucose levels frequently. In the ambulatory care setting this is something that usually needs to be done by the patient or a

family caregiver who is not a healthcare professional. This, of course, necessitates a blood-testing meter (glucometer), test strips, and other supplies—and using them all properly.

Who advises the patient which brand to buy and how to use it? What do you need to know about these devices to fulfill your role as patient educator? Are these products as easy to use as advertised, often with such catchy advertising phrases as "Easy to use as 1-2-3"? (To answer this question you may need to borrow an instruction manual for one or several of these devices or do a Web search to locate an online manual. This exercise is well worth the effort!)

19. Hop on the Web and find out when troglitazone was approved for use in the United States and when it was pulled from the market—and why. What does this information suggest about the drug approval process in "recent times?" Go back to Chapter 3 and review the importance of Phase IV (postmarketing) drug surveillance. What lessons are there to learn from the troglitazone situation? Do they apply to the remaining agents that are classified like troglitazone?

CASE STUDY

Gus Cone, 38 years old, has type 1 diabetes. He is admitted to the hospital in diabetic ketoacidosis. He is hot, flushed, and diaphoretic. He complains of nausea and abdominal pain. His pulse is 110/min but regular; BP is 96/68. Urine is colorless and positive for acetone and sugar. Mr. Cone responds somewhat to verbal and tactile stimuli, but he is lethargic. According to a family member, Mr. Cone has had diabetes for 6 years and takes Humulin N 15 units and Humulin R 5 units every morning and Humulin N 7 units at bedtime. His wife said he has stopped exercising this week, he no longer rides his bike, and he's been too sick and tired to take his insulin for the last 2 days. She said he woke up this morning and acted extremely sleepy and "out of it."

Here are some of Mr. Cone's lab results on samples taken and measured right after he arrived at the emergency department:

Serum glucose: 355 mg/dL

BUN: 25 nmol/L (normal, 8–16.4 nmol/L)
Serum osmolality: 410 mmol/kg water (normal, 285–295)
Creatinine, serum: 180 mmol/L (normal, 50–110)
Sodium, serum: 90 mmol/L (normal, 135–145)
Urine: positive for ketones, glucose

1. Describe some basic epidemiologic and pathophysiologic differences between type 1 and type 2 diabetes. In your answer, state how the underlying pathophysiology affects which antidiabetic drug(s) is/are appropriate for managing each type.

The new young physician states that Mr. Cone is in hyperosmolar diabetic ketoacidosis.

2. Why are there ketoacids (acetone, etc.) in Mr. Cone's blood and urine? From what metabolic source do they arise?

3. Could we have used urine "dip sticks" (test strips) to make initial and reasonably correct diagnosis of diabetes and ketoacidosis before we got the blood test results from the lab?

4. Blood tests show that Mr. Cone's serum sodium concentration is very low. State (a) *why* it is low and (b) how it *can* be low, given the fact that the patient's plasma osmolality is so high.

5. Why are Mr. Cone's BUN and creatinine levels so high?

6. What accounts for the very low blood pressure we measured in this patient? Which of Mr. Cone's signs and symptoms are likely to be caused by this hypotension? What other findings noted in the scenario are almost certainly contributing to his problems?

The MD orders 50 U of regular insulin, to be given IV, and insists that you draw the drug from an ampule of U-500 insulin, stating "We need to get the patient's blood glucose down stat." He also wants you to start an IV infusion of "free water"—sterile water with no salts or other additives in it. The purpose, he explains, is to quickly lower the osmolality of Mr. Cone's blood ... to make it more dilute ... and quickly.

7. What is wrong with the doctor's orders?

Mr. Cone hasn't had a really good medical work-up for quite a while before this hospital admission. Not surprisingly, his blood pressure is elevated, and it's been elevated throughout his entire hospital stay, even after his blood glucose levels are brought under control with insulin. The physician feels it is necessary to begin drug therapy for what is classified as Stage 2 essential hypertension.

8. As you may recall, four main groups of drugs are generally considered reasonable first choices for starting treatment of this degree of hypertension: thiazide diuretics, beta-adrenergic blockers, calcium channel blockers, and angiotensin-converting enzyme (ACE) inhibitors. Comment on the pros and cons of each of those drug groups as they apply to Mr. Cone and his diabetes.

Mr. Cone ultimately gets his blood glucose and blood pressure under control. It's time to discharge him, and as you might imagine a lot of patient education needs to be done. Among the issues are the following.

9. Mr. Cone asks you about the insulin he takes at home. He states that the injection sites on his legs have fat deposits. He also states that he gives himself two separate injections every morning because he was prescribed two "kinds" of insulin. What important aspects about insulin therapy in regard to rotating sites and mixing insulins should Mr. Cone have been taught from the outset?

10. Mr. Cone states that his "doc" mentioned he has "insulin resistance." Mr. Cone asks what that is, and what's a good way of managing it. Your thoughts? What is the most common cause of insulin resistance, and what is probably an excellent way to manage it (in addition to proper drug therapy)?

Drugs for Thyroid Disorders

KEY TERMS

agranulocytosis
cretinism
euthyroid(-ism)
exophthalmos
goiter
Grave's disease
Hashimoto's disease
iodism
myxedema (and
  myxedema coma)
Plummer's disease
T_3

T_4
thioamine (thioamide;
  drug class)
thyroid-binding globulin
  (TBG)
thyrotoxic crisis
  (thyrotoxicosis;
  thyroid storm)
toxic nodular goiter
TRH (thyrotropin-
  releasing hormone)

OBJECTIVES

After reading and studying this chapter you should be able to:

1. Give a reasonably accurate summary of the biosynthesis of thyroid hormones and the processes involved in regulating synthesis, release, and feedback regulation of both.
2. Compare and contrast T_3 and T_4 in terms of relative abundance, biological activity, and onsets and durations of action.
3. Describe the physiologic actions of thyroid hormones on basal metabolism, cell growth, and regulation of adrenergic receptor activity.
4. Compare and contrast the effects of dietary iodine/iodide deficiency, normal dietary intake, and high-dose iodine supplementation on thyroid hormone status and thyroid gland function.
5. Describe signs and symptoms typically associated with hypothyroidism and with hyperthyroidism.
6. Compare and contrast the biologic activities of thyroid hormone replacement products; which is generally preferred for management of hypothyroidism; and why.
7. Describe the imminent dangers of the two extremes of thyroid hormone status—myxedema coma and thyrotoxicosis/thyroid storm—and summarize a reasonable treatment plan for each.

8. Discuss drug treatments usually used in preparation for thyroidectomy, and explain why this/these drug(s) are used.
9. Describe the uses of and contraindications for radioactive iodine in terms of diagnosing or treating disorders of the thyroid.

CRITICAL THINKING AND STUDY QUESTIONS

1. Is there a linear or direct relationship between dietary iodine intake and thyroid hormone levels—that is, the greater the iodine intake, the greater the circulating hormone levels? What are the clinical consequences of inadequate and excessive iodine intake?

2. During which trimester of pregnancy is it most important to ensure a euthyroid status in a hypothyroid mother, and why?

3. Why are measurements of serum TSH levels considered more sensitive than measurements of serum T_3 or T_4 for diagnosing hypothyroidism, and how do results of measuring TSH help one establish the etiology (i.e., primary vs. secondary hypothyroidism)?

157

4. Hypothyroid patients often have deficiencies of both T_3 and T_4. Why, then, is supplementation with only T_4 (levothyroxine) usually the preferred approach? What pharmacokinetic property(ies) of therapeutic T_4 affect its onset and duration, and how are those properties both a benefit and limitation of replacement therapy.

5. By definition the signs and symptoms of hyperthyroidism are almost exclusively due to an excess of thyroid hormones, which overstimulates receptors for those hormones.

   Why then do adrenergic receptor blockers play a crucial role in managing thyrotoxic crisis? Which class of adrenergic blocker is used? What is the main purpose for giving them? How do they work? What adjustments to the dosages of the adrenergic blocker need to be made as a euthyroid status is reached?

6. A patient with undiagnosed hypothyroidism requires warfarin therapy for long-term anticoagulation. Compared to a euthyroid patient, would you expect his warfarin dosages to be higher, lower, or the same in order to achieve a target INR and a low risk of experiencing either intravascular clotting or spontaneous bleeding? Why? What, if anything, will need to be done to the warfarin dosage if and when hypothyroidism is diagnosed and treatment for it started with T_4?

7. When we think of altered thyroid hormone status as it affects the actions, half-lives, and dosage regimens of other drugs, we tend to focus on those drugs that are very dependent on hepatic metabolism for elimination. After all, thyroid hormone status affects metabolism of many medications. Assume a patient is taking a medication that isn't metabolized; instead, it's eliminated only by renal excretion. Might any dosage adjustments be needed for it? To simplify things, assume that the drug has a low margin of safety,

and consider myxedema or thyrotoxic crisis as extremes of altered thyroid status.

8. You and your SN2 colleague are on your first day of a rotation in the hospital's endocrinology section and you're reviewing the charts of two patients who had hyperthyroidism from a thyroid tumor about 2 years ago. One is a 21-year-old woman who had a thyroidectomy for her tumor. The other is a 66-year-old man who received high-dose radioiodine (^{131}I) therapy for his tumor.

   What is the most likely explanation for the different approaches to managing what amounts to the same endocrine condition?

   Your colleague is confused about follow-up management. Both patients are receiving supplemental T_4. He says, "This is crazy! These patients were hyperthyroid, and now they're receiving T_4? I thought T_4 was for treating hypothyroidism!" Clear up his confusion.

9. What is the current status (or belief) concerning bioequivalence of various levothyroxine products? What is the main apparent benefit of Synthroid over the alternatives?

10. You know from the text (and see question 5 above) that beta-adrenergic blockers play important roles in managing severe, acute hyperthyroidism. Why aren't oral antithyroid drugs such as propylthiouracil (PTU) used as the sole therapy? After all, they are efficacious inhibitors of thyroid hormone synthesis, and excessive thyroid hormone effects are the crux of the problems.

11. Head to the grocery store and look at the boxes of table salt. No doubt you'll see such comments as "iodized salt" or see that iodine/iodide has been added to the product. Why?

CASE STUDY

Helen Thomas is a 35-year-old mother of 5-year-old twins. She notices that she is gaining weight and complains of unusual fatigue, lethargy, and intolerance to cold. She visits her family physician who, after doing appropriate lab studies, determines that she is hypothyroid and starts her on levothyroxine (Synthroid).

1. Before any drugs are prescribed, what laboratory tests are done to determine the status of her thyroid?

2. What does the thyroid gland do for the body?

3. What symptoms does she have that are consistent with hypothyroidism?

4. What adverse effects should Mrs. Thomas know about when taking levothyroxine?

5. Discuss how thyroid hormone replacement therapy will be evaluated.

6. Mrs. Thomas asks the nurse how long it will take before her thyroid hormone level is normal and she will no longer need medication. How would you answer?

7. Mrs. Thomas tells the nurse that her sister has asked for some of her thyroid pills to help her lose weight. Mrs. Thomas wants to know if this would be a problem. How should the nurse respond?

8. Assuming the half-life of the levothyroxine is about 7 days, how long does it take for the plasma levels to reach a plateau (steady state)? What's the easy and usually reliable way to estimate this?

9. What information does Mrs. Thomas need to take her medication correctly?

evolve To check your answers, go to http://evolve.elsevier.com/Lehne/ for Study Guide Comments from the author.

Drugs Related to Hypothalamic and Pituitary Function

KEY TERMS

acromegaly
adenohypophysis
cachexia
diabetes insipidus
(hypothalamic and
nephrogenic)
dwarfism
epiphyses (of bone; and
epiphyseal closure)

galactorrhea
gigantism
insulin-like growth
factor-1 (IGF-1)
lyophilized
negative feedback loop
neurohypophysis
Turner's syndrome

OBJECTIVES

After reading and studying this chapter you should
be able to:

1. Discuss the general pathways and mechanisms by
which the pituitary, hypothalamus, and many
endocrine glands in the periphery work in concert
to regulate blood hormone levels.
2. Summarize the main consequences of growth
hormone deficiency and excess, comparing and
contrasting what you are likely to find in the way
of clinical presentation depending on whether the
dysfunction occurs before or after puberty.
Include in your summary expected effects on protein and carbohydrate metabolism.
3. Describe the main actions and regulation of
release of prolactin; summarize the main clinical
findings in hyperprolactinemia and how we may
manage it.
4. Explain the main systemic effects of antidiuretic
hormone (ADH) and the expected effects of
hypersecretion and hyposecretion and how we
manage it.
5. Demonstrate a basic but correct understanding of
the similarities or differences between vasopressin, ADH, and oxytocin in terms of what they
are and what their main physiologic or pathophysiologic effects are.

Note: This chapter in the text emphasizes three hormones (growth hormone, antidiuretic hormone, and
prolactin) and three hypothalamic-releasing factors
(growth hormone-releasing hormone, thyrotropin-
releasing hormone, and gonadotropin-releasing hormone). We will do the same here ... after some initial
questions about the overall organization of the hypo-
thalamic-pituitary "axis."

But be sure to get the big picture—other hor-
mones, releasing factors, and effects. That includes
(but is not limited to) integrating content from
Chapter 55 (*Drugs for Thyroid Disorders*), Chapter
58 (*Androgens*), Chapters 59 and 60 (*Estrogens and
Progestins and Their Use in Hormone Replacement
Therapy* and *Drug Therapy of Infertility*), Chapter 62
(*Drugs That Affect Uterine Function*), and Chapter
70 (*Drugs Affecting Calcium Levels and Bone
Mineralization*).

CRITICAL THINKING AND STUDY QUESTIONS

1. Are all hormones regulated through interactions
involving the pituitary-hypothalamic axis? If
not, can you name two or three of them?

2. The anterior pituitary synthesizes and releases
relatively many hormones. The posterior pituitary (neurohypophysis) releases only two. What
are they, and where are they actually synthesized?

3. Compare and contrast the effects of growth hormone (GH) on protein and carbohydrate metabolism. Consider what happens normally (physiologically) in persons who do not have pathologic growth hormone deficiency or excess and who do not have diabetes mellitus.

4. What is the primary physiologic event that prevents an increase in growth (height) in people who develop pathologic growth hormone excess in later life? (It is the event that leads to gigantism when GH excess occurs in children.)

5. A 9-year-old child with documented GH deficiency is a candidate for replacement therapy with somatropin. At the time of diagnosis, when somatropin therapy was started, he was in the 8th percentile of height for boys his age. The short height was the main (and indeed only) reason his mom wanted hormone replacement therapy. About 6 months later he develops asthma, and the respiratory disorder quickly progresses to *severe and recurrent*. In fact, over the last year he's been hospitalized twice and intubated once for the asthma. Can you envisage how and why therapy of one of these disorders can complicate treatment of the other?

6. The text notes that one of the handful of approved uses of GH is to treat Turner's syndrome. Do you know what that is?

7. Your text notes that "GH is dispensed as a lyophilized powder for reconstitution..." What does lyophilized mean? (It's pronounced ly-**oph**-i-lized, by the way.) I'll bet many of you have consumed something that was lyophilized and reconstituted. In fact, I'm having some as I write this. Can you guess what that may be?

8. What is the significance of dopamine with respect to regulation of prolactin release? When a patient presents with hyperprolactinemia, why do we not manage it with dopamine? What drug can be used for this purpose, how does it affect prolactin levels, and what is the main clinical use of that drug nowadays?

9. A patient with a posterior pituitary tumor has extraordinarily high serum ADH levels.

A. What are the expected changes in plasma and urine osmolality, and how do they occur? A colleague states that excess levels of the hormone are activating specific ion pumps in the renal tubules to change urine volume and composition. Do you agree? Why or why not?

B. Is there *any* hormone that affects the way the kidneys regulate ion movements and that directly or otherwise affects urine and blood osmolality? If so, what is it, what does it do, what is its physiologic source, and what is the physiologic "trigger" for its release?

10. How do the main signs and symptoms of hypothalamic diabetes insipidus differ from those that occur with nephrogenic diabetes insipidus? How do the two conditions differ in etiology and clinical management? (P.S.: Common synonyms for hypothalamic diabetes insipidus include *neurogenic* or *central* diabetes insipidus.)

11. In Chapter 17 (*Adrenergic Agonists*) we identified such drugs as phenylephrine and norepinephrine. We called them vasopressors or said that they have vasopressor effects. Are they vaso*pressins?* Do they and vasopressin have similar mechanisms of action? Are they all used interchangeably?

CASE STUDY

Michael (he prefers to be called Mickey) Mause is a 47-year-old man. Very pleasant, but with a rather unique squeaky, high-pitched voice. Three years ago he had surgery to remove a large astrocytoma that invaded much of his posterior pituitary gland. He's received radiation therapy and seems to be doing fine now. Of course, he now lacks both endogenous oxytocin and ADH.

Mr. Mause was placed on intranasal desmopressin ("DDAVP") postoperatively.

1. What are some of the likely reasons for picking desmopressin as opposed to vasopressin (Pitressin)? And what's one "problem" with the drug?

2. A colleague looking over Mr. Mause's chart notices the operative history and the reason for it. He comments that without his pituitary, Mr. Mause is not releasing any oxytocin, yet he's not on oxytocin supplements. Why not?

Mr. Mause travels out of town—to your city—for a weeklong business trip. As you learn from him later, almost as soon as he got off the plane he developed what he thought were cold-like symptoms—nasal congestion and what he refers to as the "worst non-stop runny nose" I've ever had. He was achy and feeling "crummy," but didn't think he had a fever.

3. Could this horrible rhinorrhea have been caused by the desmopressin nasal spray?

After 3 days of coping with the nasal congestion and runny nose, Mr. Mause heads to a local pharmacy and asks the pharmacist for "the strongest nasal decongestant spray" they have.

4. What do you think the "horribly runny nose" and then the "strong nasal decongestant" he started taking could do to affect his desmopressin therapy?

Mr. Mause presents in your hospital's urgent care facility. He's been drinking copious amounts of water because he's been "thirsty all the time" and is doing the same in terms of putting out urine. And the night before he was sitting at the hotel bar watching Monday Night Football—and drinking a beer during every commercial break.

He is coherent enough to say that he's had a cold, he's been taking decongestants, and is on intranasal desmopressin since he had a brain tumor removed several years ago.

5. A sample of his urine is sent off to the lab to check, among other things, the urine's specific gravity and osmolality. The results come back: Specific gravity is 1.001 (normal minimum is about 1.003); osmolality is 20 mOsm/kg water (20 mmol/kg water; normal minimum is about 286). What does that mean? What is the specific gravity of plain distilled water?

6. Could Mr. Mause's night-before alcohol consumption have caused his present problems?

7. Normal plasma osmolality is 286–295 mOsm/kg water. Normal hematocrit is for an adult male is 40–54 mL/dL (0.40–0.54 volume fraction). In which "direction"—if at all—would you expect these values to change in Mr. Mause, given his acute and significant ADH lack?

8. Upon seeing some of the lab test results, the first-year house officer orders an "otherwise right" dose of IV heparin because he's worried about venous thrombosis. Should he be worried?

9. Really concerned about the very high plasma osmolality and hematocrit, the house officer orders an IV infusion of sterile water to "dilute" the blood. He wants 100 mL infused over an hour. What would you expect this to do?

An attending physician, overhearing the house officer's comments, comes in and asks the HO to go to the exam room next door and take care of the patient with the infected hangnail. He then orders an

initial SC dose (the "right" dose) of vasopressin (Pitressin).

Shortly after the vasopressin injection, Mr. Mause's blood pressure goes up "significantly" and he complains of crushing chest discomfort.

10. What might the intense chest discomfort indicate, and what should you do in terms of assessing and managing things?

11. Before, and then after, giving the vasopressin, do we want to be aggressive with our IV fluid and electrolyte infusions?

evolve To check your answers, go to http://evolve.elsevier.com/Lehne/ for Study Guide Comments from the author.

57

Drugs for Disorders of the Adrenal Cortex

KEY TERMS

Addison's disease
adrenal crisis
adrenocortical
   insufficiency, primary
   and secondary
circadian rhythm
Cushing's syndrome
dexamethasone
   suppression text

gluconeogenesis
glycogenolysis
pharmacologic dose or
   effect (of
   corticosteroid)
physiologic dose or
   effect (of
   corticosteroid)

OBJECTIVES

After reading and studying this chapter you should be able to:

1. State the three classes of steroid hormones produced by the adrenal cortex, and describe in general terms how their physiologic effects differ.
2. Compare and contrast glucocorticoids and mineralocorticoids in terms of which substance(s) and processes in the body they mainly regulate. State why labeling a corticosteroid drug as either a glucocorticoid or a mineralocorticoid is, to a degree, an oversimplification.
3. Describe the physiologic processes and pathways (central nervous system and peripheral) that regulate cortisol production and release. Compare and contrast that with how aldosterone production and release are regulated physiologically.
4. State three basic ways that hormones or drugs with glucocorticoid activity promote carbohydrate availability to the brain and other essential tissues and organs. In addition, state the expected effects these agents have on protein and lipid metabolism.
5. Describe the signs and symptoms of insufficiency and excess of cortisol and of aldosterone. State the main lab test alterations that would be consistent with a diagnosis of the above conditions,

applicable diagnostic tests, and a reasonable treatment plan.
6. Describe how glucocorticoid administration at *pharmacologic* doses affects the hypothalamic-pituitary-adrenal cortical axis (HPA), the signs and symptoms and relative duration of withdrawal, and some strategies to minimize suppression of the HPA.

Be sure you eventually integrate content from this chapter with information presented in Chapter 68 (*Glucocorticoids in Nonendocrine Diseases*) and Chapters 58 (*Androgens*). (*Drugs for Disorders of the Adrenal Cortex* and *Androgens*). Review relevant content in Unit VI, *Drugs that Affect Fluid and Electrolyte Balance,* with a focus on spironolactone. Be sure, too, to become familiar with ketoconazole and other azole antifungal agents (see Chapter 87).

CRITICAL THINKING AND STUDY QUESTIONS

1. What is the direct impact of adrenal cortical hyperfunction or hypofunction on circulating levels of epinephrine?

2. What are the main differences among hydrocortisone, prednisone, and methylprednisolone in terms of the effects they cause, how they are used, and factors that would go into selecting one over another.

3. A patient with recurrent, severe asthma (a common nonendocrine disorder for which glucocorticoids are very beneficial) has been on high doses of oral prednisone for 6 months. Highly dissatisfied with weight gain and mood changes, he abruptly stops taking the steroid altogether. Aside from potential pulmonary problems (exacerbation of the asthma), what is likely to occur, what are the likely signs and symptoms, and how is it managed?

4. A colleague says that hydrocortisone is superior to cortisol, the naturally occurring and main glucocorticoid hormone, because hydrocortisone is synthetic and "more pure." Do you agree? Why?

5. The most common approach to managing many glucocorticoid deficiency syndromes (replacement therapy) and many other conditions that are responsive to glucocorticoids involves administering synthetic glucocorticoids. So long as the patient has a functioning adrenal cortex, why not treat with corticotropin (or cosyntropin) instead, thereby making use of the body's own glucocorticoid supply?

6. A young child has congenital adrenal hyperplasia. How do we treat this pharmacologically? After all, we are saying that cells that make up the adrenal cortex are hyperplastic.

CASE STUDY

Jim Kale, 35, describes symptoms of lethargy, fatigue, and muscle weakness. However, he tells you he thinks the symptoms are due to his stressful job. He also states that he loves salty food and eats at least one bag of potato chips daily. He states that he has experienced impotence on occasion, along with anorexia and nausea. You notice that he has increased pigmentation around the face and hands and a decrease of body hair. Blood work indicates hypoglycemia, decreased sodium, increased potassium, and increased blood urea nitrogen (BUN). He

is prescribed hydrocortisone (30 mg/day), and fludrocortisone (1 mg/day) for additional mineralocorticoid activity.

1. Of the endocrine disorders discussed in this chapter, what is the most likely diagnosis for Mr. Kale?

2. How would you describe this disorder to him?

3. What should Mr. Kale's love of salty foods tell you?

4. What main serum electrolyte abnormalities can you expect to find in Mr. Kale before he is treated? Why?

5. If Mr. Kale requires surgery, what would be the concern of the healthcare team?

6. When instructing Mr. Kale about the administration of the glucocorticoid therapy, it is important to discuss the need to carry a significant amount of extra drug when on trips. Why?

58

Androgens

KEY TERMS

anabolic (drug or effect)
"andro"
androgen (drug or effect)

erythropoiesis
virilization

OBJECTIVES

After reading and studying this chapter you should be able to:

1. Discuss the physiologic effects of androgens in both males and females. Consider in your discussion likely effects in utero, during childhood growth and development (e.g., infancy through puberty), and in later life.
2. Summarize the expected beneficial actions of androgens used to manage hypogonadism in adult males. Include comments on the key physiologic and psychologic signs and symptoms that might lead to a diagnosis of male hypogonadism and a decision to begin testosterone therapy.
3. Summarize our current knowledge (as described in the text) about use (misuse and abuse) of androgens by athletes. Include in your summary key points about the hoped-for (and sometimes clinically proven) physical, metabolic, and psychologic effects of these drugs and the types of adverse responses that pose risks with such use. You should also comment on basic legal or other regulatory points concerning anabolic steroid use.

CRITICAL THINKING AND STUDY QUESTIONS

1. A nosy and not too bright member of your class glances over your shoulder as you're making and reviewing your personal notes on this chapter. He sees that you've penciled in the terms FSH and LH. "Silly you," he says, "FSH and LH are female hormones. Androgens are male hormones! FSH and LH have nothing to do with guys." How would you respond (pharmacologically, that is)?

2. Androgens are, of course, automatically considered "male" hormones. Why then is gynecomastia a potential side effect of these drugs? Isn't gynecomastia a term applied only to women?

3. What is unique and clinically important about the 17-alpha-alkylated androgens, such as methyltestosterone? What points should come to mind immediately when you hear that someone will be, or is, taking these compounds?

CASE STUDY

Max Giles, 16 years old, has come to his healthcare provider with his dad. Max's concern, and his parents' too, is his small testes and penis.

He is 6 feet 6 inches tall and weighs 160 pounds. His legs are unusually long for his trunk. He tells you that he has always been in trouble in school but will finally be a freshman in high school this year.

Further evaluation indicates the absence of sperm in the semen and the presence of two extra X chromosomes. The diagnosis of Klinefelter's syndrome is made.

As the nurse, you know that this is not so rare (occurs in 1 of every 500 live male births) but it is

166

often not discovered until the male comes in for an infertility work-up.

The MD plans on administering the long-acting parenteral (IM) preparation of testosterone enanthate, 100 mg every 3 weeks for at least 3 years.

1. Mr. Giles asks you what his son can expect from these "shots" How would you respond?

2. Max asks, "Why can't I take a pill? Isn't there any way to take this medicine without having to take the shots so often?" How would you respond?

3. Max tells you that some of his friends on the high school football and wrestling teams are taking androgens to enhance their athletic performance. What is your response to this?

4. Max tells you that he's been doing a lot of reading about "these hormones" and knows that pro

athletes have been using "andro." "It's a vitamin," he says, and adds that he went to the big health-food store at the mall and found it there. "Why shouldn't I just take them instead of these expensive drugs my parents are gonna have to pay for? After all, the health-food store sells the stuff so it's gotta be healthy, and natural—and good—for me. And I won't have to take those darned shots, either."

5. Max's dad listens to your comments and then asks how the health-food stores can sell this stuff if it doesn't do what it's assumed to do, and especially since there might be some adverse effects in the long run. How would you explain things?

6. Max's mom happens to be an RN, currently licensed in the state. If the physician chooses to go with an injectable androgen, and Max agrees to taking that dosage form, can his mom help out?

evolve To check your answers, go to http://evolve.elsevier.com/Lehne/ for Study Guide Comments from the author.

Estrogens and Progestins and Their Use in Hormone Replacement Therapy

KEY TERMS

corpus luteum

Heart & Estrogen/progestin Replacement Study (HERS)

hormone replacement therapy (HRT)

nidation

selective estrogen receptor modulators (SERMs)

Women's Health Initiative (WHI; clinical study)

OBJECTIVES

After reading and studying this chapter you should be able to:

1. Discuss the menstrual cycle in regard to phasic changes of hormone levels and their effects on other body systems. Identify the major triggers (regulatory stimuli) for these changes.
2. Summarize the main physiologic effects of estrogen and progesterone.
3. Compare and contrast the benefits and adverse effects of estrogen and progesterone hormones as replacement therapy, compared with the risks and benefits of not replacing them with prescribed drugs. In your comparison, consider such important outcomes as breast cancer, ovarian or endometrial cancer, and menopause (including a common consequence of it, osteoporosis). Consider both signs and symptoms of hormone deficiency as well as long-term and more serious consequences.
4. Describe premenstrual syndrome (PMS) and summarize the effects and actions of drugs that are deemed effective for it.
5. Discuss, based on current evidence, the benefits and risks of hormone replacement therapy (HRT) for postmenopausal women. Related to this, give a succinct but accurate description of the aims of

HERS I and II) and the WHI study, and the major findings of each.

Notes: Be sure to integrate information from this chapter with information in Chapters 60 and 61 (Birth Control, and Drugs for Infertility, respectively). Also be sure to refer to this chapter when you read about the selective estrogen receptor modulators (tamoxifen, raloxifene) in their uses for certain cancers (see Chapter 99) and for management of osteoporosis in menopausal and postmenopausal women.

CRITICAL THINKING AND STUDY QUESTIONS

1. A patient tells you she's heard that the use of therapeutic doses of estrogens alone may increase the risk of endometrial cancer and that adding a progestin to the regimen increases the risks even more. Explain and clarify the situation.

   ESTROGEN CAN CAUSE PROLIFERATION OF HYP WHICH CAN LEAD TO CANCER. PROGESTERIN ANTAGONIST HYPERPLASIA WHICH REDUCES THE RISK.

2. Why is it acceptable (or, at least, more acceptable) to administer estrogens without supplemental progestins to an older woman who has had a hysterectomy? BECAUSE ESTROGEN ONLY THERAPY TENDS TO CAUSE ENDOMETRIAL HYPERPLASIA PRECURSOR TO CANCER THIS CANNOT HAPPEN IN WOMEN W/O A UTERUS.

3. Your text describes the WHI clinical trial as a "primary prevention" study. The HERS trial was referred to as a "secondary prevention" study. Such approaches to gaining information about preventing certain disorders are quite common—used for a variety of diseases and drugs or other preventive measures. In simple terms, what are the basic differences between primary and secondary prevention clinical trials? Who were the main subjects in WHI and HERS? How, medically, did they differ? What were the basic questions the investigators were asking?

PRIMARY CONDUCTED IN PEOPLE W/O SYMPTOMS. WILL HRT PREVENT THE DEVELOPMENT OF HEART DISEASE.

4. What changes in bone metabolism usually is associated with the estrogen loss that occurs with menopause? Summarize the role(s) of estrogen (more specifically, estrogen deficiency) in a process that often leads to osteoporosis in women.

ESTROGEN SUPPRESSES BONE BREAKDOWN WHEN ESTROGEN ↓ BONE ABSORPTION ↑ (OF OSTEOCLASTS) CAUSE BONE WEAKENING ↓ FRACTURES

CASE STUDY

Sonia Bradford is a 52-year-old woman whose menses stopped 18 months ago. She has experienced hot flashes and palpitations for the past 2 years. Recently she has begun to notice vaginal dryness that interferes with her ability to enjoy intercourse. She makes an appointment with her gynecologist to discuss hormone replacement therapy. During the office visit her physician notes that her vaginal tissues appear thin and dry. The physician determines that Mrs. Branford's symptoms are related to menopause and prescribes conjugated estrogen (Premarin) 0.625 mg PO for the first 25 days of the month and medroxyprogesterone (Provera) 10 mg PO to coincide with the last 10 days of the estrogen.

1. What is the rationale for taking both estrogen and progesterone replacement for menopausal symptoms?

PURPOSE IS TO REPLACE ESTROGEN LOST IN MENOPAUSE. PROGESTERIN COUNTERACTS THE RISK OF ESTROGEN INDUCED HYPER PLASIA ✓ CANCER

2. What common mild side effects may be expected with estrogen replacement?

COMMON MILD SIDE EFFECTS SUCH AS NAUSEA ✓ HEADACHE.

3. What benefits are documented and which are under investigation that Mrs. Bradford might expect in addition to relief of her menopausal symptoms?

↓ HOT FLASHES, ↓ INCONTINENCE, VAGINITIS, PREVENTION OF OSTEOPOROSIS ✓ PROTECTION AGAINST CORONARY ARTERY DISEASE BUT CAN ↑ CANCER RISK.

4. Mrs. Bradford asks whether her menstrual periods will reappear while she is on hormone replacement therapy.

YES, SHE WILL HAVE SOME MENSTRUAL BLEEDING DURING HRT.

Identify the phases of the menstrual cycle and describe the roles of estrogen in relation to that cycle.

5. In addition to evaluating her relief of menopausal symptoms with the hormone replacement therapy, what additional health screening measures should be incorporated into Mrs. Bradford's plan of care?

SHOULD HAVE FOLLOW UP BREAST EXAMS EVERY YEAR, ✓ A ENDOMETRIAL BIOPSY 2-3 YEARS.

6. Does Mrs. Bradford have any contraindications to hormone replacement therapy? What are some of the main contraindications?

PROGESTERON IS CONTRIDICTED IN PRESENCE OF UNDIAGNOSED VAGINAL BLEEDING, THROMBOPHLEBITIS, LIVER DISEASE, CANCER OF RED ORGANS, AVOID AT PREM

7. Mrs. Bradford tells you that it is really difficult for her to swallow pills. She wants to know whether she can take the drug any other way. What is your answer?

AN ESTRADIOL TRANSDERMAL SYSTEM IS AVAILABLE. STICK THE PATCH ON THE SKIN FOLLOW THE INSTRUCTIONS ✓ MORE TIMES THAN NOT THINGS WILL WK FINE.

Birth Control

KEY TERMS

abortifacient (drug or effect)
depot (preparation of drug)
minipill

monophasic (and biphasic and triphasic) oral contraceptive
nidation
Yuzpe regimen

OBJECTIVES

After reading and studying this chapter you should be able to:

1. Describe the different methods of birth control (pharmacologic or not) and their main known benefits, adverse effects, and overall contraception (or contraceptive failure) rates.
2. Discuss how oral contraceptive (OC) efficacy can be altered by interactions with other drugs. Cite specific examples of interactants and the predicted outcome. Summarize the common mechanisms by which these drugs either inhibit or increase the effects (desirable or not) of OCs.
3. Describe the general meaning of the term *minipill* in terms of the active ingredient(s) found in one. Explain what seems to be the main advantage of the minipill compared with a combination OC.
4. Identify the main contraceptive action of the combination OCs, and state two other mechanisms that are likely to occur and contribute to the overall desired effect.
5. Summarize the main features that distinguish monophasic, biphasic, and triphasic OCs. Do this with respect to the presence and dosages and cycle-related changes in the dosage(s) and changes of the ingredient(s).
6. In the context of combination OCs, state the main signs and symptoms of excess and of deficiency (of dosages in the product) of estrogen. Do the same for the progestin component.
7. Summarize the main interactions involving oral contraceptives: drugs that may lower the contraceptive effects of OCs and drugs that are targets of interactions caused by the OC. Summarize the main pharmacokinetic mechanisms that are

responsible for these interactions. Specifically, focus on:
   Warfarin
   Anticonvulsants/antiepileptic drugs such as phenytoin
   Tetracycline antibiotics and ampicillin
   Theophylline
8. Explain the Yuzpe regimen: its purpose, what drugs are used, the main way to optimize the desired outcome, and the most common side effects associated with it.

CRITICAL THINKING AND STUDY QUESTIONS

1. Table 60-2 and related text show that the method of sterilization chosen most often (by men and women combined) is sterilization: tubal ligation and vasectomy. In what way might this information be misleading? OVERALL STERILIZATION IS MOST WIDELY SELECTED, BUT CHOSEN BY OLDER INDIVIDUALS WHO HAVE HAS CHILD SO OTHER CONTRACEPTIVES ARE USED.

2. Why is personal preference (for the mode of contraception) such an important consideration in the choice and ultimate selection of which approach(es) to use?

   MUST BE USED IN OPTIMAL WAY.
   NO NEED TO USE IF NOT BEING USED CORRECTLY.

3. What one method of contraception (a single method or combination of methods)—other than total abstinence—confers the greatest chance of protecting against a venereal disease?

   ANY BARRIER METHOD COMBINED WITH SPERMICIDE.

4. Identify the main contraceptive action of the combination OCs, and state two other mechanisms that are likely to occur and contribute to the overall desired effect. THROMBOSIS OF EMBOLI IS MAIN REASON FOR CARDIOVASCULAR COMPLICATIONS OF OC. ALSO STROKE & MYOCARDIAL INFARC

5. What is the main cardiovascular complication of combination OCs? Which drug in such combinations seems to be responsible for this complication and secondary consequences of it? What factor seems to account most for the decline in this risk (but certainly not risk elimination) as combination OCs have been reformulated over the years? INHIBITS OVULATION IS MAIN ACTION. 2.) ALSO THICKENS THE CERVICAL MUCUS TO HINDER SPERM TO EGG. CAUSES AN ENVIROMENT UNFAVORABLE TO SPERM.

6. What are the main applicable precautions or contraindications to using combination OCs as they apply to the "main cardiovascular complications" noted above? THE USE OF CIGARETTES & HISTORY OF THROMBOEMBLOC DISEASE 4 RISK OF OC DEVELOPMENT.

7. Estrogen (alone or in combination OCs) is said to increase the risk of *thromboembolic* stroke. What is the presumed mechanism of that? Can you envisage a mechanism by which these drugs can increase the risk of *hemorrhagic* stroke? How do these two types of stroke differ pathophysiologically (keep it simple)? ARISES FROM OCCLUSION OF ONE OR MORE CEREBRAL VESSELS. & HEMORAGE STROKE INVOLVES HEMORAGE IN BRAIN.

8. A woman is discussing with you what she recalls from all the TV and newspaper reports about links between estrogen and breast cancer. She admits she's confused, but her impression is that for most women estrogen doesn't increase the risk of breast cancer and it doesn't worsen existing breast carcinoma. Is her impression correct? Why or why not? IN MOST WOMEN ESTROGEN DOESN'T INCREASE. THE RISK OF NEW BREAST CANCERS.

9. Now she asks about ovarian, endometrial, and cervical cancer risks. Do the data justify any major concerns? ESTROGENS EXERT A PROTELTIVE EFFECT EFFECT. CANCER OF CERVIX IS PROBABLY AN EXCEPTION.

10. A colleague is confused about what might happen if OCs are administered to a woman who happens to become pregnant. She believes that, like many other drugs she's read about (she cites some of the anticonvulsants), OCs are teratogenic. Do you agree? MAIN RISK IS NOT THE PRODUCTION OF BIRTH DEFECTS BUT RATHER AN INCREASE RISK OF CANCER IN UTERO FEMALES.

11. A young woman who has persistent atrial fibrillation starts on a combination OC product. Her MD has not done an adequate physical exam before writing the prescription. What is the most likely adverse effect this woman will experience once she begins taking her OC? ARTICIAL FIBRILATION IS USUALLY ASSOCIATED WITH THROMBI. TAKING OC 4 RISK.

12. A month's supply of many OCs consists of 21 pills that contain the active drug and 7 that have either iron or nothing in them. What is the probable rationale for having iron in 7 pills? What is the rationale for having nothing in 7 pills in some other products? SIMPLY TO 4 IRON LOST IN MENSTRATION. SIMPLY TO MAKE IT EASY BY TAKING 1 PILL

13. Anna Doolittle, 17 years old, comes to the pediatrician's office with her mom. Anna is a star athlete on her high school swim and track teams. Her mom says, "She's always practicing... a couple of hours on the track or in the pool every morning, and again in the afternoons... every

day, rain or shine." Anna is in the 40th percentile of height for girls her age. She is remarkably healthy otherwise: lean, but very healthy looking. Anna eats a well-balanced diet and doesn't like junk food at all. She denies any sexual activity. The reason for the visit is that Anna has not had a consistently regular menstrual cycle—ever. She frequently has vaginal bleeding or spotting at times that, her mom predicts, should be around the middle of her menstrual cycle.

A. Why would the MD do a physical exam that includes a check for scoliosis (aside from the fact that it's routine) and send Anna for a bone mineral density scan?

REASON TO SUSPECT THAT ANNAS EXTREME PHYSICAL BEHAVIOR HAS SUPPRESED ESTROGEN PRODUCTION.

B. What is the most likely therapeutic approach that will manage both the bone mineralization problems and the menstrual irregularities?

AN ESTROGEN - PROGESTERON ORAL CONTRACEPTIVE COMBINATION PRODUCT

C. Anna's mom says, "The doctor is prescribing a birth control pill for Anna?! I told you she's not sexually active. Don't you believe us?" Comment.

NO QUESTIONING IF ANYONE IS SEXUALLY ACTIVE BUT OC ARE BEST FOR HER THERAPY.

D. The estrogen-progestin product is being prescribed for Anna to normalize her menstrual cycles and provide some aspect of "bone health." It is not being prescribed as a means of contraception. Does that mean that we needn't do the complete work-ups that would be necessary if the drug were prescribed for birth control instead?

NO, PRETREATMENT ASSESSMENTS NEED TO BE DONE.

14. A patient who was just started on contraception with a subdermal levonorgestrel implant (Norplant) actually took the time to read the package insert. She finds that the product contains Silastic capsules. She calls, wanting to know if the Silastic is a drug too. She's never heard of it. Respond.

IT IS A SILICONE RUBBER THAT HAS LOW POTENTIAL TO TRIGGER A REACTION.

15. Misoprostol (Cytotec) is mentioned and discussed towards the end of your text chapter as one drug in a regimen used to induce abortion. What is the main use of this drug? How does it work when used for that purpose? How does the drug's ability to induce abortion relate to its use for that "other" purpose? (Admittedly, comments about misoprostol are in "small print." And if you're going through the text sequentially, you won't have come to this information yet. Nonetheless, I think the question is important and this is a good time to raise it.)

IT USED TO TREAT GASTRIC ULCER CAUSED BY ANTI FLAMITORY DRUGS.

CASE STUDY

Rita Booth is 17 years old and reports that she is sexually active. Her male partners use condoms to keep her from getting pregnant and to prevent the spread of sexually transmitted diseases.

Ms. Booth has decided to start on an oral contraceptive (OC). Her medical history includes asthma that is controlled with Theo-Dur (a proprietary formulation of theophylline), dysmenorrheal, and irregular menses.

Ms. Booth's last menstrual period was 2 months ago, but she says she "isn't concerned about being or getting pregnant because her partners use condoms."

1. Are you as confident as Ms. Booth that there's no reason to be concerned about her being or becoming pregnant? Why or why not?

THERE IS A CONCERN. FAILURE RATE OF CONDOMS IS 15 ?. SHE HAS NOT MENSTATED IN 2 MONS. AS WELL.

2. Ms. Booth is anxious and asks you about the medical exam and what procedures will be completed. Briefly describe what will be included in the preadministration assessment and how frequently she will need to have it repeated.

FOR HYPERTENSION, DIABETES, THROMBOTIC DISORDERS & CORONARY ARTERY DISEASE.

The pregnancy test is negative. Aside from the history of asthma (see below), there are no contraindications for the use of OCs. Ms. Booth does not smoke at all.

3. When educating a patient in the use of OCs, it is important to stress the need to take them as prescribed. Ms. Booth will be started on a triphasic OC. She is concerned that she may forget to take the pills consistently. Does this raise any concern? YES SHE MAY BECOME PREGNANT IF SHE DOES NOT REMEMBER DAILY.

4. What written instructions should you give Ms. Booth to follow if she misses one or more doses of her OC? Remember, we're talking about a triphasic combination OC for this patient.

IF ONE IS MISSED TAKE IT WITH THE NEXT DOSE, BUT WILL NEED TO ABSTAIN FROM SEX.

5. Might we consider a minipill for Ms. Booth, instead of a combination OC? What is the ingredient in the minipill? Why would we use it? What's the main advantage, and does it seem to apply to this patient?

MINIPILLS CONTAIN ONLY PROGESTERONE.

6. Ms. Booth's mother calls during your consultation with Rita. She wants you to tell her daughter to stop having sex. What would you do?

EXPLAIN RISK OF PREG & STI'S. BUT IT IS HER MOTHERS ROLE TO EXPRESS ABSTINENCE.

7. Rita says, "Once I start on these pills they'll not only help keep me from getting pregnant, but they'll also protect me from VD (venereal disease), right?"

WRONG, OC CONFER NO PROTECTION AGAINST STI'S

8. Knowing that Ms. Booth has asthma and is presently taking theophylline for it, what special considerations need to be taken, and why? What signs or symptoms would indicate a "problem" with the theophylline and the OC?

CAN IMPARE HEPATIC METABOLISM OF THEOPHYLINE = SLEEPY, HYPER

9. Let's assume that the physician who will be writing the prescription for the OC and who is doing the necessary preadministration work-up and follow-ups is also the physician who prescribed the theophylline for Ms. Booth's asthma. That means she (the MD) ought to be able to make medication changes better than another MD who might be treating the asthma and be unaware of OC use.

Are there other things you might consider, possibly discuss with the MD? To make things a little easier, let's assume that Ms. Brown is having spells of "bad wheezing" about once a week while on the theophylline.

A. Would it be appropriate to increase the theophylline dose since it seems not to be working as well as we might like it?

RASE THEOPHYLINE DOSE FIRST.

B. Should we leave the theophylline dose as is and hope that the interaction with the OC will raise it to an effective yet safe level?

IT'S A POSSIBILTY, BUT MUST MONITOR TOXICITY LEVEL.

C. What else might be considered? If needed, refer to the chapter on the drug therapy of asthma (Chapter 71) and review the actions and current status of theophylline as a primary (or even adjunctive) therapy for asthma—especially in someone who is 17 years old (or older).

I'D WANT TO GET HER ASTHMA UNDER CONTROL FIST.

We go back to "square one" on the asthma therapy and start Ms. Booth on a combination OC. The MD prescribes Ortho-Novum 1/35.

10. She is compliant, but after a couple of months she reports feeling bloated all the time. Indeed, she's gained a few pounds despite attempts to exercise more and cut back on high-calorie foods. Indeed, she claims she's often nauseated but isn't really sure whether the nausea is related to meals. She has some breast tenderness. What's the most likely cause?

TOO MUCH ESTROGEN IN THE OC PRODUCT SELECTED FOR HER.

evolve To check your answers, go to http://evolve.elsevier.com/Lehne/ for Study Guide Comments from the author.

CHAPTER

61

Drug Therapy of Infertility

KEY TERMS

controlled ovarian
  stimulation
endometriosis
gonadotropins
human chorionic
  gonadotropin (HCG)
hypogonadotropic
  hypogonadism

infertility
luteal-phase defects
menotropins
polycystic ovary
  syndrome (PCOS)

OBJECTIVES

After reading and studying this chapter you should
be able to:

1. Be able to give a good working definition of
infertility (subfertility) and distinguish it from
sterility.
2. Briefly summarize the essential elements or
processes of the female reproductive system that
are required for conception and the ability to
carry a viable fetus to parturition. In your summary, identify the main hormones involved and
their production or regulation by the ovaries, the
uterus, the pituitary gland, and the hypothalamus.
3. Summarize the basic medical work-up to diagnose infertility in women. Assume the cause of
infertility in a particular woman is ovulatory failure. Then discuss a typical management plan that
may involve clomiphene, menotropins, and HCG.
State the main purpose of giving each drug; the
timing of drug administration; and basic follow-
ups to track the progress, efficacy, and potential
adverse effects of the interventions.

As noted in the text, you should review key information from the previous (two) chapters, focusing on
what is going on physiologically and hormonally
during the menstrual cycle; and what estrogens,
progestins, gonadotropin-releasing hormone,
luteinizing hormone, and follicle-stimulating hormone do. Depending on your instructor's wishes,
you may need to review some information from
other chapters on the basic pharmacology of several
antidiabetic drugs (metformin and the glitazones;
Chapter 54); and of bromocriptine (Chapter 21).

CRITICAL THINKING AND STUDY QUESTIONS

1. You're in a small study group preparing for the
quiz on the material discussed in this chapter. Just
as you comment out loud that clomiphene pro-
motes follicular maturation and ovulation by
blocking estrogen receptors, the class wise-guy
walks by and says, "You're crazy! How can you
cause those effects by blocking estrogen receptors?" Explain your point for the poor dunce.
Explain further what the physiologic prerequisites are for clomiphene to increase fertility.

2. Why should blood tests to assess pituitary function be part of a complete work-up before
clomiphene is prescribed?

3. Now that we've identified the main site and
mechanism of the desired effects of clomiphene,
comment on the potential unwanted effects, particularly as they affect the ovaries and the cervix.

4. It's your first week working at a small Ob-Gyn practice. You're reviewing the records for a patient and note that she's taking metformin (glucophage) for polycystic ovary syndrome (PCOS). It was prescribed by one of the docs for whom you're working. Is your boss moonlighting as a diabetologist? What's going on?

5. The text notes that pituitary dysfunction that leads to an increase in prolactin levels can be managed with bromocriptine. Can you recall how that drug works, and what its arguably more common use is? Include in your answer the drug's main endocrine and nonendocrine effects. (It's OK to peek at the index and check; you should do that if you don't know the answer.)

CASE STUDY

Mr. and Mrs. Brooks are in their late 30s and are childless. Mr. Brooks is healthy with normal sperm count, motility, and viability. Mrs. Brooks is healthy too. Neither is taking any medications. Neither smokes; they drink alcohol only about once a month, and in moderation.

They've been trying to conceive for the past 8 years but have not been successful. During a lengthy diagnostic work-up for infertility, Mrs. Brooks was found to have no increase in her basal body temperature throughout her menstrual cycles.

1. In this scenario, what's the most likely explanation for the observation that Mrs. Brooks's body temperature doesn't rise during the menstrual cycles?

The physician diagnoses primary infertility due to anovulation and decides to induce ovulation. She prescribes menotropins (Pergonal; also known as human menopausal gonadotropin, or HMG) to be given IM for days 7 through 14 of the menstrual cycle. You provide counseling about the need for follow-up and early detection of ovarian hyperstimulation syndrome, and give an overall explanation of what is being done.

2. What are the ingredients in menotropins, and what is the overall goal or purpose of administering them?

3. How are the actions of menotropins and clomiphene alike yet different?

4. The physician will use human chorionic gonadotropin (HCG) as an adjunct to the menotropins. Mrs. Brooks asks why the HCG can't be used by itself. She's heard that it's just one injection.... A lot more tolerable than the daily menotropin injections she'll be getting. Explain the reason to her.

5. Mrs. Brooks asks whether she is more likely to have a multiple pregnancy (i.e., more than one fetus) if she takes menotropins. How would you respond?

6. Mrs. Brooks is told that she's going to need frequent blood tests and ultrasound (ultrasonogram) investigations of her abdomen once she starts the menotropin therapy. She says, "I know blood tests and ultrasounds are used to determine pregnancy, and 'look at the baby.' Am I going to get pregnant *that fast?*" Explain the need for this monitoring and why it's so important to the overall success of the fertility treatment.

7. What are the signs and symptoms of ovarian hyperstimulation syndrome, and arguably its most serious consequence?

evolve To check your answers, go to http://evolve.elsevier.com/Lehne/ for Study Guide Comments from the author.

Drugs That Affect Uterine Function

KEY TERMS

ergot alkaloid
tocolytic (drug or effect)

oxytocic (drug or effect)

OBJECTIVES

After reading and studying this chapter you should be able to:

1. Describe three major clinical settings in which use of an oxytocic is deemed acceptable.
2. Discuss the factors that should be considered in selecting a particular oxytocic drug or drug class for use before versus after delivery.
3. State the major risks of magnesium sulfate used as a tocolytic drug in terms of adverse effects on the mother, on the fetus, and on the infant shortly after delivery.
4. Classify and state the mechanism of action of ritodrine (or terbutaline), and identify the main systemic maternal adverse effects related to its primary mechanism of action.
5. Identify the three main groups of uterine stimulant drugs; compare and contrast their effects on uterine muscle tone and rhythmicity, and state why their different intensities of effects do (or don't) make them suitable for use before or after labor and delivery.

CRITICAL THINKING AND STUDY QUESTIONS

1. A woman in premature labor is given an IV infusion of ritodrine to slow uterine contractions and delay delivery. She becomes tachycardic and starts manifesting signs and symptoms of pulmonary edema. How and why do these effects occur? After all, ritodrine is classified as a selective beta$_2$ agonist and a uterine relaxant, and it is given in this situation for precisely those uterine effects? Would you expect vasoconstriction (either maternal, leading to hypertension, or placental, leading to placental underperfusion) to be

a part of the clinical picture based on how ritodrine works?

2. How are the effects of the ergot alkaloids, prostaglandins, and oxytocin on the intensity, frequency, and rhythmicity of uterine tone similar yet different? To keep the discussion simple, assume these drugs might be administered to a woman who is close to going into labor or who has just started labor. Assume further that the drugs are being used at usual recommended doses for their main indications. Since all are effective uterine stimulants, why can't they be used interchangeably at these times?

3. A pregnant woman with asthma is using very high doses of her albuterol inhaler each day to control respiratory signs and symptoms. What consequences might this have on the progression of her pregnancy, labor, and delivery? Why?

4. What adjunctive drug(s) is/are important when using tocolytics when preterm delivery seems unavoidable? (**Hint:** These drugs are given for their effects not on the mother's uterus but on the fetus.)

177

5. A pregnant woman in her third trimester who is a patient in your practice calls to report she has been having occasional headaches. She asks if it's OK to take aspirin, saying she'll faithfully follow the dosing recommendations on the package. What advice would you give her, and why?

6. The text notes that indomethacin can cause premature closure of the ductus arteriosus. What is that anatomic structure? What does it do? What is the consequence of closing it prematurely? What might we do or give when that structure *fails* to close spontaneously?

7. A woman begins labor at a stage of fetal development when there are great concerns about fetal lung development and risks of fetal respiratory distress syndrome. Ritodrine therapy is started to delay delivery as long as possible, but premature delivery seems imminent. What adjunct should be administered specifically for the purpose of reducing dire consequences of fetal respiratory system dysfunction?

8. In what other (and rather uncommon) labor and delivery scenario is magnesium sulfate infusion not only important but also usually necessary? For what purpose is it given?

CASE STUDY

Linda Moss is a 25-year-old multipara (gravida 2, para 1) who was admitted to the labor and delivery unit in early labor 7 hours ago. She was 39 weeks gestation with stable vital signs and fetal heart rate. On admission her cervix was dilated 4 cm and 90% effaced and the fetal head was at 0 station in a left occiput anterior position. Her uterine contractions were coming every 4 minutes, lasting 40 seconds, and of moderate intensity.

Four hours after admission, the nurse noted that the contraction pattern had changed to contractions every 6 to 8 minutes, lasting 30 seconds, and of mild intensity. No cervical changes were found at that time. Ms. Moss was encouraged to walk in the hallway. When a poor quality and frequency of uterine contractions persisted 1 hour later, without any change in the cervix, the obstetrician decided to augment labor with oxytocin. An intravenous infusion of 10 units of oxytocin in 1000 cc of 5% dextrose and 0.5 normal saline was piggybacked (via a secondary line) into her primary infusion line. The oxytocin infusion was regulated by an infusion pump and was initiated at 1 mU per minute.

1. Why is the oxytocin infusion piggybacked into the primary infusion line?

2. What is the usual protocol for advancing the oxytocin infusion rate?

3. What specific observations must be made of the mother and fetus during oxytocin augmentation?

4. Ms. Moss has suddenly started having contractions lasting 90 seconds every 2 minutes. What would you do?

5. When is oxytocin augmentation of labor contraindicated?

6. Ms. Moss has delivered a 3-kg boy. She is to receive methylergonovine maleate (Methergine;

0.2 mg PO, q 6 hr for 3 days). Identify the purpose for this drug. Identify the main situations in which it should not be given and another class of drugs (specify) should be used instead.

evolve To check your answers, go to http://evolve.elsevier.com/Lehne/ for Study Guide Comments from the author.

63

Review of the Immune System

KEY TERMS

antibody
antigen
apoptosis
B lymphocytes
basophil
cell-mediated immunity,
  cell mediated
complement system
cytokine
hapten
humoral (as in humoral
  factor)
immunity, acquired
immunity, antibody-
  mediated (humoral)
immunity, natural
immunoglobulin(s) (esp.
  IgE and IgG)
interleukins

lymphokine
major histocompatibility
  complex (MHC)
mast cell (compare with
  basophil)
membrane attack
  complex (MAC)
monocyte (compare with
  macrophage)
monokine
opsonization (as of
  bacteria)
phagocytosis
stem cell
T lymphocytes, cytolytic
  (CTLs)
T lymphocytes, helper
tumor necrosis factors
  (TNFs)

OBJECTIVES

After reading and studying this chapter you should be able to:

1. Compare and contrast antibody-mediated immunity (humoral immunity) and cell-mediated immunity. Include in your comments general mechanisms of antibody production and how they exert their host-defense actions; and state the origins and roles of helper T lymphocytes (CD4 cells), macrophages, and cytolytic T lymphocytes (CD8)

2. State the main roles of the following cells that are important in the immune response:
   B lymphocytes (B cells)
   Cytolytic T lymphocytes (T cells, CD8 cells)
   Helper T lymphocytes
   Macrophages/monocytes
   Mast cells/basophils

3. Explain the general role(s) of the immunoglobulins, and give a brief explanation of why there are five major classes of them.

4. Explain what the major histocompatibility complex (MHC) is and what its main functions are. Consider the functions in terms of autoimmune diseases (protection against) and organ/tissue/cell transplantation.

5. Compare and contrast the basic mechanisms and outcomes of delayed vs. immediate hypersensitivity reactions. In your comparison of delayed hypersensitivity, integrate general concepts about cell-mediated immunity.

6. Summarize the main purpose of the classical complement pathway and how, eventually, its activation leads to cell death.

Notes: This is an extremely comprehensive (and well-done) chapter on the immune system. However, unless your instructor tells you otherwise, I'd urge you to get the big pictures on the various components of the immune systems—how they may work together; and how in a general sense they go about their business—and not get so bogged down in details that you don't see the "big picture." The *Key Points* summary at the end of the textbook chapter is particularly useful in terms of getting the broad overview of this material.

You will also see that some cells, and their mediators, go under several names. That can be (heck, it is) confusing. Ask your instructor about the term he or she prefers. It's probably fair to have you realize that mast cells and basophils are the same thing, or that the same applies to monocytes and macrophages. It's probably important to know that, for example, humoral immunity means antibody-mediated immunity. But then we get into cytolytic T cells (a.k.a. CD8 cells, cytolytic T lymphocytes) and others. A whole exam can be constructed on these synonyms, and you can remember them all if you try, but you'll come away with a very poor grasp of the more important stuff—the big picture that we note above.

Should you learn the main functions and locations of all five of the major immunoglobulins? Learn what the dozen or so interleukins do? I think not. Indeed, we seldom go into this much detail with our medical students; they often come away with "can't see the forest for the trees" syndrome;

180

and return in a few years to ask why they had to "learn all that stuff when they've never put it to clinical use."

CRITICAL THINKING AND STUDY QUESTIONS

1. How does one develop specific acquired immunity?

2. What is the difference between cell-mediated immunity and antibody-mediated (humoral) immunity?

3. What are the major cell types associated with immunity?

4. What are the three phases of the immune response? What does each one do, in simple terms? What's going on?

5. What are the five classes of antibodies and their functions?

6. Why is the thymus gland so critical to the function of the immune system?

7. The text, including Figure 00-1, mentions pluripotent hematopoietic stem cells. What does pluripotent mean? (**Hint:** A dollar bill might help you figure this one out.) Legal and ethical issues aside, why is stem cell research such a hot topic in medical research nowadays?

8. What are the critical roles of helper T lymphocytes in the immune system, and why are they of particular importance to people with HIV/AIDS? Do they just "help out?"

9. An antidote of sorts for massive overdoses of digoxin (a drug widely used for chronic heart failure (see Chapter 46) is called digoxin immune Fab (and it's marketed as Digibind). What does the term *Fab* mean? How (in the most basic sense) do we get them? How do they work?

10. Why do you think that chemotherapy for cancer is often associated with such other problems as bleeding disorders, immunosuppression, and the increased risk of opportunistic infections?

11. Two of the "characteristic features of the immune responses" described in your text are *memory* and *time limitation*. What is generally going on in the development of memory? Why is it important? How does it relate to time-limited aspects of immune responses? In what one area of pharmacotherapeutics—perhaps more than any other—do these concepts come into play? (You might want to start your comments on this by thinking about how you learn and

then memorize things and what the benefits of memorizing things are.)

12. A classmate is arguing with you. He says that antibodies, immunoglobulins, and gamma globulins are completely different things in terms of what they are and what they do. Do you agree?

13. In reading and hearing about immunology and immunopharmacology, you'll often encounter the term **hapten?** What is that?

14. Why are such disorders as rheumatoid arthritis, systemic lupus erythematosus (SLE), type 1 diabetes, and myasthenia gravis mentioned in and relevant to a chapter on immunology?

15. A classmate states that the major histocompatibility complex (MHC) is a set of antibodies that are unique in every (or nearly every) individual. Do you agree?

16. Before we select an organ (or bone marrow) that will be transplanted into a recipient, we check blood types and the MHC to get as close a match as possible between recipient and donor. Yet, we also use immunosuppressant drugs (see Chapter 65) as part of the overall treatment plan. Why?

17. Your colleague, who has been "instructing" you on MHC, antibodies, immunoglobulins, gamma globulins, and the like, now spouts off about cytokines, lymphokines, and monokines. She says that they're just different words for the same antibodies. Is she right... this time?

18. You're in a continuing ed/in-service seminar. The speaker is talking about some new developments in immunology and immunopharmacology. She casually refers to the classical pathway of the complement system, a "cascade," and MAC. What is all this about, in general terms? What's the complement system? What's a cascading system? What (or who) is MAC?

19. Your annoying know-it-all classmate is back. This time he's trying to tell you that macrophages and monocytes are the same thing. Same goes with mast cells—they're the same thing as basophils. Is he wrong again?

Can you guess where (in what chapter) we'll be spending more time visiting the importance of mast cells and basophils because they play unusually critical roles in the pathophysiology of a particular (and particularly common) disease?

20. In the discussion of how the immune system recognizes and attacks virus-infected cells, the term **apoptosis** (which means "programmed cell death") is noted. Just to round out our study questions to a nice number (20), do you know how to pronounce *apoptosis?*

evolve To check your answers, go to http://evolve.elsevier.com/Lehne/ for Study Guide Comments from the author.

Childhood Immunization

KEY TERMS

antitoxin
immunity (active, passive)
immunization (compare
    with vaccination)

toxoid
vaccination
vaccine (killed,
    attenuated, live)

OBJECTIVES

After reading and studying this chapter you should be able to:

1. Describe the role of vaccines in maintaining health.
2. Differentiate between active and passive immunity; explain how vaccines work.
3. List the three main contraindications that apply to administering any vaccine.
4. Know where to look for current information on the vaccinations that are required or recommended for children, and when and how they should be given.
5. Explain why we give multiple doses of vaccines, not just one, for a given preventable infectious disease.

Notes: I do not think you should have to memorize all (or any) of the pediatric immunization schedules as they apply to each vaccine or illness. These recommendations change, and what you learn now may soon be out of date. You need to know and understand the basic *concepts.*

This is not a supplement to a pathophysiology or infectious diseases text. It's pharmacology. The chapter in Lehne is basically short in terms of critical information, and I will keep my study questions short and focused on the pharmacology of drugs used for diseases that are really best learned somewhere else.

CRITICAL THINKING AND STUDY QUESTIONS

1. Three pieces of information that must go into some sort of permanent record of immunizations is the vaccine type, lot number, and expiration date. Why so much detail?

2. On what data do the Centers for Disease Control and Prevention (CDC) depend to determine if an outbreak of a vaccine-preventable disease (or any disease for that matter) has occurred, and how do they decide whether and how to develop strategies to prevent more cases?

3. When you look at Table 64-2 in your text you'll see that vaccines for any preventable disorder are given more than once. Why can't we give each one just once? Why doesn't immunity necessarily last "forever" or be fully induced with just one vaccine injection?

4. If a child developed chills, fever, and other flu-like signs and symptoms after a vaccination, why not recommend aspirin? Aspirin is still extremely cheap. Or would you? If not, what would you recommend, and why? Your colleague says not to recommend aspirin because it causes asthma and suppresses the immune system.

5. Your prof wants you to memorize the current recommendations for pediatric immunizations (Table 64-2 in your text). Aside from the fact that this will gobble up zillions of cells in your brain's memory bank, why *shouldn't* you be advised to do this?

evolve To check your answers, go to http://evolve.elsevier.com/Lehne/ for Study Guide Comments from the author.

Immunosuppressants

KEY TERMS

allograft
calcineurin

cytotoxic drug (in the context
of immunosuppressive therapy)

OBJECTIVES

After reading and studying this chapter you should
be able to:

1. Identify the two most common clinical uses for
   immunosuppressive drugs.
2. Explain why immunosuppressants can be considered both a blessing and a potential curse to the
   host.
3. Summarize the main mechanism of action, pharmacokinetics, toxicity, and drug-drug interactions
   involving cyclosporine. Do this in the context of
   a holistic care plan that will maximize the drug's
   desired effects while minimizing the risks of
   adverse responses or drug interactions.
4. Name some of the common autoimmune disorders for which immunosuppressants are used.

Be sure to consult Chapter 68 for more thorough
information on glucocorticoids, with particular
emphasis on their basic mechanisms of action and
adverse effects; and review information on
methotrexate, cyclophosphamide, and azathioprine.
This might also be a good time to integrate information here with that which you will find in Chapter 90,
which deals with human immunodeficiency virus
(HIV) and AIDS.

CRITICAL THINKING AND STUDY QUESTIONS

1. Cyclosporine's main targets are helper T cells
   (lymphocytes). How does that primary effect get
   translated into a suppressed immune response?
   How does that effect alter bone marrow function?

2. A colleague says, "There's always one big trade-
   off to using immunosuppressants to reduce the
   risk of organ transplant rejection or to manage
   such autoimmune disorders as rheumatoid arthritis." To what fundamental concept is she referring?

3. What *organ* is the main target of cyclosporine
   toxicity? Is this toxicity common or rare? Is it the
   result of immunosuppression? How can it be
   monitored? How and when might the signs and
   symptoms of that organ-specific toxicity be confused with rejection of the transplanted organ?

4. One of the first (if not the first) drugs to be linked
   to the "grapefruit juice effect" was cyclosporine.
   What is that effect?

5. The text notes that some degree of hypertension
   occurs in about half of the patients who receive
   cyclosporine. How might this finding be linked to
   the adverse renal effects of the drug or to kidney
   rejection?

6. How might glucocorticoids, which are often adjuncts to such drugs as cyclosporine, contribute to hypertension—perhaps making the cyclosporine-induced problem even greater? What other unwanted effect caused bycyclosporine might be worsened by a glucocorticoid? (**Hint:** I'm thinking about a problem with a very important nonelectrolyte.) What electrolyte imbalance that may be caused by cyclosporine (and moreso by tacrolimus) might be counteracted by a glucocorticoid?

7. Your text notes that there are two main cyclosporine products: Sandimmune and Neoral. There are two oral formulations of both (capsules and solutions). The text notes that these two products are not bioequivalent. A colleague states that one is better (more effective) than the other. I say they *are* bioequivalent; they just have different bioavailabilities. Who (if anyone) is right? Why?

8. Tacrolimus is an alternative to cyclosporine for some patients. What is its main perceived advantage, and what is its main disadvantage compared with cyclosporine?

9. The text notes that the effects of most cytotoxic immunosuppressant drugs are nonspecific—they act on virtually all *proliferating* cells. What are the major cytotoxic immunosuppressants, and what are the adverse host effects of their nonspecific actions? Where do these host toxicities place the cytotoxic agents in terms of preferred treatments for suppression of allograft rejection? To which other large group of drugs are the host toxicities of the cytotoxic agents quite similar?

CASE STUDY

Alan Dean is a 30-year-old who had a kidney transplant 2 years ago, after being diagnosed with end-stage renal disease. He visits the transplant team monthly for blood work (and, if needed, biopsies) to monitor rejection status, kidney function, and overall health. He was originally discharged on cyclosporine, azathioprine (Imuran), and prednisone.

Alan has only been on cyclosporine and azathioprine for the past year because he has shown no sign of rejection. He is very active. He no longer has fatigue and is thrilled that he is no longer "hooked up to the dialysis machine." He performs well at work and at home; he has more time to play with his kids; he's taken up golf and "heads to the links" every weekend. He's a friendly guy and urges you to call him by his first name.

After a recent trip to a national park, Alan developed fatigue and appeared tired.

Blood work done back home indicated evidence of macrophages and monocytes beginning the rejection process. He was hospitalized with evidence of transplant rejection.

1. As Alan's nurse, what is your first priority aside from the organ rejection?

2. What was the fundamental reason that Alan was placed on multidrug therapy to ward off rejection in the first place? Why not just give one drug and increase its dose as needed?

3. With Alan now apparently in very early stages of rejection, what medication is likely to be added?

4. While we haven't stated the type of infection that Alan has (and that determines which antibiotic drug we'll use), there is a concern about potential interactions between one of his drugs and one main class of antibiotics. What is that? Why are we concerned? Let's assume Alan has developed a bacterial infection. That's a reasonable assumption.

C. Why should Alan's mention of flu-like symptoms pique your interest?

5. Two of your clinical teammates are arguing. Both say that Alan will be at increased risk of infection now that his treatment will be changed. One says it's because of the prednisone. One says it's because of the cyclosporine, which was the problem in the first place. Do you agree with one or the other? Why?

7. Alan occasionally gets heartburn, saying (with a smile) that his wife's cooking could be better. He sometimes takes an antacid combination product. His favorite is Maalox. Do you have any issues with that?

8. You ask a little more about Alan's heartburn. He admits that he's getting heartburn often, and it's not really his wife's cooking. Anything he eats can cause it. In fact, he's switched from an antacid to OTC cimetidine (e.g., Tagamet HB). Are you concerned now? What might you recommend for Alan?

Alan says that he gets headaches about every few months. For one reason or another he doesn't "like" aspirin (it makes him wheeze a little). And he says that acetaminophen never gets rid of his headache, no matter how much he takes. So he uses OTC ibuprofen for his occasional headaches, colds, and flu-like symptoms. He swears he follows the instructions on the ibuprofen package label about maximum dosages and how long to take the drug except on the advice and supervision of an MD.

6. A. Do you see any particular and major concern with Alan's use of ibuprofen occasionally? Why?

9. Why should you ask about Alan's alcohol intake? Yes, we know that drinking too much, too often, is bad. But let's focus on the fact that he's also taking cyclosporine.

B. If Alan said that he has frequent headaches and takes a lot of ibuprofen "all the time," would you have any concerns?

evolve To check your answers, go to http://evolve.elsevier.com/Lehne/ for Study Guide Comments from the author.

Antihistamines

KEY TERMS

allergic release (of histamine, other mast cell mediators)

antihistamine (first-generation, second-generation)

H_1 receptor

H_2 receptor

mast cell

rhinitis, allergic

rhinorrhea

triple response of Lewis

urticaria

OBJECTIVES

After reading and studying this chapter you should be able to:

1. State the body's richest physiologic source of histamine and part(s) of the body where they are found in abundance; describe the two main processes by which this chemical can be released from these structures.
2. Summarize the main effects of histamine on airway smooth muscle tone; arteriolar and venular tone, gastric acid secretion, and the heart (e.g., rate); identify the receptor(s) involved in these effects.
3. Identify the receptors that are blocked by a typical first-generation antihistamine, especially as they relate to clinical uses and precautions for their use; state whether and how a typical second-generation antihistamine differs from the older agents.
4. Compare and contrast the effects of first- and second-generation antihistamines on the CNS; assume they are given at "usual therapeutic doses."
5. Summarize the benefits or limitations of antihistamines (and specify the types thereof) for managing anaphylaxis, signs and symptoms of the common cold, allergic rhinitis, and asthma.

CRITICAL THINKING AND STUDY QUESTIONS

1. Diphenhydramine, arguably the prototype of all the older antihistamines, is prescribed for managing some cases of Parkinson's disease. That's a disorder that (as far as we know) has nothing to do with histamine. Why, then, is the drug sometimes used for this purpose?

2. You may have heard some people say, "If aspirin were a new drug, it would never get approved [by the FDA], at least not as an OTC drug, because of its many side effects and contraindications." Some have said the same about OTC diphenhydramine. Why might that be?

3. We now have second-generation antihistamines appearing on the OTC market (loratadine [Claritin] appeared in late 2002). Compare and contrast their effects (desired and otherwise), precautions, and contraindications, with those of a typical first-generation agent. Given your comparison, and considering your comments to question 2 above, does it seem suitable to have the newer agents available to the general public without prescription? Is there now any reason to buy one of the first-generation agents, now that we have a new kid on the block? Why?

4. A friend who has a history of severe reactions to bee stings (laryngeal edema and difficulty breathing, light-headedness from hypotension, etc.) tells you she's going off on a camping trip. Bees and wasps will be there, for sure. Not wanting her to be drowsy during the trip, her doctor writes a prescription for one of the new second-generation antihistamines, to take "just in case" she gets stung. If you could, what advice would you give her?

5. Why might physostigmine be used as an adjunct for managing life-threatening overdoses with diphenhydramine? Would it be beneficial, or even necessary, for massive overdoses of a second-generation antihistamine?

6. For nearly all the many widely advertised brand-name OTC cough and cold remedies and hay fever remedies (with an antihistamine in it), various chain stores have their own alternatives. They contain identical dosages of identical ingredients, often at much lower cost per dose. Are these alternatives really "equivalent"? Is it worth spending the extra money for brand-name meds?

7. Ranitidine (Zantac), available by prescription and OTC, is indicated for managing some disorders associated with excessive gastric acid secretion. It works by blocking histamine receptors. If a patient took the recommended dose of ranitidine for heartburn and the recommended dose of diphenhydramine (you can assume a usual 25 mg OTC dose) for allergic rhinitis, what would the consequences be, say, in terms of overdose?

8. Discuss the potential benefits and risks of taking a first-generation antihistamine (use diphenhydramine as your example) for asthma, either as primary therapy or as an adjunct. Would a second-generation antihistamine be better or worse, and why?

9. In what ways does a simple mosquito bite demonstrate the many effects of histamine, albeit on a tiny scale?

CASE STUDY

Your 65-year-old dad comes for a visit. He has a bad cold and tells you he's thinking of taking some Benadryl; he has a bottle of the product, purchased over the counter at the neighborhood drug store.

Comment on the following, knowing that you're not going to prescribe for your dad, and knowing that the best advice might simply be to advise him to see his physician.

1. What do the histamine receptor–blocking actions of diphenhydramine do, beneficially, based on your understanding of the underlying pathophysiology of common cold symptoms?

2. You've tried to convince your dad that getting some sleep and drinking some homemade chicken soup might do more for his cold symptoms than the diphenhydramine. He tells you that he's "taken the same stuff for a cold long ago, and it works!" Assuming he wasn't dealing with a placebo effect, how might the diphenhydramine have provided symptom relief?

3. Given your dad's age (and sex), what other conditions might he have (perhaps undiagnosed) that may be worsened by diphenhydramine? What effect of diphenhydramine is responsible for these potential unwanted effects?

4. Dad says, "Easy for you to tell me to get some sleep! I can't. I'm gonna go out and buy some Nytol." Do you think this is a good idea? Why, or why not?

evolve To check your answers, go to http://evolve.elsevier.com/Lehne/ for Study Guide Comments from the author.

Cyclooxygenase Inhibitors: Nonsteroidal Anti-Inflammatory Drugs and Acetaminophen

KEY TERMS

antipyretic (drug or effect)
APAP (abbreviation)
arachidonic acid
COX-1
COX-2 (and its inhibitors)"-coxibs"
cyclooxygenase(s)

nonacetylated (type of salicylate)
NSAID
Reye's syndrome
salicylate
salicylism
tinnitus

OBJECTIVES

After reading and studying this chapter you should be able to:

1. Describe the similarities or differences between the cyclooxygenase-1 and -2 pathways, and state which (patho)physiologic process is mainly responsible for the following: analgesia, anti-inflammatory activity, antipyresis, bleeding tendencies (antiplatelet effects and the related beneficial prophylaxis against myocardial infarction), and gastric mucosal damage. From this you should be able to predict the beneficial or unwanted effects of nonselective inhibition of COX-1 and COX-2 vs. selective COX-2 inhibition, as well as identify key drugs that cause those effects.
2. Discuss the beneficial and adverse actions of nonsteroidal anti-inflammatory drugs (NSAIDs) and the basic mechanism(s) by which they arise.
3. Identify situations (whether the presence of comorbid conditions or use of interacting drugs) when aspirin should not be used, even for relief of mild or episodic headache or fever; state which of the alternative OTC analgesic/antipyretic drugs would be a more acceptable alternative to aspirin, and explain why.

4. Compare and contrast the signs and symptoms of acute poisoning with aspirin and with acetaminophen, the time-course of the signs/symptoms and underlying causes, and management.

Consult content from other chapters, particularly Chapters 69 (*Drug Therapy of Rheumatoid Arthritis and Gout*), 68 (*Glucocorticoids in Nonendocrine Diseases*), 71 (*Drugs for Asthma*) and 73 (*Drugs for Peptic Ulcer Disease*), and integrate it with the material presented in this chapter.

CRITICAL THINKING AND STUDY QUESTIONS

1. The text notes that aspirin has a half-life of about 15 to 20 minutes. Why, then, do we typically administer the drug every 4 or 6 hours, and many of the effects of just a single aspirin dose seem to last much longer? Indeed, your text notes that just a single dose of aspirin can *permanently* inhibit cyclooxygenase that's involved in activating platelet aggregation. What are the explanations?

2. For patients with a history of hypersensitivity reactions to "plain aspirin," who are at risk of gastric ulcers, or who are taking drugs that are known interactants with this prototypic NSAID, which other formulation of the drug is recommended—buffered aspirin (tablets or solution), enteric-coated tablets, timed-release tablets, or rectal suppositories?

191

3. You may have seen the ads on TV. A man has a heart attack, which may have been prevented by use of aspirin. The manufacturer of the aspirin brand being sold claims, "Only OUR aspirin has been clinically proven to reduce the risk (of a heart attack)." Does this mean that other aspirins won't work or that they'll work less well than the brand-name product? Why haven't manufacturers of other brands gotten the same clinical "proof"?

4. When reading about a drug that may be unfamiliar to you, you should be alert to key phrases that describe the drug's properties and may predict significant interactions with other medications. What descriptive phrase about other meds should get your attention about a potential interaction with aspirin? (***Hint:*** It relates to one of the four main pharmacokinetic properties of nearly all drugs).

5. The text lists several conditions that predispose people to hypersensitivity reactions to aspirin: asthma, hay fever, chronic urticaria, and nasal polyps. By far the most significant (and common) predisposing condition is asthma, especially if the patient has "triad asthma" (which is defined as asthma plus nasal polyps plus aspirin sensitivity).

   Why *is* aspirin so dangerous for patients with asthma? We're not asking for the signs, symptoms, and possible outcomes, but how the problems are thought to arise.

6. Choline, magnesium, sodium salicylate, and salsalate are *nonacetylated* salicylates. What does this mean in terms of their desired or untoward effects on or in (1) platelet function, (2) the GI mucosa, (3) children at risk of Reye's syndrome, and (4) patients with a history of hypersensitivity reactions to aspirin?

7. You'll note from the text that salicylic acid is the "active metabolite" of aspirin. Does salicylic acid itself have any therapeutic uses? (You should check the index of the textbook for a little help on this.) And there's another salicylate you might like to know about. That's methyl salicylate, from which aspirin can be synthesized. Do you know what its common name is or anything about its pharmacology? I'll bet all of you have taken a tiny amount at one time or another. (You may have to do a search on the Web for more information, but we'll give you some idea in the comments for this question, which you'll also find on Lehne's website.)

8. We mentioned above that methyl salicylate (oil of wintergreen), the active ingredient in many topical pain-relief creams, lotions, and other formulations, acts as a counterirritant. What does that term mean?

9. Your dad, who is also your best tennis and jogging partner, complains of sore muscles and joints after a day of unusually vigorous exercise. He tells you he's gone to the supermarket and bought a tube of cream that "smells like wintergreen." Obviously it contains methyl salicylate. He wants to "boost" the product's relief by wrapping his painful elbow in an elastic bandage (e.g., an Ace bandage) right after he applies the medication. What advice would you give your dad about this?

10. Several students on a shopping trip for some OTC analgesics are arguing over three ibuprofen products on the OTC med shelves. One is generic ibuprofen, another is a brand-name ibuprofen product, and the third is Midol 200. A quick look on the label indicates that each contains 200 mg ibuprofen per tablet. Will any one of these be superior to or safer than another for managing mild pain or fever or for relieving discomfort of dysmenorrhea? Which product would you buy if OTC ibuprofen were indicated, and why?

11. Several other colleagues are arguing about which OTC pain reliever is "best" for relieving their occasional, simple (nonmigraine) headaches. One claims that Drug X works best, Drug Y doesn't work at all. Another claims just the opposite when the drugs are used in the recommended dosages at the recommended intervals. Still another student says, "Only Brand A of Drug Z ever works for me." What is the likely explanation?

12. Other than the risk of gastric ulceration, what is the main concern for most "otherwise healthy" people who use high doses of ibuprofen, naproxen, and other OTC analgesics long-term and almost daily?

13. What's the most basic reason why aspirin, or *most* of the other common NSAIDs, are not suitable substitutes for an opioid analgesic (e.g., morphine) for, say, a patient with severe postoperative pain?

14. Some patients are prescribed both warfarin and aspirin. Others are given such instructions as, "Don't take aspirin if you have a headache, fever, or mild joint pain" (if you're taking war-

farin). Why the apparent inconsistency in these diverse opinions? What problems might arise from giving aspirin to a patient who is taking warfarin, and how do they occur?

15. Indomethacin is arguably one of the most efficacious nonselective NSAIDs, and as you'll learn in Chapter 69, it's one of the preferred agents for symptom relief in acute gout. However, there are side effects and adverse responses that make it poorly tolerated by many patients. What are they?

16. For some cases of postoperative pain, ketorolac seems to be about as effective as morphine. What adverse property (properties) of morphine, or other opioids, does this NSAID lack—properties that accounted for such widespread popularity for this drug soon after it was approved? (Yes, you may need to refresh your knowledge about opioids; Chapter 27.) What adverse property does ketorolac cause—one that necessitated label changes and reigning in excessive use of the drug at healthcare agencies?

17. A mom calls the pediatrician's office in which you work "just to let you know" that her 8-year-old son swallowed "a bunch" of acetaminophen tablets a day ago. She reports that he was "pretty sick" overnight but he's "feeling much better now." What's your interpretation of this information and your advice to this mom?

18. In Chapter 48 we noted that one lipid-lowering drug, niacin, tends to cause cutaneous flushing and other disturbing signs and symptoms. We also mentioned that taking aspirin before taking the niacin can reduce the severity of many of the unpleasant responses to the lipid-lowering

agent. Knowing what you know now about how aspirin causes its main therapeutic effects, speculate on what is involved in the side effects to the niacin.

19. Someone writes an order for "650 mg APAP; take by mouth every 4 hours, up to 4 times a day for 3 days, for fever." What is the APAP to which this order refers?

20. Consider acetaminophen to be the most widely used pain- and fever-reducing medication for children. There are many OTC products available for administration to "children."

A. Take a look at your local pharmacy or consult some drug handbook or website, and tell us why having so many different products and so many different formulations can actually make it difficult for some parents or other caregivers to administer these products optimally and safely.

B. Tell us why just telling a parent "Give your child Tylenol" isn't a wise or safe instruction at all.

C. Tell us why giving a parent or guardian instructions to "Give acetaminophen, 10–15 mg/kg/dose every 4 hours, up to 5 doses per 24 hour period" might be giving very *explicit* instructions yet instructions that are totally meaningless or useless to many people.

21. What is the chemical basis by which acetaminophen destroys hepatocytes? What is "nature's endogenous protective chemical" against this "attack"? What is the generally accepted antidote for acetaminophen poisoning, and how, in general terms, does it work?

22. Is acetaminophen (e.g., Tylenol, the major OTC nonaspirin product for headache, fever, and pain) an absolutely safer alternative to aspirin for warfarin-treated patients? Why or why not?

CASE STUDY

A patient presents in the ED after a known and potentially lethal overdose of aspirin. You know that blood acid-base and electrolytes imbalances are important indicators of the severity and stage of aspirin poisoning.

1. Initial blood tests in the patient reveal a very alkaline blood pH. What causes it? Should we administer, intravenously, an "acidifying salt" such as ammonium chloride?

2. The early stages of aspirin poisoning are characterized by ventilatory stimulation, and your patient is clearly hyperventilating. Should you administer a respiratory depressant drug (e.g., morphine) to combat it and normalize ventilatory rate and depth?

3. Another measurement of blood pH (and oxygen, CO_2, and electrolytes) is taken an hour or so later. The results indicate that the patient's blood pH is now normal. Is that a good sign, and why? Should you be worried? If so, about what?

4. What changes should you expect next, assuming the overdose was, indeed, potentially lethal? What interventions would you anticipate being needed to treat the patient? Why, how, might they be effective in saving the patient?

5. Since your patient is now experiencing ventilatory depression, should you administer a respiratory stimulant at this time?

6. Your severely poisoned patient has a profound fever. Should you manage this with an antipyretic drug (e.g., acetaminophen), being quite aggressive with the dosing of the fever-lowering agent while you're at it?

7. Why is IV administration of sodium bicarbonate an important element in treating the later stages of severe (or life-threatening) salicylate poisoning?

8. We've been focusing on blood gas and pH (acid-base) changes. What other aspects of aspirin poisoning do we need to expect, assess for, and be prepared to manage? Why?

Through considerable skill and effort of the health-care team, and a bit of luck, it's clear the patient will survive. Moments later another OD patient is brought into the ED. It's a massive acetaminophen overdose that, according to the patient's mother, occurred "sometime yesterday." She goes on to say, "He was pretty sick after he took all those pills. But he started feeling better so I waited. Now he's real sick again."

9. A colleague who was working on the aspirin overdose patient proclaims, "That aspirin poisoning was tough. This acetaminophen poisoning should be easy to manage. After all, there's an antidote for acetaminophen poisoning."

   What are your feelings about your colleague's enthusiasm and optimism? Why? What *is* that antidote, by the way?

---

evolve To check your answers, go to http://evolve.elsevier.com/Lehne/ for Study Guide Comments from the author.

Glucocorticoids in Nonendocrine Diseases

KEY TERMS

allograft
intra-articular (mode of
    injection)
pharmacologic dose (as
    of glucocorticoid)

supraphysiologic (dose
    or effect)
systemic lupus
    erythematosus

OBJECTIVES

After reading and studying this chapter you should
be able to:

1. Review the feedback loop (and its components)
that regulates physiologic glucocorticoid secretion.
2. Describe the general mechanism by which glucocorticoids cause their biologic effects. Compare
the cellular site of glucocorticoid receptors with
those of typical agonists such as epinephrine and
acetylcholine.
3. State and describe the main therapeutic uses of
glucocorticoids for nonendocrine disorders.
4. State in terms of mechanisms and targets of
action why glucocorticoids exert greater anti-
inflammatory activity than nonsteroidal anti-
inflammatory drugs (NSAIDs; see Chapter. 67)
such as aspirin or the more efficacious by-pre-
scription-only NSAIDs.
5. State and describe the potential adverse effects of
administering pharmacologic doses of glucocorticoids on the following:
    Regulation of endogenous glucocorticoid
      synthesis
    Blood glucose regulation and levels
    Blood fluid and electrolyte balance (with
      special regard to Na and K)
    Bone integrity (density and strength) and
      metabolism
    Skeletal muscle integrity
    Gastric and duodenal defensive mechanisms
      (against ulcerogenesis)

    Growth (when glucocorticoids are adminis-
      tered to children)
    Endogenous defenses against infection
    Eye function (vision and intraocular pressure)
    (This should be old information to you since it is
    presented thoroughly in Chapter 57.)
6. Describe issues related to the timing of glucocorticoid administration, particularly as they relate to
maximizing therapeutic responses and minimizing adverse responses during corticosteroid
administration and discontinuation.
7. Describe the potential risks to, and relative glucocorticoid requirements of, patients who are under
stress (e.g., physical) during discontinuation of
pharmacologic doses of systemic glucocorticoids.
8. Discuss issues and concerns related to administering pharmacologic doses of glucocorticoids to
women who are pregnant or are breast-feeding
their infants.

CRITICAL THINKING AND STUDY QUESTIONS

1. Virtually all the drugs you've learned about so far
that act as agonists have receptors on cell membranes. Do glucocorticoids differ? How? Trace
the steps from glucocorticoid interaction with its
receptors to their final effects on regulatory proteins.

2. What are the potential "added" risks of using
pharmacologic doses of systemic glucocorticoids
for a patient with symptoms of heart failure who
is receiving digoxin? Are the risks different, or
changed, if the patient were also taking a diuretic
to manage edema? Does it make a difference
which diuretic is used?

affected joint(s) (intra-articular injections). The assumptions here are that the drug is placed directly where it is needed most and systemic side effects are reduced. Are these assumptions correct? Do you have any concerns about this administration route and the frequency with which it may be used in a given patient?

3. You are debating the actions and uses of corticosteroids for nonendocrine disorders with a couple of classmates. One says he's under the impression that since these drugs are being given for disorders that don't involve "deficiencies" in the body's endocrine system (e.g., adrenal cortical insufficiency), they won't cause endocrine effects. Comment on this.

4. Classmate 2 states emphatically that in order for corticosteroids to cause their desired effects, no matter what the nonendocrine use or indication is, they must be absorbed. What are your thoughts? Give some examples.

5. A patient who is taking oral prednisone (you pick the indication for which it is used; it doesn't really matter) gets depressed and takes 15 days' worth of medication all at once. No other drugs have been ingested. What one drug can we administer to antagonize the effects of this steroid overdose—to manage the signs and symptoms of acute overdose by blocking the effects of the drug?

6. How might systemic corticosteroid therapy reduce a patient's responses to some vaccines yet increase the risk of infection as a result of other vaccines?

7. Some patients with recurrent arthritis receive frequent injections of a glucocorticoid into the

CASE STUDY

Lynn How is a 35-year-old woman who was diagnosed with systemic lupus erythematosus (SLE) 2 years ago. She has been in remission for more than 6 months. Lupus is a connective tissue disease that progressively gets worse. It appears to be an autoimmune process in which antibodies are produced and then react with the person's own tissues. Fever and arthritis-like symptoms tend to appear early on. But eventually there's damage to such organs as the heart, liver, and kidneys.

Ms. How comes in today because of a fever. She also complains of generalized weakness and fatigue. Overall she's very concerned that her lupus is worsening.

1. A nursing intervention for patients diagnosed with SLE is to enhance drug therapy. What type of environmental conditions and activities can trigger exacerbations and what realistic interventions can the nurse suggest?

2. A usual drug treatment is systemic glucocorticoids. What do these do?

3. Ms. How asks what the advantages of glucocorticoids are if they don't cure the condition.

4. What diet should Ms. How follow while on chronic glucocorticoid therapy?

7. What assessments need to be made when Ms. How comes in for her healthcare visit?

5. What adverse effects can occur with the glucocorticoid therapy?

8. Ms. How states she is planning to get pregnant. What counseling might she require?

6. What are the nursing interventions for each adverse effect?

evolve To check your answers, go to http://evolve.elsevier.com/Lehne/ for Study Guide Comments from the author.

Drug Therapy of Rheumatoid Arthritis and Gout

KEY TERMS

cyclooxygenase
DMARD
gout (and gouty arthritis)
hyperuricemia
nitritoid crisis
osteoarthritis
ototoxicity
podagra
purine degradation
    (metabolism) pathway
rheumatoid arthritis
tophaceous gout
uricosuric (drug or
    effect)
xanthine oxidase

OBJECTIVES

After reading and studying this chapter you should be able to:

1. Compare and contrast the etiologies, contributing pathophysiology, clinical presentation (signs and symptoms), and long-term complications of osteoarthritis, rheumatoid arthritis, and gouty arthritis. Based on these, compare and contrast the usual therapeutic approaches and goals or objectives for each.
2. Discuss the classes of drugs used in the treatment of osteoarthritis, rheumatoid arthritis, and chronic gouty arthritis. State why drug therapy may differ for each, even though all three disorders are called "arthritic" and all the drugs can be called "antiarthritic."
3. Discuss the usual treatment sequence for rheumatoid arthritis, starting with OTC drugs and working on up to prescription NSAIDs and then DMARDs.
4. Summarize the main adverse effects of the drugs used for arthritis therapy. Compare the "special" or extra monitoring that is required when a DMARD is used. Select several DMARDs (your choice) so you can identify their unique toxicities.
5. Give an overview of the metabolic pathway by which uric acid is formed, starting with the main original source, ATP; name the enzyme involved in the conversion of hypoxanthine to xanthine, and xanthine to uric acid; and compare and contrast the solubility of hypoxanthine, xanthine, and uric acid in body fluids (e.g., urine, synovial fluid).
6. Summarize the mechanisms of action of allopurinol, probenecid, and colchicine in the context of hyperuricemia, gout, and gouty arthritis. State where each "fits" in a treatment plan for asymptomatic hyperuricemia, treatment of acute gout, and prophylaxis of recurrent attacks; and when each should not be used (and why).
7. Describe the dose-dependent effects of aspirin on renal handling of uric acid, and discuss the roles of this "most commonly used" NSAID in the therapy of asymptomatic hyperuricemia and gout.

Be sure you review content from other chapters, particularly Chapters 67 (*Cyclooxygenase Inhibitors*) and 68 (*Glucocorticoids in Nonendocrine Diseases*), and integrate it with the material presented in this chapter.

CRITICAL THINKING AND STUDY QUESTIONS

1. Aspirin is an effective drug for many patients with rheumatoid arthritis. However, it is relatively uncommon for a physician to prescribe therapeutic (antiarthritic) doses of this medication as initial therapy for many patients diagnosed with this disorder; a prescription drug is ordered instead. Why might this be?

2. Is aspirin suitable for all the main types of arthritis: rheumatoid arthritis, osteoarthritis, and gouty arthritis? If not, why not?

199

3. How do NSAIDS differ from such drugs as methotrexate, gold salts, and penicillamine in terms of their effects on the signs and symptoms and clinical course of the underlying pathophysiology of rheumatoid arthritis?

If the patient is receiving methotrexate, what would you advise about using aspirin to manage headache, fever, or other conditions for which aspirin would be appropriate?

4. What information or evidence, even if it is indirect, supports the notion that for some patients, rheumatoid arthritis is due to an autoimmune disorder?

8. Not all that long ago, DMARDs were considered second-line drugs, or even drugs of last resort, for managing rheumatoid arthritis. Why might that be, and what accounts for the "paradigm shift" such that these agents are being prescribed much earlier in the treatment plan?

5. A student friend says that acetaminophen is an NSAID. Do you agree? Is this drug suitable for managing arthritic disorders, even as an adjunct? Would it be acceptable to use acetaminophen for mild headache or fever that develops during therapy of arthritis? Does it depend on which type of arthritis the patient has?

9. A colleague is arguing with you over therapy for a patient with severe hyperuricemia and poor kidney function. She says that probenecid would be a preferred drug for this individual. After all, it lowers serum uric acid and does so by helping the kidneys get rid of it. Is she right or wrong, and why?

6. What is the main claimed advantage of COX-2 inhibitors over traditional NSAIDs when used for arthritis? Do current data definitively support this claim? What are some recent concerns about risks associated with long-term COX-2 inhibitor use?

10. Using only your powers of observation and information from an adult patient's medical history, can you make a diagnosis of acute gout and be reasonably certain that you are not dealing with rheumatoid arthritis or osteoarthritis instead? Formulate your reply in the form of questions, and for each give an explanation of why you posed that question.

7. A patient is diagnosed with moderate to severe rheumatoid arthritis. The plan is to begin therapy with methotrexate (MTX) at a usual starting oral dose, 10 mg once weekly. Are there any medications that should be part of this plan? Why? Why is it important to determine whether the patient has normal renal function? What pregnancy-related questions should be asked, and answered, before the drug is prescribed?

CASE STUDY

Sam Beatty, 62 years old, is a carpenter. He has been treated for heart failure for the last 5 years. Therapy includes digoxin, furosemide, and sprinolactone (assume each is being given at an effective and otherwise proper dose). He's also taking a "statin" for elevated cholesterol levels. At the last appointment

Mr. Beatty's heart failure signs and symptoms were wholly acceptable to the MD; lipid levels were "right where they should be." The doctor noted, however, that Mr. Beatty's serum uric acid level was at the high end of the normal range. His blood glucose levels were "a bit high" too," but not to the point that a diagnosis of diabetes mellitus would be made, nor would any treatment other than diet and exercise be started for it.

Mr. Beatty feels he's "doing so well" that he visits his physician only once a year for a checkup, and apparently the MD can't convince Mr. Beatty to come in for an evaluation more often than that.

About a month after his last doctor's visit, Mr. Beatty develops some mild aches and pains in the joints of his fingers and hands and concludes that he has "a touch of arthritis." After all, on the previous doctor's visit the MD suggested that indeed he might be developing rheumatoid arthritis. Mr. Beatty begins to self-medicate with aspirin, taking two regular-strength tablets (325 mg each) morning and night.

After 2 weeks on aspirin Mr. Beatty goes to a party with his buddies. It's a hot Saturday; plenty of hot dogs and beer; and he participates in a rather long-lasting softball game.

First thing Monday morning Mr. Beatty hobbles into the emergency department of his local hospital. He's in such excruciating pain that he didn't even want to try to get an appointment with his personal physician. One of his big toes is red and swollen, and it "hurts just to look at it." He couldn't even put a shoe on his "bad foot." Based on a visual assessment, no other joints seem to be affected, nor does Mr. Beatty complain of any discomfort in them.

1. What's the likely diagnosis? What elements of Mr. Beatty's clinical presentation might lead you to this conclusion?

2. What aspects of Mr. Beatty's history over the long run, and medications he has been taking, would be consistent with this?

3. What recent events might have occurred and triggered Mr. Beatty's signs and symptoms? How would they contribute?

4. When a "mild" gout attack occurs various processes are triggered, and more often than not they "amplify" the underlying pathophysiology such that a "major attack" soon develops. Explain the pathophysiology that accounts for this. (Start by assuming that "just a little" uric acid has crystallized in a joint of a hyperuricemic patient.) What property of uric acid accounts for this and explains why an acute gout attack differs from an acute attack of rheumatoid arthritis or osteoarthritis?

The ER physician suspects gout and now will attempt to confirm the diagnosis.

5. What will a blood test to measure serum uric acid levels (very easy to do), taken during the height of the attack, be likely to show? How important is that blood test for confirming the diagnosis of gout?

6. What information is necessary to "prove" this is a gout attack? How, drug-wise, will you prepare the patient for gathering this proof?

The diagnosis of gout has been confirmed. There are three main classes of antigout drugs: anti-inflammatory agents such as colchicine (or some other approved NSAIDs), allopurinol, and probenecid. Explain which should be administered right away, and why (or why not)?

7. Which should be administered right away for fastest symptom relief? (Note that currently Mr. Beatty is taking no antigout medication.) Which should *not*?

ure. However, one of those medications may have contributed to the hyperuricemia. Which one? What other medication may be added to control the hyperuricemia? How does it work? When should it be started?

8. The physician decides to start therapy with oral indomethacin rather than colchicine (which is often considered the prototype anti-inflammatory drug for gout. Why? How do colchicine and indomethacin differ in terms of mechanisms of action, and does that explain the reason for using the indomethacin instead of the colchicine?

10. You've realized that Mr. Beatty's aspirin consumption may have helped raise his serum urate levels. Should Mr. Beatty develop a headache or mild discomfort from the flu, what OTC headache and fever-relieving medication would you recommend? Would buffered aspirin or enteric-coated aspirin, instead of the plain aspirin tablets he used before, be a reasonable choice?

9. Mr. Beatty's physician feels it is necessary to continue the current drug therapy for heart fail-

evolve To check your answers, go to http://evolve.elsevier.com/Lehne/ for Study Guide Comments from the author.

Drugs Affecting Calcium Levels and Bone Mineralization

KEY TERMS

bisphosphonate
calcitonin
calcitriol
hydroxyapatite
osteoblast
osteoclast
osteoid
osteomalacia
osteoporosis
Paget's disease (of bone)

parathormone
    (parathyroid hormone)
resorption (as of calcium
    from bone)
rickets
selective estrogen
    receptor modulator

OBJECTIVES

After reading and studying this chapter you should be able to:

1. Briefly describe the roles of parathyroid hormone and vitamin D as they affect absorption of dietary calcium and bone mineral metabolism.
2. Briefly describe the roles of osteoblasts and osteoclasts in bone formation and resorption.
3. Compare and contrast the benefits, limitations, and risks of estrogen replacement therapy with those of raloxifene in terms of their effects on (a) bone metabolism and integrity, (b) risks of breast and endometrial cancer, (c) menstrual bleeding; (d) other signs and symptoms of menopause, (e) the incidence of thromboembolism, and (f) fetal development if the patient receiving the drug is or might be pregnant.
4. Describe the typical etiologies and characteristic signs, symptoms, and lab abnormalities that are associated with hypocalcemia and with hypercalcemia.
5. Describe drug therapies and non-drug interventions that are indicated for osteoporosis. Be sure to distinguish between prophylaxis and treatment of the disease once it's been diagnosed.

CRITICAL THINKING AND STUDY QUESTIONS

1. What are the two main thyroid and parathyroid hormones that are important in systemic calcium regulation? Are their effects similar or different? How?

2. Aside from demonstration of low serum calcium levels in a blood sample, what are the typical signs and symptoms of hypocalcemia?

3. What is the primary metabolic deficiency in rickets? Why might inadequate exposure to sunlight be a cause? Why is it correct to say that the biochemical processes that are triggered in rickets do one "good" thing with respect to body calcium, but they do it at the expense of another process that contributes to signs and symptoms of rickets?

4. Does the pathophysiology (or underlying biochemical problems) in osteomalacia differ from that of rickets?

5. When vitamin D mobilizes calcium from bone and increases serum calcium levels, it also mobilizes and raises serum levels of what?

6. Give a simple explanation of why osteoporosis is more prevalent in and associated with menopause and the years beyond.

7. A rather callous and uninformed person comments on osteoporosis saying, "So, you break an arm... put on a cast; break a leg, do the same thing. What's the big deal?" So, what is the "big deal"?

8. A postmenopausal woman is watching TV and sees an ad for a new state-of-the-art diagnostic facility that offers, among other things, bone mineral density scans (BMD). It's quick and painless, the person on TV says! She has some extra change, so she gets the scan done. The results of the BMD scan, she's told, indicate that she's at "very low risk" of developing osteoporosis. But are there other factors that go into estimating risk—ones that weren't mentioned above?

9. You have a patient with osteoporosis. A bisphosphonate has been prescribed. You've explained to your patient, in a way that she obviously understands, the basics of mineral metabolism (as it relates to bone health) and what the osteoblasts and osteoclasts are and do in terms of bone formation and bone dissolution (resorption).
    Now give her a simple explanation of how a bisphosphonate works to help the altered bone

status. It's her understanding that these new drugs help the body make new, stronger bones.

10. A patient with severe pain from bone cancer is started on etidronate. A colleague states that that drug, and the bisphosphonates in general, are effective analgesics. What are your comments on that? Why do we use that drug?

11. Your text often mentions Paget's disease of the bone. What is it? What is its main cause? Is it common?

12. How might a bisphosphonate cause hyperparathyroidism and possibly hypocalcemia? What might we do to reduce these risks? Consider bisphosphonate therapy of Paget's disease as the situation in which this is occurring.

13. A patient presents with severe, acute but non-life-threatening hypercalcemia. The MD chooses not to use EDTA (edetate disodium, a highly effective calcium chelator).

    A. Why might the physician want to avoid using EDTA?

B. The physician orders intermittent, slow infusions of furosemide (Lasix). A colleague says that that is done for two reasons: (1) the patient has, or is likely to develop soon, edema and heart failure and (2) the drug has EDTA-like calcium chelating activity, although of a milder and safer degree. Comment on this.

C. If we were to use furosemide, are there any other concerns you should anticipate and be prepared to deal with because of this particular drug?

D. Another colleague, somewhat familiar with the use of furosemide for managing hypercalcemia, recalls a situation in which there were some "very bad" effects of the drug on the patient's blood pressure and electrolytes. He suggests using a "milder" drug instead and cites chlorothiazide. That's the thiazide diuretic (prototype is hydrochlorothiazide; see Chapter 39) that is available in an injectable preparation. Do you agree that this would be a good idea? Why or why not?

14. Some will argue that calcitonin-salmon is a very "attractive" drug for managing osteoporosis. What is so attractive about it? How does the drug work? Are there limitations, for example when it seems to afford its benefits? (***Hint:*** Consider its possible use in both prophylaxis of osteoporosis and management of the clinical disease itself.)

15. Recently studies have provided data that will (are) causing a dramatic decline in the routine use of estrogen for replacement therapy after menopause. Simultaneously there is an increased use of raloxifene or other drugs for osteoporosis prevention or treatment as the use of estrogen declines. A colleague says that that is because the new data definitively show that estrogen does not significantly reduce the risk of bone fractures and does not significantly increase bone mineral density. Is this impression correct?

16. A patient who has recently entered menopause has been keeping up with the "latest medical news" in the papers and on TV. She's been taking estrogen for replacement therapy. She admits, "With all the conflicting advice out there I'm confused, but I do know I want to stop taking the hormone supplements." She wants to start on raloxifene instead. Tell her what she can, and cannot, expect from this switch. Explain which current or potential problems might be helped, or perhaps worsened, by switching therapies.

17. A friend who wants to "maintain strong, healthy bones" consumes Tums (or Rolaids, or any of the many other OTC calcium supplements that are being touted in commercials nowadays). He takes a lot of them, but you've calculated the daily and long-term intake and are satisfied that he isn't at risk of developing hypercalcemia. In fact, he had his serum electrolyte levels checked recently, and "all's well."

Sometime later this patient develops an infection for which antibiotics are indicated. Do you have any concerns about the use of calcium supplements in this setting? Any antibiotics in particular about which you have special concerns?

18. A somewhat savvy patient knows that OTC products like Tums and Rolaids are promoted as a *good source of calcium* (italics mine). She also knows that Tums and Rolaids can alleviate occasional heartburn or "acid indigestion." She, however, uses Maalox for her indigestion. (Pick any of many other OTC antacids... Mylanta, Gelusil, and others.) She asks whether that's a good source of calcium too. Your response?

CASE STUDY

Joan Smith, a 50-year-old woman who is going through menopause, had a total thyroidectomy earlier today. She has just come to you from the postanesthesia care unit (PACU).

1. The literature says to be sure calcium is available postoperatively for injection. Why?

2. You now recall that calcitonin comes from the thyroid gland. You remember something about its role in calcium metabolism. What is that role? How does the hormone work? Does removal of the thyroid, and hence the source of calcitonin, eliminate the need to "have calcium handy postoperatively"?

3. What signs and symptoms, over and above a blood test that shows low serum calcium levels, might prompt you to consider the need for intravenous calcium gluconate?

4. If you need to administer calcium intravenously, for what do you monitor?

5. If Mrs. Smith were taking digoxin for heart failure and that drug wasn't discontinued in the perioperative period, what effect(s) might you anticipate if she became hypocalcemic? If she became hypercalcemic from an overdose of IV calcium used in an attempt to manage acute, severe hypocalcemia?

6. Because Mrs. Smith is at high risk for osteoporosis (she is going through menopause and her mother has severe osteoporosis) and she is prone to hypocalcemia from her endocrine surgery, it is a good idea to develop a plan to help her prevent this problem as well as possible. What different aspects of the plan should you discuss with her (nondrug and drug therapy)?

7. What calcium-rich foods would you recommend, perhaps in addition to oral calcium supplements? What foods should be avoided, and why?

8. Mrs. Smith can't wait to get home. It's springtime and she and her older sister are going to cook up some rhubarb pies. Sounds good? Or does it? Any concerns about the rhubarb, or any other foods? Why?

9. You're laughing about the rhubarb pie as you chat with a technician on the venipuncture/phlebotomy team. She says, "Yeah, I know all about that." How might she know it?

10. Mrs. Smith's mother has severe osteoporosis and was treated last year for a fractured hip. Her mom developed thrombophlebitis during her hospital stay. She was placed on alendronate (Fosamax) 10 mg PO daily. What is the main risk from taking this drug?

11. Mrs. Smith is cautioned to remain standing or sitting for 30 minutes after taking the Fosamax. She says that instruction is really odd. She's never heard of such advice given for any other drug. Explain the reason to her.

12. And Mrs. Smith finds it odd that you emphasized taking the medication first thing in the morning, on an empty stomach, and before consuming any breakfast or even a glass of juice or coffee. Explain the rationale to her.

13. In talking with you about her potential for osteoporosis and noting that her mother (and sisters too) have it, she says, "How come it seems that only women get osteoporosis." How would you reply?

evolve To check your answers, go to http://evolve.elsevier.com/Lehne/ for Study Guide Comments from the author.

Drugs for Asthma

KEY TERMS

anhydrous theophylline
asthma
inspissation
leukotriene(s)
mast cells (and mast cell
 stabilizers)

metered-dose inhaler
 (MDI)
methylxanthine
mucolytic (drug or effect)
rescue therapy
theophylline *salt*

OBJECTIVES

After reading and studying this chapter you should
be able to:

1. State a reasonably accurate definition of asthma
   that includes your understanding of the roles and
   involvement of airway smooth muscle hyper-
   responsiveness and inflammation in the disease.
   Describe the typical signs and symptoms that
   would lead to the diagnosis of a respiratory disorder as asthma.
2. State the criteria used to classify asthma (e.g.,
   mild, moderate, etc.) based on symptom severity
   and frequency.
3. Summarize the mechanisms of action, roles, and
   limitations of the following drugs in the therapy
   of long-term and acute asthma:
   - Beta-adrenergic agonists (inhaled, oral, par-
     enteral and rapid-acting agents vs. long-act-
     ing agents such as salmeterol)
   - Corticosteroids (inhaled, oral, and parenteral)
   - Methylxanthines
   - Mast cell stabilizers such as cromolyn or
     nedocromil
   - Leukotriene synthesis inhibitors and
     leukotriene-receptor blockers
4. Explain what a theophylline *salt* is and how theophylline salts are similar to or different from one
   another and from anhydrous theophyllline.
5. State characteristics of inhaled sympathomimetic
   use for rescue therapy that might constitute overuse.
6. Identify and describe the drugs indicated for
   status asthmaticus, how they are used, and what
   they do.

7. Compile a list of drugs or drug groups that are
   relatively or absolutely contraindicated for
   patients with asthma, and state what their main
   problems are.
8. Discuss some nondrug interventions that might
   be used to decrease the frequency and severity of
   asthma attacks.

CRITICAL THINKING AND STUDY QUESTIONS

1. Why are therapies aimed only at dilating the
   bronchi, whether by activating adrenergic receptors or blocking muscarinic receptors, often
   doomed to failure over the long run?

2. For decades, until the last 5 to 10 years or so,
   hospitalizations and deaths from asthma (even in
   Western societies) have been skyrocketing. This
   is despite the fact that some of the best and most
   sophisticated drugs and healthcare services have
   been available during that time. Why is this?

3. How does salmeterol differ from albuterol (or
   terbulaline or metaproterenol) pharmacologically and pharmacokinetically? If a patient has a
   flare-up of asthma symptoms and has no rapidly
   acting sympathomimetic available for rescue,
   can salmeterol be used instead?

208

4. Since epinephrine is one of the most efficacious bronchodilators available, why is it seldom prescribed for asthma? What properties of inhaled epinephrine seem to account for its popularity as an OTC asthma remedy?

A. Beta-adrenergic agonists (inhaled, oral and rapidly acting agents vs. long-acting agents such as salmeterol)

B. Corticosteroids (inhaled, oral, and parenteral)

5. An asthma patient who has been on oral prednisone for 4 months now has good symptom control. We decide to stop the prednisone and start the patient on an orally inhaled steroid. How should the switch be made? Why, or doesn't it matter?

C. Methylxanthines

6. In relative terms, compliance with instructions to use inhaled sympathomimetics is "good." In contrast, it is difficult to achieve compliance with inhaled steroids, especially when they are started. Why might this be?

D. Cast cell stabilizers such as cromolyn or nedocromil

7. Two healthcare providers are arguing over the use of oral drugs with atropine-like activity for ambulatory patients with asthma. One says these drugs are good: "After all, we're blocking the bronchoconstrictor effects of acetylcholine." The other says they're bad. Who is right, and why?

E. Leukotriene synthesis inhibitors and leukotriene-receptor blockers

9. An asthma patient who has been overusing a sympathomimetic inhaler presents in the emergency department with status asthmaticus and profound respiratory distress. The physician orders an IV injection of isoproterenol at the "usually effective" dose. What would you expect, and why? What dangers should you be aware of? What is the proper therapy for this patient?

8. On which of the following self-administered meds can an asthma patient rely most for prompt relief of asthma symptom flare-ups? Why? Assume no drug tolerance has developed.

10. Atropine, administered with a nebulizer, is becoming a routine adjunctive intervention for hospital management of acute asthma. Given the concerns of using antimuscarinic drugs in ambulatory patients with asthma (see comment 6), why would this very class of drugs be safe during life-threatening asthma attacks?

11. A patient with status asthmaticus presents in the emergency department. He is hyperventilating and anxious. The new intern orders IV diazepam to "calm the patient down and slow the ventilatory rate" while waiting for the proper meds, and the respiratory therapy team, to arrive. Comment on this order.

12. A mother brings her 12-year-old to the physician's office. She reports that for the last 6 months the child has had a hacking cough that may last just a day or for several days in a row, then it disappears for days or weeks, and then it returns. She has not heard any wheezing nor seen any breathing difficulty. Auscultation of the child's chest in the exam reveals no abnormal ventilatory sounds. What might this be?

13. State why and how the following drugs can cause harm to asthma patients, and state the types of medications in which they are commonly found (i.e., their main clinical uses).

A. Cholinergic (muscarinic agonists)

B. Acetylcholinesterase inhibitors

C. Aspirin and many other nonsteroidal anti-inflammatory drugs

D. Beta-adrenergic blockers

E. Tubocurarine

F. Antipsychotic drugs (typical ones, e.g., phenothiazines)

G. Diuretics

CASE STUDY

Karen Gold is an 18-year-old college freshman who was diagnosed with asthma when she was 10 years old. Since that time her primary therapy has been theophylline.

1. What are the goals for drug therapy in the treatment of asthma? Which pathophysiologic process is the crux of all the signs and symptoms?

2. How is theophylline classified? What are its main expected effects in asthma and what are the common side effects, adverse responses, and other therapeutic problems associated with the drug? Is oral theophylline suitable for rescue therapy?

3. If a patient were receiving a methylxanthine for asthma, would it be appropriate to substitute the various brand-name products (salts) for one another or for anhydrous theophylline on a milligram-for-milligram basis? Why or why not?

Karen's mother states that when Karen was 10, the doctor wanted to start her on oral prednisone. The mother refused the therapy, stating that it would stunt her daughter's growth.

4. Comment on the pros and cons of using oral steroids for a young child with asthma and on Mrs. Gold's likely concern for her daughter.

Karen has been hospitalized for acute asthma 3 times in the last 7 years. All the hospitalizations have come during the winter months. On the last admission she had to be intubated and was in the hospital for a week.

5. What does this history tell you about Ms. Gold's prognosis?

6. How would you counsel Ms. Gold about her use of cola and coffee?

7. What is the likely ingredient in the OTC remedy that Ms. Gold takes to relieve her asthma and keep her awake? How is it classified? How well does it work for asthma? What other properties of this medication should you be concerned about?

8. What are the main ingredients in the OTC oral and inhaled meds for asthma? Why are they not used by physicians to treat asthma?

9. Give your personal thoughts about the availability and use of OTC asthma remedies, whether oral meds or inhalers.

Ms. Gold realizes that while her prescription and OTC meds help her stay awake to study, she can't fall asleep. So she often takes an OTC sleep aid; her favorites are Nytol and Unisom.

10. What are the active ingredients in Nytol and Unisom? What are the potential benefits and risks for a patient with asthma? (Focus on the airways, not on the CNS-depressant effects.)

Karen studies for long periods at a time. Her snacks usually consist of cola or coffee. She found an OTC medicine that is advertised as "good" for asthma, and it also keeps her awake, which is helpful when she wants to study.

Karen likes to jog in the spring and winter, but has "some" breathing problems when she runs. She also likes to swim laps at local indoor pools and seems to have few problems doing that unless they've just added chlorine to the pool.

11. What might contribute to the variability in symptoms during these different types of exercise?

14. What would you consider to be a complete and effective medication plan for Ms. Gold, assuming that her current therapy is inadequate and not safe?

Once Karen became old enough to use an MDI properly, she was prescribed an albuterol MDI with instructions to use it as needed. All the pertinent information was discussed with Karen and her mother.

12. How is albuterol classified? What are its expected effects in asthma? What are the common side effects or adverse responses associated with the drug? Are there any potential benefits or problems associated with using it with theophylline? If so, what are they?

15. Karen's mom comes back to you, quite angry at the poor healthcare she thinks her daughter has been getting. She's heard that if her daughter has an acute and severe flare-up of asthma, all she needs to do is take a prednisone pill. She looked on the Internet and found that the onset of action of oral prednisone is "almost instantaneous" and the drug's peak effects occur in about 1 to 2 hours. She's also discussed this with another doctor who not only confirmed that information but also said, "Come see me if your daughter seems to be getting a cold. I'll prescribe an antibiotic." Karen's mom says, "You are perpetuating bad information and it's killing thousands of asthma patients." Your thoughts?

Karen states that for the past 6 months or so she has been having to take 4 or 5 puffs from her inhaler at least 5 times a day, and 1 or 2 puffs every other night or so just so she could breathe without too much difficulty.

13. What are your interpretations of this information? What fundamental problem does it reflect?

evolve To check your answers, go to http://evolve.elsevier.com/Lehne/ for Study Guide Comments from the author.

Drugs for Allergic Rhinitis, Cough, and Colds

KEY TERMS

antihistamine
antitussive (drug or effect)
conjunctivitis
expectorant (drug or effect)
hay fever
mucolytic (drug or effect)

quaternary (referring to chemical structure of drug)
rebound (nasal) congestion
rhinitis, seasonal and perennial
sympathomimetic

OBJECTIVES

After reading and studying this chapter you should be able to:

1. Review the basic pharmacology of sympathomimetics that are used for nasal decongestion and rhinitis signs and symptoms; H_1/histamine blockers (antihistamines), and corticosteroids. Apply that knowledge to the content of this chapter.
2. Summarize the roles of antihistamines, glucocorticoids, and sympathomimetic decongestants in terms of managing the signs, symptoms, and underlying causes of the common cold.
3. State the role of antibiotics in managing allergic rhinitis and the common cold.

Note: Be sure to refresh your memory about the actions, properties, and uses of drugs noted in objective 1.

CRITICAL THINKING AND STUDY QUESTIONS

1. There's good evidence that intranasal steroids relieve symptoms of allergic rhinitis better, over the long run, than oral or topical sympathomimetics or oral antihistamines. They also probably cause fewer side effects, which may be important for some patients. Why, then, does there seem to be greater use of the sympathomimetics and antihistamines by the lay public?

2. A patient with a seasonal allergy is given a prescription for an intranasal steroid. She experiences no side effects, but after a couple of days she stops taking the medication anyway. What's the most likely reason?

3. In very general terms, compare and contrast the onsets, durations, and intensities of action of sympathomimetic nasal decongestants administered intranasally (e.g., as nasal sprays) vs. those taken orally.

4. The text notes that rebound nasal congestion can be a problem with intranasal sympathomimetics. This can lead to dependence on and the need for progressively increasing dosages of the medication, and for quite a long time. If these drugs are to be used, what are two ways to minimize the risks of this (other than not using these products at all)?

213

5. The text notes that some intranasal sympatho-mimetics are linked to rebound nasal congestion. It states that "with oral administration, responses are delayed, moderate, and prolonged."

   One implication of this is that systemic administration of sympathomimetics are associated less with the rebound phenomenon. Do you agree with that notion?

   Another implication is that oral sympatho-mimetics are, therefore, preferred to intranasal preparations. Comment on that, too.

6. You're watching prime-time TV. The inevitable commercials include ones about drugs for your bladder or your bowels, but sooner or later there's an ad for an oral cold or allergy remedy "you just gotta take." The ad says, "This stuff won't keep you up all night." What does this really mean, and what's the most likely "won't keep you up all night" ingredient?

   The next ad touts a product that won't make you drowsy. Again, what does this probably mean, and what's the most likely ingredient in this product?

7. I have hypertension. It's amply documented in my medical history. I also have rather bothersome symptoms of a seasonal allergy. My nasal passages are really congested. I can't stand the stuffiness. I come to you and say, "I'd like to take one of those decongestant pills or nasal sprays (a sympathomimetic). What do you think?" Well, what do you think? Is there one answer that fits all hypertensive patients who ask you this question? Wear two hats when you answer this question: the nursing professional dealing with a patient and a son or daughter of someone asking for your advice.

8. You're on a shopping trip with a classmate. Both of you have a cold, and decide that an OTC anti-histamine is what you want (whether that's a correct choice is debatable). You say you both should buy one of the older, cheaper first-generation antihistamines. Your classmate admonishes you, saying that loradatine (Claritin) is now on the OTC market. "It's new, it's better for a cold," she says. How would you respond (other than by saying "Get whatever turns you on")?

9. Now that you've clarified things with your classmate, he says that you have to buy one of the nationally known brand name products—not one of those "cheap knockoffs" that the store sells under its own label. You pick up a package of the brand-name product and one of the store's alternatives. What are you likely to find, what are you likely to do (if you're smart)?

10. The text notes five different ingredients (drug classes or drugs), several or more of which you'll frequently find in combination cold remedies. What are they? What other drug is also found in some these products? (*Hint:* focus on liquid preparations.)

11. Now that you have a good understanding of the drugs discussed in this chapter, especially the multi-ingredient products for the signs and symptoms of a cold, how confident do you feel that you can go to the local pharmacy or grocery store and purchase what's "precisely right" for your symptoms or for your child who has these symptoms?

Drugs for Peptic Ulcer Disease

KEY TERMS

acid-neutralizing capacity
acute stress ulcer
adsorb (adsorption)
antacid (drug or effect)
gastroesophageal reflux
  disease (GERD)
Helicobacter pylori

parietal cell(s)
pepsins
proton pump (and
  inhibitors; PPIs)
systemic antacid
Zollinger-Ellison
  syndrome

OBJECTIVES

After reading and studying this chapter you should be able to:

1. State what peptic ulcer disease is and do so in terms of a "battle" between protective and destructive factors focused on the GI mucosa. In your summary you should state the contributions of histamine, gastrin, and acetylcholine to overall gastric acid secretion; explain why gastric acid is a necessary but not sufficient (by itself) cause of peptic ulcers and how (and how well) they are targets of drug therapy; and debunk the notion that common gastric and duodenal ulcers are invariably caused by excess gastric acid secretion.

2. In the context of the above, summarize the benefits and limitations of drug therapy targeted at those mediators; their abilities to achieve those goals, and how well and how quickly they do so; and identify which drugs or drug groups truly alter the underlying disease process(es), rather than creating a local environment that is conducive to "natural" ulcer healing.

3. Discuss short-term and long-term goals of therapy for acid peptic disease, and identify one or more drugs or drug groups that can meet those goals quicker or better than others can.

4. State conditions for which a trial of OTC drug therapy might be indicated for either PUD or GERD. Recommend a treatment plan that involves OTC drugs. Related to this, highlight the limitations and potential dangers of self-medication with OTCs, and state findings that would lead you to direct a patient to see a physician.

5. Identify the four main chemicals in single-ingredient antacid products and the major benefits or limitations associated with them. State the ingredients typically found in proprietary antacid combination products and the rationale for using them as opposed to single-ingredient products. Include in your discussion the main expected effects of single-ingredient antacids on gut motility. State why even OTC antacids may pose a risk of interactions with certain other oral drugs, and describe the mechanisms by which they might do that.

6. State when and how OTC drugs for acid peptic disorders can play an important, if not helpful, role in managing these conditions. Conversely, state why the availability of OTCs for these potentially serious conditions may pose a risk for some patients.

7. Compare and contrast the H_2 blockers in terms of efficacy, side effects, and drug-drug interactions. Be able to argue for, or against, the selection of a particular H_2 blocker over another.

8. State the role of antihistamines such as diphenhydramine in the management of PUD.

9. Prepare a short list of drugs or drug groups (classes) that are ulcerogenic.

Note: As needed, be sure to integrate content of this chapter with pertinent information in other chapters about histamine antagonists (see Chapter 66), amoxicillin (see Chapter 80), clarithromycin and tetracyclines (see Chapter 82), and metronidazole (see Chapter 87).

CRITICAL THINKING AND STUDY QUESTIONS

1. Explain why reducing gastric acidity slightly (say, from a normal of 1.2 to about 3), whether by using antacids that neutralize acid or any of the various drugs that inhibit gastric acid secretion, can do more harm than good.

215

2. Discuss the cost/benefit issues surrounding the use of eradicative therapy of ulcers aimed at killing *H. pylori* vs. the use of other regimens that don't use antibiotics. Assume the hypothetical patient you are discussing has *H. pylori* infestation. Be sure that your discussion of cost includes not only financial cost but also costs in terms of the patient's long-term well-being.

3. Compare and contrast cimetidine with the alternative H_2 blockers. State one reason that prescribing cimetidine would be preferred instead of any of the others.

4. Drug companies have developed a drug, pirenzepine, that rather selectively blocks the muscarinic receptors that mediate gastric acid secretion that is triggered by acetylcholine. Given the other drugs we have available nowadays for inhibiting gastric acid secretion, would you think this atropine-like drug has a bright future in terms of clinical utility?

5. What is the relationship between gastrin production and gastric acid production? What does gastrin do to the gastric mucosa and the parietal cells of the stomach? Think of this in terms of "complete" gastric acid suppression caused by such drugs as esomeprazole and omeprazole (the PPIs).

6. Why is sucralfate an "easy" drug to take? If the patient taking it were to consume antacids in an attempt to quell gastric pain quickly, would that help or hinder sucralfate's action, and how? What other aspect of sucralfate action needs to be considered when the patient is taking other oral meds?

7. What is the sole FDA-approved use for misoprostol? How does its mechanism of action relate to its main clinical use and to the main contraindication for its use?

8. Why is quick relief of ulcer or esophagitis pain and discomfort a potentially great hindrance to compliance with long-term therapy?

9. A patient presents at the physician's office with signs and symptoms consistent with peptic ulcer disease. The patient reports being very stressed at work for the last 6 months, during which time the abdominal discomfort developed and worsened. The physician prescribes alprazolam, a benzodiazepine (see Chapter 34) often recommended for anxiety disorders, and recommends that the patient take a combination antacid product (the usual magnesium-aluminum formulation available OTC) as needed. Your comments?

10. Your text describes systemic antacids as those drugs that can alter blood pH. Which antacid(s) meet that criterion? Use a more liberal definition of the term *systemic* to include agents that contain an ion that can be absorbed into the bloodstream, regardless of whether they affect blood pH. Which antacids now would be considered systemic? What are the major contraindications or precautions related to their use because of their systemic effects?

11. You remember from chemistry class that calcium carbonate is insoluble in water, and your prof demonstrates this by sticking a piece of chalk in a glass of water. How then can calcium carbonate (e.g., taken as an antacid) cause hypercalcemia? Not all that long ago, OTC antacids that contained only calcium carbonate were advertised for relief of heartburn. Now they are more extensively advertised for something else. What is that, and how can that be used as proof that calcium carbonate is, indeed, absorbed?

CASE STUDY

Mike Harmon is a 62-year-old man who just moved "back home" after his wife died. He comes to the physician's office with a chief complaint of a 6-month history of searing abdominal pain that "comes and goes." And he says he has heartburn that's especially bad when he goes to bed too soon after eating, which he seems to do often.

His history reveals that he is a pack-a-day smoker, and the doctor in the town from which he moved had him taking pills for what was described to him as emphysema (chronic obstructive pulmonary disease). You check and learn that the medication was theophylline.

Mr. Harmon takes extra-strength aspirin about 3 times a week for joint pain. He states he is a moderate drinker. He self-medicates daily with Tagamet HB, an OTC formulation of cimetidine.

1. Given the history, what are reasonable diagnoses?

2. What factors in Mr. Harmon's life-style probably contributed to his symptoms and the underlying disorders?

3. How is cimetidine classified, and what is its main expected action for this patient? Assuming an OTC drug of its class were indicated for Mr. Harmon, which would be most (or least) preferable? Why?

4. If Mr. Harmon had occasional allergy symptoms (including wheezing) too, would the cimetidine be of benefit for that also?

The physician passes an endoscope and sees multiple gastric ulcers and mild erosion of the lower esophagus. A dual diagnosis of PUD and GERD is made. Breath, stool, or blood tests for H. pylori are not done. She prescribes an 8-week trial of esomeprazole at the usual recommended dose.

5. Explain how the action of omeprazole (Prilosec) differs from H_2-receptor antagonists. Is it more or less efficacious, and why?

6. Mr. Harmon is concerned about taking his medication because a friend of his developed enlarged breast tissue while taking his ulcer pill. What might account for this?

7. Mr. Harmon asks why he is not on a special diet. He has heard that ulcer patients should eat bland foods and drink a lot of milk. How would you respond?

8. Mr. Harmon says he read that certain bacteria can cause ulcers. How would you explain this to him? What is the current drug treatment for bacteria-causing ulcers?

9. If Mr. Harmon continues to have ulcer and GERD discomfort (although with decreasing frequency and severity), what would you recommend as capable of relieving the discomfort the fastest? Be specific in terms of the ingredient(s) in that medication.

10. If Mr. Harmon had poor renal function, which common antacid ingredient might be particularly problematic for him? What if he had hypertension or edema from heart failure?

11. If Mr. Harmon had HTN or edema from heart failure, would it be acceptable to recommend any antacid combination product, so long as it was one of the usual magnesium-aluminum mixtures?

evolve To check your answers, go to http://evolve.elsevier.com/Lehne/ for Study Guide Comments from the author.

Laxatives

KEY TERMS

bulk-forming (type of
   laxative)
cathartic (drug or effect)
constipation

laxative (drug or effect)
surfactant (type of
   laxative)

OBJECTIVES

After reading and studying this chapter you should be able to:

1. State the relative importance of stool frequency vs. stool consistency in arriving at a definition of constipation, and state recommendations for treatment (if drug therapy actually is indicated).
2. Describe the main criteria used to group laxatives and cathartics according to (1) the mechanism(s) by which they work, (2) whether they simply soften the stool or cause a more watery and more complete bowel evacuation, and (3) their valid uses based on the characteristics summarized in (2). You should be able to name the main agents (drugs) that are generally suitable for the uses stated in (3).
3. Describe a general sequence of events that leads to chronic, repetitive misuse of laxatives or cathartics; state the potential physiologic consequences of such continued use. State how the misuse of antidiarrheal drugs might become part of the cycle.
4. Describe some effective nondrug methods that help normalize bowel function in an individual who develops a period of bowel irregularity (with respect to either the frequency or consistency of stool).
5. As a knowledgeable healthcare provider, describe information you would pass on to a patient, friend, or family member who is literally deluged with television ads about laxatives, cathartics, and other GI drugs, and now may feel they "need one" when it is actually not medically necessary or even safe.

Note: I advise you *not* to memorize the drugs discussed in this chapter according to the number of the group in which they have been placed—Group I, II, and so on. It is extremely unlikely that you will ever hear a clinical medical professional refer to a Group I agent, ask you the group to which a particular agent belongs, or say "order a Group III drug" for a patient. But you *will* need to know whether, for example, a particular drug causes a prompt, watery evacuation of the bowel; what the clinical implications, both good and unwanted, of such a drug can be; and whether it is the appropriate drug or type of drug for the job at hand.

CRITICAL THINKING AND STUDY QUESTIONS

1. In very general terms, how can laxatives or cathartics alter the bioavailability (and therefore the effects) of many other drugs that are administered orally at more or less the same time?

2. You have an elderly patient who is taking multiple oral drugs. You advise her, verbally and in writing, to avoid taking laxatives; you've also asked her to tell you what over-the-counter medications she takes. She tells you she never takes laxatives but frequently she takes milk of magnesia for her heartburn. Any concerns?

219

3. Bisacodyl enteric-coated tablets (for oral administration) are fairly popular OTC laxatives, and they are also prescribed for certain purposes by physicians. What are the two main reasons that some oral medications (bisacodyl and many others) are formulated as enteric-coated tablets? What instructions should be given to the patient taking one of these products (just focus on the bisacodyl), and why? What are the likely consequences if this advice to the patient is ignored?

4. The text does a nice job of stating how laxative/cathartic misuse can lead to dependency on those drugs. Can you envision a way in which abuse of antidiarrheal drugs can become part of the problem, leading to what amounts to a laxative-antidiarrheal drug cycle that's hard to break?

CASE STUDY

Bev Allen is a spunky 64-year-old widow who lives alone. She has a history of systolic hypertension and two "mini-strokes" (transient ischemic attacks, or TIAs) over the last 5 years. There is some age-related cognitive dysfunction, but no specific or unusual CNS impairments that might be the result of her mini-strokes. Her blood pressure has been stable, at 150/90, for the last 6 years as a result of her antihypertensive medication.

During a routine physical examination at the office, you discover that Mrs. Allen uses several OTC laxatives every day, allegedly in order to have a daily bowel movement.

She says that if she doesn't use a laxative, she really has to "push hard" to force herself to defecate. She's admitted that a couple of times when she's done this she's gotten light-headed; at other times she's developed a terrible headache; a couple of times she's passed out on the toilet.

1. What additional information do you need to know about Mrs. Allen before you can address her issues of laxative abuse?

2. What aspects of normal bowel function will we need to address with Mrs. Allen to reduce or eliminate her use of or dependency on laxatives or cathartics?

3. What may cause Mrs. Allen to get light-headed or get headaches when she strains to defecate? A colleague says that she's performing the "Valsalva maneuver" when she defecates. What is the Valsalva maneuver, and how (if at all) does it relate to Mrs. Allen's history or to other specific physical findings you might encounter in any patient? And finally, how do these issues relate to the issue of laxative use?

4. Given the above, which type of laxative or cathartic may be helpful to reduce Mrs. Allen's cardiovascular consequences of defecation?

5. Mrs. Allen tells you that she was "raised on laxatives." Her parents gave laxatives to her all the time, even if she had a cold. Comment on this.

6. One of Mrs. Allen's most remembered remedies when she was young was Haley's M-O. It was a combination of drugs that included mineral oil (the M-O part). She's taken that for years and wishes to continue using mineral oil as a laxative. What would you advise her?

7. When, in general, are laxatives contraindicated? After all, you need to know this for Mrs. Allen and many other patients.

8. Mrs. Allen asks whether all the laxatives and cathartics are alike, especially in terms of the problems they may pose for her (i.e., what you might consider contraindications or special precautions). How would you respond?

evolve To check your answers, go to http://evolve.elsevier.com/Lehne/ for Study Guide Comments from the author.

Other Gastrointestinal Drugs

KEY TERMS

"nonspecific" (antidiarrheal drug or effect)

"specific" (antidiarrheal drug or effect)

antiemetic (drug or effect)

cannabinoid(s)

chemoreceptor trigger zone (CTZ)

cholelithiasis

Crohn's disease

diarrhea

emesis (and anticipatory, delayed emesis)

emetogenic (drug or effect)

gastroparesis (e.g., diabetic)

irritable bowel syndrome (IBS)

prokinetic (drug or effect)

traveler's diarrhea

ulcerative colitis

OBJECTIVES

After reading and studying this chapter you should be able to:

1. Discuss the (patho)physiologic mechanisms by which emesis is triggered and the main neurotransmitters that participate (and that can be blocked to cause antiemetic effects) in triggering the signs and symptoms. Conversely, identify some drugs that often cause emesis, mainly because they activate one or more of those receptors. Do the same in the context of motion sickness.
2. Describe the drugs that are used as antiemetics and summarize their main mechanism(s) of action, if known.
3. Describe a care plan for managing cancer chemotherapy–induced nausea and vomiting. It should include interventions and drugs that would be suitable for the three main types of emesis in this setting (anticipatory, acute, and delayed) and considerations for effective administration routes.
4. State the criteria that must be met, the adverse effects that might be expected, the associated contraindications, and the generally accepted "risk management program" when we consider using alosetron.
5. Describe the etiology and symptomatology of Crohn's disease. Describe the drugs that are used

to manage it and how those drugs (and their main mechanisms of action) are consistent with the notion that Crohn's disease is an autoimmune disease.

Several drugs or drug groups highlighted in this chapter are discussed in more detail elsewhere. Be sure to review the basic and clinical pharmacology of the antimuscarinic drugs (e.g., atropine; see Chapter 14), phenothiazine and butyrophenone antipsychotics (see Chapter 30), the opioids (see Chapter 27), and the older antihistamines (H₁ blockers) such as diphenhydramine (see Chapter 66).

CRITICAL THINKING AND STUDY QUESTIONS

1. Your text notes that H-HT₃ blockers such as ondansetron don't block dopamine receptors and so don't cause extrapyramidal side effects associated with antiemetics that do block dopamine receptors. With what disorder do we typically associate extrapyramidal effects, whether drug-induced or idiopathic?

2. Phenothiazines and butyrophenones were identified as being used as antiemetics. Do you recall what their main other uses are? How is the antiemetic action of these drugs likely to participate also in one of the most common neurologic adverse responses when these drugs are used long-term?

222

3. As noted in your text, parenteral diphenhydramine can be used to manage acute extrapyramidal reactions caused by those antiemetic drugs (e.g., metoclopramide and others) that activate dopamine receptors. How does this work?

4. Your text notes that oral therapy won't work for acute emesis. Why not?

5. What type of extra monitoring is particularly important before and while a patient receives droperidol (a haloperidol-like drug) for emesis control?

6. Some people with frequent nausea and vomiting from chemotherapy swear that smoking marijuana is the only way they can stay comfortable. Some AIDS patients smoke marijuana to improve their appetite (some may refer to this as the "marijuana munchies," a common term for the desire to eat after using the drugs). Skeptics say these individuals are just using their symptoms as an excuse to "get high." Social and legal issues aside (and they are important issues), how would you respond to either side in the controversy?

7. Based on our current understanding of how the brain works, what are the main differences between motion sickness and vomiting, as the former often leads to the latter? Focus mainly on the neurotransmitters involved, which affects the types of drugs we use.

8. An elderly man, one of your patients, is going on a cruise and has heard of scopolamine patches that have worked for his friends. He asks for a prescription. What underlying medical conditions should be ruled out first, and why? Provided there are no contraindications identified in this man, when would you advise him to first apply the patch?

9. You've won the lottery. You got enough money to buy a very nice, very big (and expensive) boat. Unfortunately, you have no money left over to hire anyone to clean up any messes your guests might make on it. You take some of your friends out for a sail. The seas are rough, and you warn them about seasickness. One person responds, "Don't worry, I have one of those scopolamine patches. If I start feeling bad, I'll stick it on." How will you reply?

10. A patient with a week-long history of diarrhea asks for a prescription for some remedy. The doctor takes a good history and does an adequate work-up for a diagnosis, then he writes a prescription for an OTC medication. The patient calls from the pharmacy and says, "What's up? The label on this stuff says it's a 'bulk-forming laxative!' I have diarrhea!" What is the likely explanation to this apparent paradox or medication error?

11. How can habitual misuse of antidiarrheal drugs be caused by the use of laxatives, such as milk of magnesia?

12. One specific type of GI disorder discussed in this chapter is managed in a way that is analogous to "replacement therapy" for such endocrine disorders as hypothyroidism and diabetes mellitus: adequate doses of the missing endogenous substance are administered therapeutically. Can you identify what GI disorder that is and what its primary management is?

13. What are the main concerns with administering alosetron—the ones for which the drug was originally pulled from the market? In light of these, what are the rather stringent limitations on its use, now that it is approved again can be prescribed for specific situations? What is that limited approved use?

14. Metoclopramide suppresses emesis, yet it has the ability to increase motility of the upper GI tract. This seems odd because one can imagine that by increasing upper GI tract motility, the drug would cause emesis. Explain this paradox.

CASE STUDY

John Xi is doing research in Central America for the summer and is taking his family along. His family doctor prescribes ciprofloxacin and Lomotil to take as soon as he gets on the airplane "just in case he develops" traveler's diarrhea.

1. What is the typical cause of traveler's diarrhea?

2. What types of medication are available for the treatment of diarrhea?

3. What are the ingredients (individual generic drugs) in Lomotil? Does each contribute to the antidiarrheal actions of the product?

4. Since Lomotil contains an opioid, does it pose a risk of opioid-like physical and psychologic dependency? Is it likely that an individual will habitually consume large doses of this product for the typically sought-after CNS effects of an opioid (e.g., euphoria)?

5. Given the non-opioid ingredient in Lomotil, are there any side effects to be expected or contraindications that you should rule out before Mr. Xi takes the combination product? What are they, and why?

6. Why might you have concerns overall with the physician's recommendation to start taking the antibiotic and the Lomotil as soon as the patient hops on the plane? Are there any tips that could be given to Mr. Xi and his family to reduce their risks of getting traveler's diarrhea and perhaps the need to take any medications for it?

evolve To check your answers, go to http://evolve.elsevier.com/Lehne/ for Study Guide Comments from the author.

Vitamins

KEY TERMS

adequate intake (AI)
antioxidant
B-complex vitamins
beriberi
estimated average
requirement (EAR)
fat-soluble vitamin
hypervitaminosis
osteomalacia
pellagra

recommended dietary
allowance (RDA)
scurvy
tolerable upper intake
level (UL)
vitamin
water-soluble vitamin
Wernicke-Korsakoff
syndrome

OBJECTIVES

After reading and studying this chapter you should be able to:

1. State the overall functional role of vitamins in maintenance of good health, i.e., what basic metabolic processes require them.
2. In general terms, compare and contrast recommended dietary allowance (RDA), adequate intake (AI), tolerable upper intake level (UL), and estimated average requirement (EAR), as those terms apply to vitamin intake.
3. Identify the two major vitamin groups or classifications, and what factor(s) place a vitamin in one of those groups.
4. Recognize the common synonyms or alternative terms (or common pharmaceutical products) for the following vitamins:
    niacin - nicotinic acid, nicotinamide
    vitamin A - retinol
    vitamin B_1 - thiamin
    vitamin B_{12} - cyanocobalamin
    vitamin B_2 - riboflavin
    vitamin B_6 - pyridoxine
    vitamin C - ascorbic acid
    vitamin E - alpha tocopherol
5. State the main biochemical roles of the following vitamins, and the clinical findings or consequences of inadequate or excessive levels of them:
    vitamins A, C, K; B_1, B_6, B_{12}, niacin, folic acid

Note: Be sure to consult previous chapters for more information on the roles of Vitamin K as a regulator of blood clotting factor synthesis and in the clinical response to warfarin; information regarding the use of niacin as a lipid-lowering agent; and information on the roles of vitamin D in the regulation of calcium and phosphate. There are two chapters of particular importance to discussions here of vitamin B_{12} and folic acid: Chapter 52 (Drugs for Deficiency Anemias); and Chapter 23 (Drugs for Epilepsy).

CRITICAL THINKING AND STUDY QUESTIONS

1. A patient asks you about a new super-multivitamin supplement advertised in a magazine. The ad says "our product is a novel source of energy for you body's health." It further insinuates that taking this product, in lieu of eating a balanced diet, will keep you in "tip top shape." "and correct spacing so sentence reads" Explain the truth to the patient (i.e., what is it that vitamins actually do in/for our bodies).

2. If you could remember the members of one group of vitamins, you could know "automatically" that other vitamins are in the other class. Can you think of an easy way to do this so you don't get faked-out on an exam question about this?"

3. A patient with a certain medical condition develops chronic steatorrhea—the production of stool that is rich in fats. Over the long-run, which class of vitamins is likely to be depleted, causing deficiencies of them?

4. Compare and contrast water-soluble and fat-soluble vitamins in terms of the degrees to which they are stored in the body. What are the implications of this in terms of our daily needs for these vitamins, and the overall risk of toxicity should intake of these vitamins be excessive for a prolonged time.

5. Match the following descriptive phrases with the proper vitamin.

A. critical for synthesis of certain clotting factors in the liver; deficiencies increase the risk of spontaneous or excessive bleeding; excesses counteract the desired effects of warfarin, which makes the vitamin also suitable for managing excessive responses to warfarin

B. abundant in citrus juices and fruit; has antioxidant activity; facilitates iron absorption from the gut; clinical deficiency leads to scurvy; touted as a "cure" for the common cold, cancer, and asthma

C. important for "eye health," especially good vision in low light levels; highly teratogenic when consumed in excess during pregnancy; chronic overdoses may cause severe liver damage; only clinical use is for replacement therapy in deficiency

D. found in many food sources; deficiency leads to dermatitis and various CNS and GI symptoms; used therapeutically, in high doses, to lower serum lipid levels; oral administration of large doses tends to cause significant vasodilation and consequences of that (e.g., facial flushing, dizziness)

E. an activated form is crucial for normal carbohydrate metabolism; most common clinical presentation of deficiency affects the CNS and includes such signs and symptoms as nystagmus, double-vision, and ataxia, and is seen most in chronic alcohol abusers; suspicion of this condition warrants prompt parenteral administration of the vitamin

F. an activated form is important for normal protein metabolism; skin, blood, and CNS responses develop with deficiencies; deficiency common with chronic alcoholism, but may also be induced by the important tuberculosis drug, isoniazid

G. deficiencies of either or both of these can cause megaloblastic anemia and/or neurologic damage; therapy with many anticonvulsant drugs during pregnancy can cause deficiency leading to neural tube defects (e.g., anencephaly or spina bifida) in the fetus, and so supplementation of the mom is almost always indicated

CASE STUDY

Leon Roberts, a 46-year-old man, has been admitted to a medical unit after four days in an alcohol detoxification center. He was admitted because of complaints of extreme weakness and an unsteady gait. His history reveals that his alcohol intake has steadily increased since he lost his job three years ago. For the past six months he has been living on the street and drinking 1 to 2 quarts of fortified wine daily. His response when asked about his diet is, "Whatever I can get—mostly donuts, chips, and candy bars." His physical assessment reveals ataxia, edema of the lower extremities, dry skin with cracks in the corners of his mouth, and multiple bruises. He is anorexic; he sips small amounts of fluid and eats only a few bites of his lunch. He complains that his mouth is too "sore" to eat much. Endoscopy reveals severe gastritis with no obvious bleeding.

1. What symptoms and aspects of the history led to a diagnosis of vitamin deficiency, and which vitamins are probably deficient?

Mr. Roberts is diagnosed with multiple vitamin deficiency and started on an IV drip with one ampule of vitamin C and B complex per liter.

2. What is wrong with the order for "one ampule" of the medication(s)?

3. What is the most likely explanation for Mr. Roberts's bruising? Does it likely reflect inadequate dietary intake of a particular vitamin, or something more serious?

4. Mr. Roberts' blood studies show that he has anemia, based on a very low total hemoglobin level. Which vitamins are essential in red blood cell production?

5. Mr. Roberts' wife has agreed that he may come home with her after his discharge from the hospital as long as he continues to stay in an outpatient rehabilitation program and does not drink. She asks you to tell her some of the foods she should prepare to be certain Mr. Roberts gets the necessary vitamins. What foods or food groups would you suggest to her to ensure adequate intake of the following vitamins: A, C, niacin, riboflavin, thiamine, and pyridoxine?

6. Mrs. Roberts asks you whether it would be a good idea to go to the health-food store and buy Mr. Roberts some high-dose vitamin pills with "all" the vitamins included. What is your best response?

Enteral and Parenteral Nutrition

KEY TERMS

aspiration pneumonitis
blood urea nitrogen
    (BUN) levels
enteral nutritional
    therapy
glucose intolerance
hyperalimentation (e.g.,
    fluid)

inflammatory bowel
    disease (IBD)
osmolarity (osmolality)
parenteral nutritional
    therapy
"tube feeding"

OBJECTIVES

After reading and studying this chapter you should
be able to:

1. Define enteral nutritional therapy in terms of its
   general indications, the typical methods of enteral
   feedings that are used, the typical ingredients in
   enteral nutritional preparations, and major complications. Compare and contrast it with parenteral nutritional therapy in terms of general
   indications and methods.
2. Identify the "core components" of fats, carbohy-
   drates, and amino acids in a parenteral nutritional
   regimen, and state the main roles of each class of
   ingredients.

Note: The chapter in Lehne does an excellent job of
presenting this information. However, such issues as
modes and methods of delivery of enteral nutrition
therapy are important, but they go beyond the traditional scope of pharmacology and are more appro-
priately medical-surgical nursing matters. Thus we
limit our comments below to more pharmacologic
aspects of the chapter.

CRITICAL THINKING AND STUDY QUESTIONS

1. A patient with type 1 diabetes (see Chapter 54)
   becomes critically ill and requires enteral nutritional therapy. Will his requirements for glucose
   (how much is present in the solution that is
   administered by a feeding tube) increase,
   decrease, or stay the same, and what do we do
   about it? How do we know?

2. A patient with type 2 diabetes becomes critically
   ill and requires parenteral nutritional therapy,
   Will her requirements for glucose (how much is
   present in the solution that is administered IV)
   increase, decrease, or stay the same, and what do
   we do about it? How do we know?

3. What is the one nutrient that generally is present
   in *in*sufficient amounts in enteral nutrition fluids?

4. What is the main electrolyte imbalance to be considered when a patient is receiving parenteral
   nutrition therapy that includes glucose? It is a
   concern if the patient has no history of diabetes
   mellitus or is not receiving insulin. It is of greater
   concern if the patient is receiving supplemental
   insulin. Why does this problem occur?

5. In some clinical situations we administer relatively large amounts of fat emulsions. We also may administer dextrose. When we are trying to manage essential fatty acid deficiency we boost the amount of fat emulsion and lower the amount of dextrose we give. Why?

6. When a patient requires a parenteral nutrient mixture that is hypertonic, what measures should be used to reduce risks of giving it?

7. For whatever reason, a patient receives an excessive amount (volume) of a hypertonic parenteral nutrient solution. The plasma osmolality is excessively and dangerously high. The physician orders an infusion of sterile water to "dilute the blood." What are your thoughts about this order?

CASE STUDY

Ann Wall is a 21-year-old college student who is admitted to your unit for a severe, acute flare-up of inflammatory bowel disease (IBD). She was diagnosed with IBD 2 years ago, but until now has had no episodes that required hospitalization. She tells you that her food intake has been limited for the last month due to cramping and diarrhea and that for the past week she has taken in only small amounts of liquids throughout the day. She does not show signs of severe dehydration, but she is very thin (she is 5 feet 6 inches tall and weighs 98 pounds) and extremely weak. Her physician starts a central line and orders hyperalimentation fluid and fat emulsion to be given through a Y-connector. She is being evaluated for resection of the small intestine.

1. Why is parenteral nutrition ordered instead of enteral feedings?

2. What nutrient deficits are likely to account for Ms. Wall's thinness and weakness?

3. Describe the risks of attempting surgery before Ms. Wall's nutritional status is improved.

4. Describe the purpose of each of the following components in Ms. Wall's parenteral nutrition solution: amino acids, dextrose, and fat emulsion.

5. Discuss the purposes of collecting the following laboratory data: levels of blood urea nitrogen (BUN), potassium, hemoglobin, blood glucose, and triglycerides.

6. What endogenous factor is essential for Ms. Wall's body cells to incorporate and metabolize the glucose? If Ms. Wall doesn't have adequate levels of this agent, supplemental doses may need to be administered to her.

7. Assume Ms. Wall also has type 2 diabetes. What oral medication should be ordered to manage the hyperglycemia she has or may develop in response to the glucose in the parenteral nutrition solution?

8. If we were to administer insulin to Ms. Wall, what main serum electrolyte change should we expect and so monitor for? How does it arise?

9. What observations, specific to Ms. Wall's parenteral therapy, would you include in your frequent assessments?

evolve To check your answers, go to http://evolve.elsevier.com/Lehne/ for Study Guide Comments from the author.

Drugs for Obesity

KEY TERMS

anorexigenic (drug or effect)
bariatrics (e.g., bariatric surgery)
body mass index (BMI)

gastric bypass surgery
obesity
serotonin syndrome
vertical banded gastroplasty

OBJECTIVES

After reading and studying this chapter you should be able to:

1. State the common comorbidities associated with obesity, and describe how obesity can aggravate them.
2. Give a general overview of the importance of the body mass index (BMI), waist circumference (WC), and other comorbidities in determining whether or how we initiate weight-loss therapy.
3. Discuss the management of obesity. Include in your discussion the benefits, risks, and limitations of lifestyle changes, drug therapy (both prescription and OTC), and surgery. Identify the healthcare profession that is most likely to be of benefit to the patient, and to you, for a nutrition consultation.
4. Identify the main pharmacologic classes and mechanisms of appetite suppressants and the common medical or psychologic conditions they may aggravate, even if they do lead to a reduction of body weight.
5. Describe the serotonin syndrome (signs and symptoms, etiology), the weight-loss medication that is most likely to trigger it, and the interacting drugs that certainly increase the risk of this serious response.
6. Summarize the main calorie-lowering actions of and indications for orlistat. Identify its main site of action with that of such drugs as sibutramine or amphetamines, and describe the clinical consequences of that different site of action.
7. Identify the main drug (or drug class) used in many (if not most) OTC weight-loss aids, the adverse peripheral autonomic effects it could

cause, and common and important contraindications to use of such aids.

CRITICAL THINKING AND STUDY QUESTIONS

1. Even though it's not listed specifically in your text, and many advertisements would lead you to believe otherwise, what is the one and only way to lose weight.... Period?

2. What are the main nondrug treatment approaches we should use and try first before resorting to drug-assisted weight reduction? Why do we too often turn to the drugs first?

3. Of late there's been a change in thought among many weight-loss experts: Treat long-term rather than for short periods of time. What's the main reason for that?

4. We tend to focus on fats as the "bad guys" in weight gain. Why?

5. Ideally, to whom should the patient who needs to alter his or her diet in a dramatic but healthy way be referred?

6. Just as there have been changes in the goals of medical therapy of obesity, so have there been changes in the surgical approach. Compare the goals of "then" and "now."

7. The text describes sibutramine's (Meridia's) actions as due to an anorexigenic effect as a result of blockade of neuronal serotonin and/or norepinephrine reuptake. This is a good time, therefore, to review some basic pharmacology:

A. What are the physiologic sources of the serotonin and norepinephrine, whose reuptake is blocked by the sibutramine?

B. What is the physiologic importance of the reuptake process? What are the consequences of blocking it?

C. Can you name another essential neurotransmitter, the actions of which are *not* terminated by reuptake?

D. We've stated that the actions of sibutramine are due to inhibited serotonin and norepinephrine reuptake. What other class of drugs exerts the same actions on both neurotransmitters, although it's used for a different clinical purpose? Are there any drugs that selectively block reuptake of just one of these neurotransmitters? What are they, and what are they used for?

8. Why can sibutramine tend to cause some elevations of blood pressure and tachycardia? And why is it so crucial to monitor for these changes and rule out relevant contraindicating conditions (e.g., coronary artery disease, heart failure, etc.) when or before using the drug?

9. Products that contain ephedrine (ephedra; ma huang) are popular weight-loss aids. Explain how the drug works (in terms of weight loss and other important pharmacologic effects), and summarize the risks of using ephedrine-containing products. What co-existing disorders, or other meds the patient may be taking, pose added (and sometimes lethal) risks? What related precautionary instructions should you give to your patients?

10. Orlistat often causes a fatty stool in greater than normal frequency (steatorrhea). Why is this important in terms of the patient's overall nutritional status?

CASE STUDY

Martin Langer is 48 years old, weighs 440 pounds, and is 5 feet 2 inches tall. His waist circumference is 54 inches.

He has just moved to your town, so this is his first visit to your office. He's there for a mandatory physical to gain health insurance for a new job and to finally "get his health issues addressed."

Mr. Langer's total cholesterol is 330 mg/dL. He states he has a history of high blood pressure and diabetes (blood glucose levels averaging 220 mg/dL; history and physical indicate it's type 2), but he's never done anything about either.

Mr. Langer denies any chest discomfort, whether at rest or on exertion. He's had "bad headaches" and is still taking "something" for it—something prescribed by his doctor in the town from which he moved. He has no idea of what the medication is, and despite your best efforts you can't figure out what it is either.

He describes himself as a teetotaler and not at all the type of person who would use any illegal or illicit substances. He states that he's never been married, nor has he been "serious" with anyone. You suspect some element of depression in Mr. Langer, simply based on his responses to your questions and his overall demeanor and affect. In fact, you don't get a good sense that he's fully forthcoming about his medical or medication history.

The physician for whom you work has proposed a program of diet, exercise, and drug therapy.

1. Convert Mr. Langer's weight and height to metric units, and calculate his body mass index (BMI).

2. Determine Mr. Langer's overall risk status and the factors that go into your determination.

3. Among many things, Mr. Langer's diabetes needs to be addressed. Assuming he has no specific contraindications to any oral antidiabetic medications, is there one that might be given a trial first? Why?

4. Mr. Langer is placed on sibutramine (Meridia) 10 mg PO daily. Identify the most common and the most worrisome adverse or side effects of this drug and why they occur.

About a month after Mr. Langer started the sibutramine, your office gets a call from the local hospital's emergency room. Mr. Langer has been admitted with severe tachycardia, severe anxiety, and what appears to be acute psychosis (he is hallucinating), and intermittent myoclonic seizures. He is diaphoretic and febrile too. He is so impaired that he cannot communicate anything about his health and medication history, so they've asked you for insight.

5. You do a quick but careful check of Mr. Langer's history, as far as you have it documented. What two or three causes of his presentation should come to mind in terms of a possible diagnosis? How might you help the ER staff figure out what might be going on? Go back to your notes (the brief comments we made above) and start preparing a list.

evolve To check your answers, go to http://evolve.elsevier.com/Lehne/ for Study Guide Comments from the author.

Basic Principles of Antimicrobial Therapy

KEY TERMS

anaerobe (anaerobic; and aerobic)
antibiotic
antimetabolite
antimicrobial
bactericidal
bacteriostatic
broad- (and narrow-) spectrum antibiotic
broth dilution procedure (for determining antibiotic susceptibility)
chemotherapy
conjugation (as a process in bacterial resistance)
empiric therapy (as of microbial infections)

Gram's stain (and gram-negative, gram-positive)
host
minimum bactericidal concentration (MBC)
minimum inhibitory concentration (MIC)
nosocomial (infection)
R factors
selective toxicity
spontaneous mutation
suprainfection (superinfection)
virulent (to describe a pathogen or an infection from one)

OBJECTIVES

After reading and studying this chapter you should be able to:

1. Define selective toxicity as it applies to the general mechanisms by which antibiotics work against invading pathogens but not against host cells.
2. Give a working definition of narrow- and broad-spectrum antibiotics, and state when one or the other would be preferred as a therapeutic approach, and why.
3. Explain the fundamental difference between bactericidal and bacteriostatic drugs and state what host-related factor(s) is required for successful therapy with a bacteriostatic agent.
4. State the main mechanisms by which microbes develop resistance to antimicrobial drugs. (At this time you do not need to match drug groups with each mechanism, but be sure you learn that

information as you work your way through the individual chapters in this unit.) Be sure you address the important issues of spontaneous mutations and R factors in your comments.
5. Familiarize yourself with the "12 action steps" that are part of the Centers for Disease Control and Prevention campaign to limit the problems of nosocomial infections. (Unless your instructor tells you otherwise, you should not rotely memorize each step, in order.)
6. Understand the general concept and purpose of broth dilution procedures to determine the susceptibility of bacteria to antibiotics. In all likelihood you will never have to perform this test, so just having a grasp of the generalities should be sufficient and informative.
7. Discuss the general rationales and needs for using antibiotics in combination, and describe situations in which antibiotic combinations should be avoided. (You should be able to answer this now, without citing specific examples... that you will learn in other chapters.)
8. Describe generally accepted indications for prophylactic antimicrobial therapy.
9. Discuss the misuses of antibiotics—general prevalence, why misuse persists as a major health problem, and consequences. Give some examples of common situations in which iatrogenic antibiotic misuse occurs.
10. Start preparing a table that you will work on as you progress through remaining chapters in this unit to indicate the following: (1) the names of each main drug class, as well as a prototype(s) and "important related drugs"; (2) whether and for what infections and infectious organisms they are considered first-line agents (or other special indications for use); (3) whether they are bacteriostatic or bacteriocidal; (4) specific and important contraindications; (5) the relative degree to which resistance develops and a general mechanism by which resistance occurs; (6) general risk of allergic reactions and whether antibiotics in other classes may cross-react to

234

trigger allergic responses; (7) any specific host toxicities (e.g., those that affect the GI tract, liver, kidney, nervous system, blood, or special senses such as hearing).

Note: For this introductory chapter, focus on the author's two main stated themes: (1) understanding how pathogenic microbes are affected by drugs and how those organisms develop resistance to antibiotics and (2) general principles regarding proper use of antimicrobials. Keep these concepts in mind as you work through the rest of this unit.

When you work through *this* chapter you do not need to memorize either the specific mechanisms by which specific antibiotics exert their desired effects or the main mechanisms that account for resistance to their actions. You will get to that learning task in short order. When you do move on, you should be able to meet most or all the general objectives listed for this introductory chapter as they apply to specific antibiotics or antibiotic groups, as well as to the treatment of such other pathogens as viruses, helminths, fungi, and the like.

As far as a *case study* goes, we'll integrate the general concepts presented here into case studies in subsequent chapters.

CRITICAL THINKING AND STUDY QUESTIONS

1. Choosing an antibiotic that is highly selective for the organism is a better treatment than simply giving a broad-spectrum agent. Why?

2. What mechanisms do antimicrobial drugs use to inhibit the growth of, or kill, bacteria? When appropriate, link these mechanisms to how antibiotics affect bacteria but not human cells. This is the concept of "selective toxicity." (Extra points: Name a class or two of antibiotics that works on each of these microbe-specific processes. And, for now, let's ignore the antiviral drugs.)

3. What are antimetabolites, in the broad sense of the term? What other important group of drugs includes some very important agents that are classified as antimetabolites? First you might want to ask, "What is a metabolite?" (If you are working through the text in sequence, you won't have come to these yet, so this is just a heads-up.)

4. Some people have called such drugs as the penicillins, the cephalosporins, and amphotericin B "bacteriolytic drugs." What might be meant by this? (***Hint:*** Look at the suffix of the word, -lytic.)

5. What general host-related factor is crucial to the success of therapy with antibiotics, especially those that are bacteriostatic?

6. State four main ways that bacteria can "fend off" the otherwise damaging or deadly effects of antibiotics. Make up a pretend microbe. Give it some make-believe antibiotic. And tell us how the ingenious bacterium can develop ways to protect itself from the very drugs we are giving to protect us from infectious disease.

7. Why does spontaneous mutation (of the bacterial genome) account for relatively slow development of antibiotic resistance and usually involve only one antibiotic drug?

8. What are R factors, and why are they important to microbial resistance to antibiotics? How do R factors contribute to multiple drug resistance (say, as opposed to the consequences of spontaneous microbial gene mutations)? Keep your answer as simple but as accurate as you can.

9. Why is the genetic makeup of bacteria so important to their life span, to how we can interrupt that process with antibiotics, and to how those bacteria can develop resistance to our drugs? In thinking about the answer to this, think about what our genes do for us. Look at some of the questions above and your answers to them, and you should get a very good idea about how to answer these questions.

10. Some have said that a main mechanism by which antibiotics cause bacterial resistance is like having a bunch of ordinary bad kids and a few *really bad and tough* kids living in your neighborhood. The antibiotics just get rid of the ordinary bad ones. Others have said that bacteria function like a bunch of people hovering around a small buffet or salad bar, trying to get something to eat. What might these strange thoughts mean?

11. For just about every infectious organism there is a list of one or two suitable drugs. However, only one or two drugs are considered to be first-line (first-choice) drugs. What characteristics of the drug usually earn it that designation?

12. What factors (other than ignorance) might lead us to prescribe a second- or third-line agent instead of one that's generally recognized as a first-choice medication?

13. A patient with a certain infection would be a candidate for therapy with a first-line bacteriostatic antibiotic. However, the physician decides to choose a second-line drug and in fact use two antibiotics. The reason, she says, is that this patient is neutropenic. What does that mean, and what is the implication of it?

14. The text succinctly cites the "first rule of antibiotic therapy." What is it, and why do we often ignore it?

15. Listed below are five common conditions. For each, millions of prescriptions have been written for patients who are not hospitalized. Take a guess about what percentage of those prescriptions has been unnecessary, irrational, or otherwise inappropriate. (You will not find this information in the text, so you'll have to just look at the answers. We ask you to guess simply so, we hope, you will be quite shocked at the magnitude of the problem concerning antibiotic misuse... and will do what you can to reduce the problem.)
    Ear infections
    Sore throat
    Sinusitis
    Bronchitis
    Common cold

16. A sample of pus is aspirated from a large abscess. It's cultured, the bacteria are identified, and an antibiotic known to kill them is administered intravenously at an effective dose—on the order of 4 to 6 times the MBC. Doses are repeated as indicated in the drug's package insert. Based only on the information given, what is wrong with this approach? How might it constitute antibiotic misuse? After all, we've matched the drug to the bug and given ample doses?

17. What are some valid indications to combine antibiotics?

18. A colleague states that combining a bacteriostatic antibiotic with a bactericidal one should be a wonderful approach to treating most infections. He argues that the bacteriostatic agent will "slow down" the bugs, making it easier for the bacteriocidal agent to "attack them and mop them up." Comment on this in general terms.

19. By now you realize that antibiotic prophylaxis is something that should be done only in special circumstances. Why is a history of rheumatic heart disease or the presence of a prosthetic heart valve one of those situations—especially in the setting of prophylaxis before even "routine" dental procedures as "innocuous" as a semi-annual teeth cleaning?

20. If a patient has a history of rheumatic heart disease or is the recipient of a prosthetic heart valve goes for a dental procedure, who prescribes the drug for prophylaxis? What must he or she know in order to do that?

21. Why is noncompliance such a major reason that outpatients fail to achieve the expected effects from their antibiotic therapy? And what is arguably the most worrisome consequence of this practice? Assume we've prescribed the correct drug for the infection, at the right dose and dose interval, and that there are no drug- or disease-related factors that will interfere with the drug's expected actions.

22. Noncompliance is common. And in some cases, patients have their antibiotic prescriptions filled, only to get a call from the MD's office saying, "The culture was negative; you don't need to keep taking your pills." Either way, many people have "leftover" pills around the house. What might be the problem(s) with this?

23. Is it likely that oral antibiotics will be approved for OTC sale in the United States? Now that you have some information about the pitfalls of antibiotic therapy, give us your two cents' worth. Also tell us how the availability in other countries of such meds without prescription may affect *our* health?

evolve To check your answers, go to http://evolve.elsevier.com/Lehne/ for Study Guide Comments from the author.

Drugs That Weaken the Bacterial Cell Wall I: Penicillins

KEY TERMS

aminopenicillin
antistaphylococcal
   penicillin
autolysins
bactericidal
beta-lactamase
clavulanic acid
extended spectrum
   (antipseudomonal)
   penicillin
hapten

methicillin-resistant
   Staphylococcus aureus
   (MRSA)
penicillinase
penicillin-binding
   proteins (PBPs)
plasmid
repository preparation
   (of a drug)
transpeptidases

OBJECTIVES

After reading and studying this chapter you should be able to:

1. Describe the basic mechanism of action of the penicillins, as a broad class. In your discussion compare and contrast the structures of gram-negative and gram-positive bacteria and show how they relate to the typical antibiotic spectrum of activity of penicillin G (as a prototype).
2. Explain in simple terms what beta-lactam is chemically; why penicillins (and cephalosporins; see Chapter 81) are called beta-lactam antibiotics; and how that relates to the vulnerability of these antibiotic classes to inactivation by certain bacteria.
3. Know that the four main classes of penicillins are the narrow-spectrum/penicillinase-sensitive agents; those with narrow spectrum of activity but resistance to penicillinase; the broad-spectrum (amino-) penicillins; and the extended-spectrum (antipseudomonal) penicillins. For each group, identify at least one member drug (prototype or at least widely used) and give an indication of the bacterial types or strains that typically are responsive to them.
4. Explain the clinical significance of various salts of penicillin G in terms of pharmacokinetics,

spectrum of activity, susceptibility to penicillinases, unique side effects or adverse reactions (and patients who are at particular risk of them), and the incidence and severity of hypersensitivity reactions in "penicillin-allergic" patients.
5. Recognize penicillins as a main cause of drug-induced allergic reactions; compare and contrast immediate, accelerated, and delayed hypersensitivity reactions in terms of time of onset and main signs and symptoms.
6. Given a patient's history of severe hypersensitivity reactions to a penicillin, state at least one other group of antibiotics that should not be administered due to risks of cross-reactivity.
7. Recognize clavulanic acid (or sulbactam or tazobactam) as penicillinase inhibitors that are combined with certain broad- or extended-spectrum penicillins; that they lack intrinsic toxicity and antibiotic effects; and that they do nothing to reduce the severity or risk of hypersensitivity reactions in susceptible patients.
8. Describe the general rationale and indications for using both an intravenous penicillin and an aminoglycoside, and state the practical and correct meaning of administering them "together."

CRITICAL THINKING AND STUDY QUESTIONS

1. Tell us a little about the overall activity of the penicillins against gram-negative and gram-positive bacteria. For now, keep this to a simple discussion of how these two types of organism differ anatomically and how that relates to penicillin activity. To make things easier, discuss this in the context of penicillin G or V.

2. When a penicillinase-sensitive penicillin is exposed to a gram-positive bacterium that's making penicillinase, where does inactivation of the drug usually occur? How about with a gram-negative organism? Answer the same questions about beta-lactamases.

3. Tell us about the site of bacterial action of drugs in this chapter and several that follow. What is crucial function of that bacterial structure in terms of their survival, and what are the two main enzymes the bacteria use to keep it intact and functional?

4. What are plasmids, and what is their connection with the bacterial response (or lack of response) to certain penicillins?

5. Complete the following table (don't peek at the rather similar table in the text). Although doing this isn't the epitome of critical thinking, it should help you see at a glance the main differences among the various penicillins... and we'll have you do the same in the next chapter, which deals with the cephalosporins.

6. There are four *salts* of penicillin G: sodium, potassium, procaine, and benzathine. What do these salts do? How do they affect the antibiotic effects of the drug of which they are a part? What other important factors relate to which penicillin salt we choose to administer, and why?

7. You're interviewing for a summer clinical job with my nurse-manager wife. You've just gotten done reviewing the chapter on penicillins. You're so geeked about those drugs that you're babbling on about several of the penicillins and their administration routes. You mention two penicillins and, trying to use a fancy word, you say that they're *repository* preparations. However, my wife is hard of hearing and she didn't turn up the volume on her hearing aids.

Class	Prototype (or Other Examples)	Response to Penicillinases	Gram-positive Activity	Gram-negative Activity
1				
2				
3				
4				

So she says, "Oh, you give those drugs *per rectum?* They must be very new penicillins." Clarify things, and tell us which penicillins you're likely referring to when you mention repository preparation.

8. What is the overall (approximate) incidence of allergic reactions to penicillin? Comment on the statement that the severity of the allergic response to a penicillin is dose-dependent.

9. A patient has had a documented anaphylactic reaction to penicillin G. Which penicillin can be used in its place? Which other class of antibiotics should be *avoided* in patients with a history of severe allergic reactions to a penicillin?

10. Have you noticed that your chapter contains little about overdoses and overdose-related toxicity of penicillins? (Sure, there's lots of information about allergic responses, injection site pain, and problems associated with some penicillin *salts*. But that's not what we're talking about.) Was this an omission? What's the deal?

11. In the days when penicillin wasn't plentiful and was very expensive, small doses of the antibiotic were administered with probenecid. What was the purpose of doing that? What does this tell you about the main pathway by which penicillins are eliminated from the body? As an aside, what is probenecid used for now? (Check the index if you don't remember.)

12. As you work your way through this unit you'll find that giving two antibiotics to a patient is sometimes necessary and beneficial. In other cases, it's dangerous or counterproductive (reduced activity of one or both antibiotics due to interaction). Comment on the use of both a penicillin and an aminoglycoside (e.g., gentamicin; see Chapter 83): good, bad, or inconsequential? Why? When might we use this combination? And if we do, do we just mix the two together and give them?

13. What characteristic of penicillin V makes it preferable to penicillin G for oral therapy?

14. What is unique about nafcillin, oxacillin, cloxacillin, and dicloxacillin, and how does this property relate to their clinical uses? Why don't we use them routinely whenever a penicillin is indicated and safe?

15. You will often read about bacteria being resistant (or not) to methicillin. That must mean methicillin is an important drug. Is it?

16. Identify one main similarity between ampicillin and amoxicillin and one main clinically important difference that relates to oral therapy. Use the word *bioavailability* somewhere in your answer.

17. The text notes that ampicillin causes two side effects or adverse reactions more often than any other penicillin causes them. What are they?

18. A colleague is commenting about what he believes to be the "magical properties" of Augmentin, saying that it contains two very effective antibiotics: amoxicillin and clavulanic acid, "all in one." Is he correct?

19. What unique side effects or adverse reactions are associated with ticarcillin more than with other penicillins, and for which patients do they pose the main risk? (**Hint:** Think "cardiovascular.")

20. Bacampicillin is a *prodrug*. What does that term mean? (You should remember this from basic material covered in Unit II, *Basic Principles of Pharmacology*.) What is the active form of bacampicillin, and why don't we just administer it instead?

21. A patient has a community-acquired pneumonia caused by *Streptococcus pneumoniae*. The physician prescribes Augmentin. He states that he chose this product specifically because it contains clavulanic acid. He says that will really boost the activity of the amoxicillin that's also in the product and simultaneously reduce the risk of an allergic reaction. Comment on this.

1. What important information should be ascertained before the penicillin is prescribed or administered?

2. To be cautious and diligent, we need to give Mary's mom some information about possible side effects and adverse reactions of the amoxicillin. What might that be?

3. If Mary has had or develops a serious allergic reaction to the amoxicillin, what alternative antibiotics can be used? Which would be preferred?

4. Mary is especially cranky and obnoxious because she just doesn't feel well. One of your colleagues is a bit cranky too. In private she says, "Just pop Mary with a dose of IM penicillin." What are your thoughts on that, pharmacologically?

5. Mary's mom now asks how long it'll take before Mary starts to feel better. What should you tell her, assuming we've made the right diagnosis and given the right drug (and dose, etc.)?

6. Mary's mother now asks whether it's OK to stop giving the drug once Mary is her perky, non-cranky self again. Your comments?

CASE STUDY

Mary is an 8-year-old diagnosed with streptococcal pharyngitis. She will be treated with amoxicillin 250 mg tid for 10 days.

evolve To check your answers, go to http://evolve.elsevier.com/Lehne/ for Study Guide Comments from the author.

Drugs That Weaken the Bacterial Cell Wall II: Cephalosporins, Carbapenems, Aztreonam, Vancomycin, Teicoplanin, and Fosfomycin

KEY TERMS

"generations" of
  cephalosporins (1st,
  2nd, etc.)
beta-lactam (and beta-
  lactamase)

carbapenem(s)
cephalosporinase
ototoxic (drug or effect)
penicillin-binding
  proteins (PBPs)

OBJECTIVES

After reading and studying this chapter you should
be able to:

1. Compare and contrast cephalosporins (as a single, large drug class) and penicillins with respect to general mechanism(s) of action and mechanism(s) by which resistance develops, and summarize the general guidelines for administering a cephalosporin to a patient with documented "penicillin allergy."
2. Identify a prototype or representative example for each of the four generations of cephalosporins, and differentiate the groups in terms of mechanism of action, spectrum of action(s), susceptibility to destruction/inactivation by beta-lactamases, and access to the cerebrospinal fluid. (See the note below.)
3. Focus on imipenem as the prototype carbapenem; recognize its broad spectrum of activity and link that to decisions about when the drug should be used, or shouldn't.
4. State the characteristics of vancomycin that make it such a critically important drug yet one we do not turn to unless the infection is very serious or,

for one reason or another, other antibiotics don't work or cannot be given to a patient.

Note: Be sure to ask your instructor for clarification about what precisely you need to know. (No, we're not asking you to say, "What do I need to know?" or "What's on the test?" This is particularly important with the cephalosporins. Should you spend hours memorizing which drugs go into which class ("generation") and get that down perfectly? Unfortunately, that information will be of little value if you don't know the essential similarities and differences among the various generations in terms of such more important things as spectrums of activity, resistance to inactivation by bacterial enzymes, main side effects and adverse responses (including hypersensitivity reactions), and the like.

CRITICAL THINKING AND STUDY QUESTIONS

1. Complete the table on the following page (don't peek at the rather similar table in the text). Although doing this isn't the epitome of critical thinking, it should help you see at a glance the main differences among the various generations of cephalosporins... and maybe help you organize the key similarities and differences. It's OK to use qualitative terms (low, high, etc).

Cephalosporin Generation	Prototype (or Other Examples)	Gram-negative Activity	Resistance to Beta-lactamases	Access to CNS (Cerebrospinal Fluid)
1				
2				
3				
4				

2. What one pharmacokinetic factor, more than any other, affects plasma half-lives and the potential for toxicity from nearly all the cephalosporins?

3. Related to the above, what is pharmacokinetically unique about cefoperazone and ceftriaxone? To which cephalosporin generation do they belong?

4. For the cephalosporins overall, what is the most frequent adverse response? Is it dose-related? What do we do about it? What other main group of antibiotics causes a similar reaction in some patients, such that patients who have experienced such a reaction should not be treated with cephalosporins?

5. What special precautions and monitoring are particularly important when we administer cefmetazole, cefotetan, or cefoperazone? Why?

6. Cefmetazole, cefoperazone, and cefotetan can cause a disulfiram-like reaction. What triggers that, and what are the key signs and symptoms of it? What factors that apply to the usual means of administering these cephalosporins makes the overall incidence of a disulfiram-like reaction probably quite low in real-world clinical settings?

10. You should never forget that vancomycin (especially when given intravenously) is potentially ototoxic. What does that mean? What other drug or drug group discussed in this unit poses a significant risk of ototoxicity? (***Hint:*** If you're following the chapters in this unit in sequence, you won't be able to answer the second question yet. So keep it in mind so you'll remember when the time comes.)

7. You and a colleague are looking at the label on a package of Primaxin powder for reconstitution. You see that it's actually a combination of both imipenem and cilastatin. A colleague states that they are both antibiotics. What's the real deal, especially the cilastatin part?

CASE STUDY

Pam Guest is a 45-year-old obese woman admitted to your unit with the diagnosis of cholelithiasis and cholecystitis. She complains of abdominal pain; she has a fever of 102° F and a white cell count of 12,000. A nasogastric tube is placed, an IV is started, and 1 gram of cefazolin (Ancef) is ordered every 6 hours. Her cholecystectomy will be scheduled when her temperature returns to normal and evidence of infection has resolved adequately. That will probably be in 2 to 3 days. Until then, her pain will be managed with meperidine (Demerol).

1. Based on the information given in the scenario, what did we *not* do that should have been done?

8. What makes imipenem an attractive choice for managing "mixed infections"?

9. Why do some practitioners refer to vancomycin as a "last resort" drug for managing most infections? A colleague of yours says it's because it just isn't very effective, and that's why it's being used less and less as time passes.

2. At this point we don't know the causative organism for what is apparently a bacterial infection. Comment, then, on the use of cefazolin or another cephalosporin in its class. To what cephalosporin class does cefazolin belong, and how does that affect the choice of this particular antibiotic?

3. Comment on your interpretation of "surgical prophylaxis" as it applies to prescribing antibiotics in general and the use of cefazolin or another drug in its class at this time. Work into your discussion the case of Mrs. Guest.

4. What are the most likely adverse effects of giving this cephalosporin intravenously?

5. How can the possibility of this "most likely adverse response" be minimized?

6. What should the nurse do if she discovers that Mrs. Guest is severely allergic to penicillin?

7. Now, for a tough question that will force you to think from the distant past. What other medication error, or medication misuse, do you see in the scenario for Mrs. Guest?

evolve To check your answers, go to http://evolve.elsevier.com/Lehne/ for Study Guide Comments from the author.

Bacteriostatic Inhibitors of Protein Synthesis: Tetracyclines, Macrolides, Clindamycin, Chloramphenicol, Linezolid, Dalfopristin/Quinupristin, and Spectinomycin

KEY TERMS

aplastic anemia
candidiasis
chelate
gray syndrome
macrolide
MRSA
myelosuppression

pseudomembranous
   colitis (antibiotic-
   induced)
R factor
superinfection
VRE

OBJECTIVES

After reading and studying this chapter you should be able to:

1. Recognize these drugs as (mainly) bacteriostatic inhibitors of bacterial protein synthesis, and be able to explain in general terms why they affect bacteria rather than host cells. (Knowing the precise biochemical mechanisms by which these drugs work—whether they affect the 30S or 50S ribosomal subunits—probably is not essential to having a good knowledge of these drugs. Ask your instructor for his or her advice on this.)

2. State the antibacterial spectrums of the drugs discussed in this chapter, and state whether and why these drugs are first-line (first-choice) agents for the stated indications.

3. Describe the mechanism and possible outcomes of interactions between oral tetracyclines and such minerals as calcium, aluminum, magnesium, iron, and zinc; and give common sources of these interactants.

4. State the drugs (and drug groups) described in this chapter that warrant special considerations for people with liver and/or renal disease, for children, and for pregnant women; explain the basis for those special considerations and the possible consequences if the stated drugs are administered to those individuals.

5. Recognize the macrolides as usually good alternatives to penicillin (e.g., penicillin G) for patients who are or may be allergic to penicillins.

6. List the drugs that should not be combined with erythromycin, and explain the basic mechanisms and outcomes of these interactions should combined administration happen.

7. State the unique adverse responses that apply to chloramphenicol and to linezolid.

246

CRITICAL THINKING AND STUDY QUESTIONS

1. Time for a quick review of principles. Your text notes that tetracyclines, and indeed all the other drugs in this chapter, are bacteriostatic. What does that mean in terms of how these antibiotics affect the growth or replication of susceptible organisms? What host-related factor is essential in order for these medications to exert their optimal efficacy?

2. The tetracyclines bind to the 30S ribosomal subunit of susceptible bacteria. In simple terms, what is the consequence of that in terms of microbial biochemistry?

3. Based on how the main drugs discussed in this chapter inhibit bacterial protein synthesis to cause bacteriostatic effects, can you conclude that all inhibitors of microbial protein synthesis are bacteriostatic? If not, what are some exceptions?

4. What process(es) enable tetracyclines to target susceptible bacteria but not host cells? How are these or other processes changed, over time, leading to tetracycline resistance? Is the resistance issue a minor one or a clinically common and important one?

5. When you think of orally administered tetracyclines you should think automatically of mineral intake. Which minerals should come to mind, where are they typically found, and what is the importance of this whole issue? Your text gives a short list of interactants. Can you add to it?

6. Comment on the suitability of administering tetracyclines to children. What problem(s) may crop up for this age group?

7. A patient with an infection that is responsive to oral doxycycline experiences significant abdominal pain and cramping. It progresses over a couple of days to a "dumping syndrome" characterized by severe, frequent diarrhea. What minor and what worrisome conditions might this reflect?

8. Although most of the tetracyclines are more alike than different, some differences lead to wider prescribing of some (when any tetracycline is indicated). A popular one is doxycycline. What's attractive about that drug, at least for some patients?

9. To which other large and important group of antibiotics is the antibacterial spectrum of activity of the macrolides most similar? When or why might we want to use a macrolide instead of an agent in that other group?

10. In several instances your text notes that food (taken with certain antibiotics) reduces the rate but not the extent of antibiotic absorption. How, then, is overall bioavailability of the antibiotic affected? What pharmacokinetic parameter(s) of the antibiotic might be affected, and how would that depend on how the body handles the specific antibiotic?

11. Your patient is taking linezolid. You've ruled out interactions with other prescribed medications, but now you need to give your patient some instructions on OTC meds and even list some foods and beverages that should be avoided. To what are we referring, and why is this important?

12. A patient taking an antibiotic develops what appears to be antibiotic-associated pseudomembranous colitis. What should be done, and done as soon as possible?

    Some quick hits... key things you must remember about specific bacteriostatic microbial protein synthesis inhibitors. For each of the antibiotics below, list one or a few "must know" points about the agent.

13. Clindamycin

14. Chloramphenicol

15. Linezolid

CASE STUDY

Patty Sims is a 30-year-old office worker who reports to the healthcare facility with a fever of 101° F and a nonproductive cough that has lasted 10 days. On physical exam her respiratory rate is 24 and nonlabored, and bilateral basilar crackles (rales) are heard.

Blood and sputum are cultured. The results indicate a respiratory tract infection with Streptococcus pneumoniae.

Mrs. Sims is advised to take acetaminophen (325 mg q 4 hr for fever until the fever is gone or for up to 7 days in a row), to drink 6 to 8 glasses of water a day, and to stay home from work for 2 to 3 days. Of course, we need to prescribe a suitable antibiotic. Mrs. Sims mentions that she's gotten hives "real bad" when she's taken penicillin before.

1. Which antibiotic might we use for her?

2. In discussing Mrs. Sims's planned therapy, she tells you that she's terrible in terms of keeping up with her medications. She's always forgetting to take her pills. What macrolide might offer some help in this regard, and why? Consider, too, that Mrs. Sims is taking theophylline, which can become an important interactant with some macrolides.

3. We learn that Mrs. Sims has recurrent asthma, for which she is taking Theo-Dur, a theophylline (methylxanthine) preparation. How would you expect her *S. pneumoniae* infection to affect her *need* for the theophylline? How might the antibiotic we just prescribed affect her *response* to the theophylline? Are there other concerns you might have about this drug combination or the use of theophylline in general? How would you assess for it? (Yes, you may have to revisit Chapter 71, *Drugs for Asthma.*)

4. How will the acetaminophen affect the underlying *S. pneumoniae* infection and the symptoms of it? How will it interact with the prescribed antibiotic?

5. Why did the physician not recommend aspirin or any of the other nonsteroidal anti-inflammatory drugs (NSAIDs) instead of the acetaminophen? (You may have to visit Chapters 67 for this information.)

6. Mrs. Sims calls the office, complaining of nonspecific but bothersome abdominal pain, nausea, vomiting, and diarrhea. What should come to mind regarding this? Briefly consider both common and relatively innocuous causes, as well as the most serious concern associated with erythromycins. Tell us what you'd be thinking if Mrs. Sims called a couple of days after she started her antibiotic and how you might change your thinking (diagnosis) if her call about GI complaints came a couple of weeks after her course of antibiotic therapy was finished.

7. Assume for a moment that Mrs. Sims is 70 years old, and instead of having a history of asthma she's been discharged from the hospital after being diagnosed with atrial fibrillation. Given her age, there were no extraordinary attempts to convert her dysrhythmia; she has been placed on prophylactic warfarin. Two weeks later she develops the *S. pneumoniae* infection. What might we do in this instance? Would erythromycin be a good choice for Mrs. Sims? Should we be managing her pneumonia on an outpatient basis?

evolve To check your answers, go to http://evolve.elsevier.com/Lehne/ for Study Guide Comments from the author.

Aminoglycosides: Bactericidal Inhibitors of Protein Synthesis

KEY TERMS

audiometry
bactericidal
otic (e.g., route of
   topical drug
   administration)
ototoxicity (cochlear and
   vestibular)

physical incompatibility
   (between two or more
   drugs)
tinnitus
trough level (of drug)

OBJECTIVES

After reading and studying this chapter you should
be able to:

1. Discuss the mechanism of action and main indications for aminoglycosides.
2. Recognize that nephrotoxicity and ototoxicity are
the two main toxicities of aminoglycosides, and
describe precautions (dosing schedules, monitoring) that need to be taken to prevent or at least
detect them.
3. Identify other drugs that increase the risk of
aminoglycoside-induced nephrotoxicity and ototoxicity, and describe the factors that should be
considered when deciding whether to use or
avoid using them when aminoglycosides are
used.

Note: Aminoglycosides almost certainly should be
tops on every nursing student's list of drugs that can
cause ototoxicity (hearing loss). Hearing loss is an
often-ignored health problem. Whether it is drug-
induced or not, more than 26 million Americans
have hearing loss, and relatively few do anything
about it. But it's rarely an issue in basic healthcare
curricula that are supposed to be "holistic." So this is
a good opportunity to learn more about drugs and
ototoxicity, and what can be done for hearing loss,
regardless of the cause. So, please, see study question 5 below.

CRITICAL THINKING AND STUDY QUESTIONS

1. A patient received a neuromuscular blocking
agent during surgery. In the recovery room, the
physician orders gentamicin 40 mg IV stat as prophylaxis against an anticipated infection. About
what should you be concerned with this combination of drugs? Why?

2. According to some authorities, some of the fluoroquinolone antibiotics (ciprofloxacin and others;
see Ch. 87) were considered mainstays of therapy
for *Pseudomonas aeruginosa.* This was not only
because of efficacy against this organism, but also
because of a relatively better safety profile, especially with respect to more severe adverse
responses. Why is there now a "rethinking" such
that at some agencies aminoglycosides, with their
known serious toxic consequences, are first-line
for this infection? What's the overall lesson that
we should learn?

250

3. Some aminoglycosides are formulated as ear drops, indicated for treating otitis caused by responsive organisms. Yet aminoglycosides are widely known as being ototoxic. Is this safe, or logical? What condition, if any, should be met (other than presence of responsive bacterial strains) in order to use aminoglycoside otic formulations safely?

4. Which other drugs or drug classes can increase the risk of nephrotoxicity during aminoglycoside therapy? Which probably poses the biggest risk, and under what administration circumstances?

5. What other medications can increase the risk or severity of aminoglycoside-mediated ototoxicity? In a more general sense, what are the other main drugs that can cause hearing loss or tinnitus, regardless of whether they're used with an aminoglycoside?

Since hearing loss is the most common and severe manifestation of ototoxicity, and the main way to help the person who becomes hearing-impaired is through the use of hearing aids, do you know anything about those devices—the various types? how they may or may not help? for which degrees of hearing loss they may be helpful? why people who might be helped by them often don't wear them? how much they cost? whether the patient's health insurance will pay for them?

As a future healthcare professional, one who is interested in the "whole patient," this is information you should want to know. Indeed, if *you* have hearing impairments to the point that you need hearing aids, can you still be a nurse?

Check out *http://www-personal.umich.edu/~mshlafer/hearing.html* and you'll find out... and find many links for more information.

CASE STUDY

Jill Brown, 30 years old, was recently diagnosed with ovarian cancer. She has been admitted to the *hospital to start her course of chemotherapy with cisplatin (Platinol AQ; see Chapter 98) for the ovarian cancer. Shortly after the start of the chemotherapy she develops a severe Pseudomonas aeruginosa infection, for which intravenous gentamicin is ordered. She is started on IV therapy with that drug at the "usually proper" dose.*

1. Briefly describe the most common serious adverse (toxic) reactions of the aminoglycosides, and state how they relate to the pharmacokinetics of these drugs.

2. Discuss the overall goal and timing of monitoring serum levels of the aminoglycoside, and why this is important.

3. What organ-specific toxicity is shared by cisplatin and the aminoglycosides? (Yes, you may have to look ahead to Chapter 98 to get some information on the cisplatin.)

4. Why might we consider using amikacin instead of gentamicin or another aminoglycoside? What are its advantages, real or otherwise?

Ms. Brown takes an unexpected turn for the worse. Septicemia develops during the combined cisplatin-aminoglycoside regimen. Cardiac output falls, and she is retaining a considerable amount of sodium and fluid. We start proper medical therapy to increase her cardiac output, but because of concerns over severe edema, and failing kidney function, one of the meds she's placed on is furosemide (Lasix; a "loop diuretic"; see Chapter 39). In Ms. Brown's case diuretic therapy must be aggressive and prompt, so parenteral administration is indicated.

5. What common dose-related toxic adverse effect is shared by all three drugs: the cisplatin, the aminoglycoside, *and* the furosemide? How do these drugs interact to increase the risk of this adverse response?

6. How do we monitor for this "common adverse" effect shared by the three drugs we've been focusing on?

7. Your text notes that the aminoglycosides can cause "high-frequency hearing loss." Do you have any idea what that entails? ...what the impact of that may be on Ms. Brown's day-to-day ability to hear and communicate?

8. Since each of these drugs can potentiate the ability of any of the others to cause this common toxicity, which should be withheld from this patient?

9. Ms. Brown knows full well that she's lost a considerable degree of her hearing. She hears sound "sort of OK," but can't understand precisely what is being said to her all the time. She has a terrible time discriminating between "sound-alike" words and doesn't enjoy listening to music anymore because it sounds "so different." Ms. Brown asks when she will get her hearing back to normal and whether there's a drug that will help her recover. What are the fundamental elements of your response to her in terms of the short- and long-term outlook?

10. Ms. Brown then asks about what might happen if she gets another infection. She's heard of people getting very sick after receiving an antibiotic to which they've had a "bad reaction" before. She says, "If I've lost most of my hearing already, and get another infection, will I have an adverse reaction to the antibiotic I get.... maybe lose the rest of my hearing?" How might you respond?

11. Your text correctly notes some concerns with ampicillin and aminoglycosides. In question 10 we said that there would be no problem if Ms. Brown got a penicillin, even ampicillin, after having a course of aminoglycoside therapy. What, then, is the "problem" with these two important classes of antibiotics?

evolve To check your answers, go to http://evolve.elsevier.com/Lehne/ for Study Guide Comments from the author.

Sulfonamides and Trimethoprim

KEY TERMS

crystalluria
dihydrofolate reductase
hematopoiesis
hyperbilirubinemia
kernicterus

megaloblastic anemia
PABA
Stevens-Johnson syndrome

OBJECTIVES

After reading and studying this chapter you should
be able to:

1. State the antimicrobial mechanism of action of
   sulfonamides and of trimethoprim and explain
   why their effects on susceptible bacteria do not
   affect human cells at the same time.
2. Describe the primary uses for sulfonamides,
   trimethoprim, and the combination of the two
   drugs.
3. Recognize the linkage between sulfonamides and
   Stevens-Johnson syndrome, hemolytic anemia, and
   kernicterus. Describe the patient populations who
   are at highest risk of these serious disorders. State
   how you might recognize Stevens-Johnson syndrome or hemolytic anemia; list their major signs
   and symptoms in the context of how we should be
   monitoring for these untoward responses.
4. Explain the general way that sulfonamide-
   induced crystalluria occurs, and state two simple
   yet usually effective and appropriate ways to
   reduce the risks, at least for certain patients.
5. Name two or three other groups of drugs that
   might cross-react and cause adverse responses in
   patients who have had hypersensitivity reactions
   to sulfonamide antibiotics.
6. Recognize that trimethoprim rarely causes megaloblastic anemia and state the patient characteristics that pose a greater risk of this potentially
   serious response. Explain the signs and symptoms of megaloblastic anemia and what to do to
   prevent it or manage it if it occurs.
7. Explain the clinical and biochemical rationales
   for the frequent combination of sulfamethoxazole
   with trimethoprim.

CRITICAL THINKING AND STUDY QUESTIONS

1. What are probably the two main reasons that sulfonamides aren't used much topically, especially
   on the skin?

2. Like many people, Joe Jingleheimer (50 years old)
   has no reliable information about his health history, particularly with respect to drug allergies.
   After going for many years without seeing a doctor for a complete physical, he has his first appointment for what he hopes will be a long-time
   interaction with his new personal physician. The
   MD makes a good diagnosis of diabetes mellitus
   (type 2), mild hypertension, and mild heart failure.

Joe is placed on tolbutamide for his diabetes and
digoxin and hydrochlorothiazide for the heart failure
signs and symptoms. The hope is that the hydrochlorothiazide will also lower Joe's blood pressure
adequately.

He travels to a remote part of the world and just as
he returns home to visit the doctor, he develops a
severe case of gastritis and urinary tract infection
with E. coli from some "bad" foods and liquids he's
ingested.

A. What are your concerns about using a sulfonamide or a sulfonamide plus trimethoprim for
   this patient?

B. Do you have any concerns about the use of a sulfonamide, or its combination with TMZ and the use of the diuretic?

Joe, despite emphatically denying any medication allergies, develops hives and other indicators of a hypersensitivity reaction once he starts his tolbutamide-digoxin-hydrochlorothiazide regimen.

C. Which, if any, of those medications may be responsible for his signs and symptoms? Why?

3. Many texts cite the use of trimethoprim (TMP) and sulfimethoxazole (SMZ) together as a great (if not best) example of a "synergistic antibiotic combination." What in general (i.e., with respect to any drug combination) is meant by the term synergistic? What is the specific synergy involving the combined use TMP + SMZ?

4. Several texts warn against administering systemic ester-type local anesthetics (e.g., procaine, tetracaine; see Chapter 25) to patients who are receiving a sulfonamide. What is the rationale for this? (Yes, this is a tough question!)

CASE STUDY

Mary Markle is a 35-year-old woman with a history of epilepsy (generalized tonic-clonic seizures) and hypertension. Her medications include phenytoin and hydrochlorothiazide. Both disorders are con- *trolled well with the medications. Mrs. Markle becomes pregnant. In the middle of her first trimester she develops an acute urinary tract infection (UTI).*

1. The physician orders trimethoprim-sulfamethoxazole, and no matter what you ask the prescription is filled and the patient begins taking this combination. Why are you concerned?

The physician responds by saying that the TMP-SMZ therapy is going to last less than 2 weeks and that it shouldn't exert any adverse fetal effects. After all, normal pregnancies last 9 months.

2. Considering this patient is taking phenytoin for seizures during her pregnancy, what nutritional supplement might (should) she be taking to reduce the risk of adverse fetal effects from her anticonvulsant? Why? Could this have an impact on her body's response to the TMP-SMZ and treating her UTI?

3. How might the TMP-SMZ affect Mrs. Markle's response to the anticonvulsant, and why?

4. You tell a colleague about your concern that Mrs. Markle might develop crystalluria in response to the TMP-SMZ. He comments that you shouldn't worry because crystalluria from the sulfonamides occurs when the drug gets concentrated in the urine. "Mrs. Markle is taking a diuretic... there's no way crystalluria can happen." Heck, let's really reduce the risk of crystalluria by having the patient take sodium bicarbonate. What are your thoughts about this?

5. Now the sodium bicarbonate issue. As you should know (see Chapter 40), the sodium in sodium bicarbonate (baking soda) is readily absorbed. When the excess sodium gets into the bloodstream, what is likely to happen to blood volume and blood pressure? Link this to the reason(s) that Mrs. Markle was taking a diuretic in the first place.

evolve To check your answers, go to http://evolve.elsevier.com/Lehne/ for Study Guide Comments from the author.

Drug Therapy of Urinary Tract Infections

KEY TERMS

bacteriuria
crystalluria
cystitis

nosocomial
pyelonephritis
urethritis

OBJECTIVES

After reading and studying this chapter you should
be able to:

1. Compare and contrast the etiologies and symptoms of acute cystitis and acute pyelonephritis.
2. Recognize *E. coli* as the main cause of community-acquired UTIs in women and an infrequent
   cause of nosocomial UTIs.
3. Compare and contrast what the text describes as
   short-course and conventional therapy for lower
   UTIs. Identify the major patient populations who
   generally are not candidates for short-course
   treatment.
4. State the key aspect of therapy (other than need
   for hospitalization) that distinguishes our pharmacologic approaches to uncomplicated lower
   UTIs vs. acute pyelonephritis.
5. Differentiate between relapse and reinfection as
   causes of recurrent UTIs, and identify the relative
   prevalence of each. State the general clinical
   approaches for each, and state the general clinical
   presentations that would warrant considering
   long-term prophylaxis.

Note that this chapter focuses on the use of urinary
tract antiseptics. Other important drugs, a variety of
antibiotics, are discussed elsewhere. Be sure to consult those sources as needed: see Chapter 80 for
information on the penicillins, Chapter 84 for the
sulfonamides and trimethoprim, Chapter 83 for
aminoglycosides and Chapter 87 for the fluoroquinolones.

CRITICAL THINKING AND STUDY QUESTIONS

1. A colleague notes that nitrofurantoin (e.g.,
   Furadantin and Macrodantin) is a broad-spectrum
   of antimicrobial action and that at sufficiently
   high concentrations it's bacteriostatic. He states
   that were it not for some significant systemic side
   effects and toxicities, it would be a great drug for
   treating systemic infections caused by multiple
   sensitive organisms. With which of his points
   would you agree and disagree? Say why.

2. Your colleague then demonstrates his further
   knowledge of macrodantin, saying that the
   macrocrystalline preparation (Macrodantin)
   causes a better, bigger therapeutic effect than the
   microcrystalline form (Furadantin). He lectures
   you: "Macro.... Big... big effect." Is he on target?

3. What are the most serious (not most common)
   adverse responses to nitrofurantoin and how do
   we monitor for them?

4. Explain why we have concerns about administering methenamine to persons with liver dysfunction. After all, the active metabolites are formed in the urine, right?

5. You have a patient who is taking methenamine. You need to caution him against taking OTC meds that can alkalinize the urine. Why? You think antacids, "Oh, my patient mentioned that he often takes Maalox for heartburn." You now wonder, "Should I tell her not to take the Maalox?" And they said something about taking OTC Zantac (ranitidine) too. Are you concerned about interactions with the methenamine?

6. The text notes that drugs that elevate urine pH inhibit methenamine's ability to form its active metabolite, formaldehyde. It specifically mentions acetazolamide. So, to tweak your memory... What is acetazolamide and the drug class to which it belongs? How does it alkalinize the urine? For what might you see the drug or another drug in its class being prescribed? Will all drugs in its class counteract methenamine's effectiveness?

7. A patient with acute pyelonephritis is under your care in the hospital. A colleague comes in and peruses the patient's chart and asks why this individual isn't being managed with a urinary tract antiseptic. Explain why, and tell us what our proper approach to this condition is.

8. Nalidixic acid (NegGram) tends to cause a rather low incidence of severe adverse reactions. It does cause photosensitive skin reactions and some transient blurring of vision, and it may exacerbate epilepsy. But for the adult population as a whole, it seems to be a "decent" drug. Why, then, don't we consider it a first-line agent? And is that "limitation" usually a problem with the drug itself?

CASE STUDY

Rick Tyson is 65 years old. His essential hypertension has been managed for about 20 years. For a while he was taking a beta blocker, but 8 years ago he was switched to an angiotensin-converting enzyme (ACE) inhibitor when his fasting blood glucose levels began creeping into a prediabetic range. However, fasting and postprandial blood glucose levels and biannual checks of glycated hemoglobins (HbA$_{1c}$) have never reached the point that the physician felt antidiabetic drug therapy was necessary. Mr. Tyson's resting blood pressure on the ACE inhibitor is now 140/80—rather typical of the systolic hypertension seen in someone Mr. Tyson's age who has antihypertensive treatment.

Mr. Tyson had acute gout about 10 years ago. After successful treatment with indomethacin, he was placed on long-term therapy with probenecid, a uricosuric drug (see Chapter 69). His serum uric acid levels on probenecid are in the high-normal range but he has had no gout attacks. Urate levels rose significantly after two attempts to discontinue the probenecid, so he remains on that drug.

Mr. Tyson had two elective surgeries for hip replacement in the last 18 months. His last surgery was 4 months ago. During both hospitalizations for surgery Mr. Tyson had some complications that required brief placement of a Foley catheter, and each time he developed an acute but uncomplicated urinary tract infection that was apparently treated successfully with a course of nitrofurantoin (Macrodantin).

Finally, there are obvious notations on Mr. Tyson's chart saying "Penicillin Allergy."

1. Mr. Tyson experienced no significant adverse effects to the nitrofurantoin, but during the first course of treatment he became alarmed when his urine turned brown, despite having an adequately copious urine output. What did the discoloration of his urine most likely reflect?

2. How is the diagnosis of UTI made?

3. Now Mr. Tyson develops a chronic UTI and goes to the physician's office. He denies any flank pain or chills. He is afebrile. If he had reported those signs and had a fever, what might you suspect?

We're comfortable with the conclusion that Mr. Tyson's UTI involves only the urethra. You do a careful check of his medication history and learn that when his hypertension was first diagnosed he was placed on hydrochlorothiazide. He developed a severe rash from it. For whatever reason, the physician tried another thiazide, and again there was what appeared to be a hypersensitivity reaction, only more severe. Then there was a short trial with furosemide, with the same outcome. Although these responses were charted, no conclusion about the cause(s) was made, or at least charted.

4. What might you conclude about these responses and how might it affect the decision about how to manage his present chronic UTI?

5. What drug(s) might we rule out for managing the chronic UTI? What might we be left with as acceptable other choices?

6. Mr. Tyson's physician elects to try a course of low-dose methenamine (Mandelamine and others). What is the active antibacterial metabolite of methenamine and what local physiologic condition must be met in order for that metabolite to be formed?

7. Do the local (urine) conditions that optimize methenamine's effectiveness affect the risks to a patient with hyperuricemia? What are those risks and why do they occur? Are there any added concerns or risks for a patient such as Mr. Tyson who is taking probenecid?

evolve To check your answers, go to http://evolve.elsevier.com/Lehne/ for Study Guide Comments from the author.

Antimycobacterial Agents: Drugs for Tuberculosis, Leprosy, and *Mycobacterium avium* Complex Infection

KEY TERMS

acetylation (as a process in drug metabolism)
Hansen's disease
mycobacteria
mycolic acids
PPD (preparation for TB skin testing)
rifamycins (e.g., rifampin)

OBJECTIVES

After reading and studying this chapter you should be able to:

1. Discuss the concept of "targeted tuberculin skin testing" for *Mycobacterium tuberculosis* in the context of who should be "targeted" and who (based on assessed risk) should be treated if a skin test is positive.
2. Describe the first-line drugs used for tuberculosis: what they are, their main individual and collective risks of toxicity to the host; and drug interactions that are likely to be encountered.
3. Describe the additional issues involved when treating patients who have tuberculosis and are HIV positive. State why it is a dilemma with no easy solution, as the text describes it.
4. Recognize that there are genetically based differences that affect how quickly a person metabolizes (acetylates) isoniazid. Given that, compare and contrast the impact of slow (and fast) acetylation on the therapeutic response to this drug (efficacy) and toxicity that affects the liver *and* other structures or functions.
5. Recognize rifampin (a rifamycin) as a classic example of a drug that inhibits the hepatic metabolism of many other drugs (including some of the

anti-TB drugs with which it is routinely used) and can cause significant rises in blood levels of those interactants (with a usual outcome being excessive or toxic effects). Also recognize the drug's hepatotoxicity and its ability to add to or potentiate hepatotoxicity caused by other drugs with that property.

CRITICAL THINKING AND STUDY QUESTIONS

1. At the very outset, the text chapter identifies several characteristics of mycobacteria, and treatment of mycobacterial infections, that make clinical management problematic. What are they?

2. Tuberculosis (TB) is a major worldwide disease and new cases globally are arising. What are the two main factors that seem to account for this?

3. What one host-related factor enables some people to harbor tubercle bacilli but not to develop clinical tuberculosis?

259

4. Aside from pulmonary dysfunction, what are the consequences in terms of the immune response and drug therapy of necrotic areas of tissue developing in the lung tissues?

5. Traditional microbiologic methods to culture and test the antibiotic sensitivity of microbes in body fluid samples usually yield results in a day or so. In terms of time needed to get this information, how does *M. tuberculosis* differ? What are the implications of that in terms of beginning therapy and the mycobacterial response to therapy?

6. Whether we look at TB patients in the United States or worldwide, we should be worried about the development of multidrug-resistant strains of mycobacteria. What is the principle cause of this alarming trend?

7. You've learned that for most bacterial infections we use a single drug (when possible) with a spectrum that is sufficiently focused (narrow) to target the bug we're trying to kill. Why do we do that? How do things differ with TB or other mycobacterial infections?

8. What is the significance of mycolic acids in the context of this chapter's main theme?

9. A colleague states that people who are *slow* acetylators with respect to isoniazid metabolism will have a reduced clinical (antimycobacterial) response to the drug, an increased susceptibility to the development of resistant strains, and a reduced risk of hepatotoxicity. Do you agree? If not, why not?

10. When rifampin (or rifapentine or rifabutin, collectively referred to as rifamycins) are administered with many other drugs, as they usually are, there are two common clinical (therapeutic) problems for which you must automatically be on the lookout. What are they, and why do those problems occur?

11. At least one widely used antitubercular drug can cause peripheral signs and symptoms that might be described as tingling, numb, or burning of the hands and feet. What is the drug associated with this? What is the underlying cause? Who seems to be a greater risk? And what can we do about it?

12. We have a patient with active HIV infection and he is among the 2% to 20% of such infected individuals who also develop TB. The text notes a therapeutic dilemma when we attempt to treat both. What is it?

13. Your text notes that such drugs as para-amino-salicylic acid (PAS), kanamycin, ciprofloxacin, and a few other drugs are considered second-line drugs for TB. Throughout the text we've been talking about why some drugs are considered first-line, others not. What is that general theme or concept?

14. There are two main classes of leprosy, based on the presence or absence of *M. leprae* in skin smears. One type is paucibacillary leprosy. What is the meaning of the prefix "pauci?" (**Hint:** You may be able to figure it out from this sentence: There is a paucity of leprosy cases in and originating within the United States, and so most nursing curricula don't include much content about it or its treatment. Therefore we won't provide any self-study questions about it either.)

15. Bonus: Can you think of another drug (in a completely different category) that is metabolized by acetylation? Its effects (good and bad) depend to a degree on whether the patient acetylates the drug quickly or slowly. It, too, causes paresthesias and other neurologic side effects that related to vitamin B_6 "deficiencies." (**Hint:** The one I'm thinking of is somewhere in the cardiovascular unit.)

CASE STUDY

Steve Evans, a homeless 45-year-old male, presents to the emergency department with weight loss, lethargy, a low-grade fever, and a productive cough streaked with blood. His chest x-ray indicates a suspicious area in the middle right lobe. He is hospitalized, and sputum cultures are ordered. The sputum cultures reveal Mycobacterium tuberculosis. His active TB is to be treated with a combination of drugs based on the sputum culture drug sensitivity. The concern with Mr. Evans is his socioeconomic status and the fact that he has no permanent address. Follow-up will be difficult, but it is essential to determine the effectiveness of treatment with the combination of drugs. Mr. Evans is started on isoniazid (INH) and rifampin in the initial phase of therapy. It is crucial that he take the medication exactly as prescribed to prevent spread of the TB to others. Mr. Evans must come to the health center monthly for sputum evaluations for at least 6 months. You also need to see all of the people who share facilities with Mr. Evans to screen them for TB and prophylactically treat them with isoniazid.

1. Why is it essential to evaluate Mr. Evans's personal contacts for TB?

2. In evaluating the contacts associated with Mr. Evans, what considerations are made to determine whether they are candidates for isoniazid prophylactic therapy?

3. Why is TB on the rise again after being controlled in the United States for many years?

4. What makes compliance to the drug therapy for tuberculosis so difficult?

5. What is the drug of choice as the primary agent for treatment and prophylaxis of tuberculosis, and why is this true?

6. What are the concerns regarding Mr. Evans taking his medications? What information do you need to help him plan for the medication protocol?

7. If Mr. Evans were found to be HIV positive, what drug-drug interactions might occur between his tuberculosis drug therapy and his HIV drug therapy?

evolve To check your answers, go to http://evolve.elsevier.com/Lehne/ for Study Guide Comments from the author.

CHAPTER 07

Miscellaneous Antibacterial Drugs: Fluoroquinolones, Metronidazole, Rifampin, Bacitracin, and Polymyxins

KEY TERMS

DNA gyrase   fluoroquinolone

OBJECTIVES

After reading and studying this chapter you should be able to:

1. Summarize the main clinical uses for the fluoroquinolones, focusing on the organisms and infections for which one of these drugs is considered first-choice therapy.
2. Describe the adverse effects of fluoroquinolones.
3. Recognize that tendon rupture is a rather unique "adverse response" associated with ciprofloxacin. You should have a simple understanding of how it can occur (impaired collagen synthesis), how the risk requires avoiding use of the drug in certain patient populations (you should know which ones), and how we should monitor for it when we do use the drug.
4. Recognize the potential of serious neurotoxicity and nephrotoxicity associated with parenteral use of polymyxin B, and that such concerns largely limit use of this drug other than as a topical anti-infective.

Note: Be sure to consult Chapter 95 for more information on metronidazole and its main use for protozoal infections. Also refer to Chapter 86 for more information about rifampin and its main use for adjunctive management of tuberculosis. Since those chapters contain more comprehensive information on those drugs, we will omit study items dealing with metronidazole and rifampin here. We'll also refer you to other related chapters where you'll find applicable case studies.

CRITICAL THINKING AND STUDY QUESTIONS

1. The text notes that fluoroquinolones exert their antibacterial effects by inhibiting DNA gyrase. What is that?

2. What general properties of the fluoroquinolones (e.g., ciprofloxacin or the group as a whole) make them such useful, and often preferred, antibiotics for a variety of infections with susceptible organisms?

263

3. When you think of orally administered fluoro-quinolones (e.g., ciprofloxacin), you should think automatically of mineral intake and simultaneous ingestion of these antibiotics. Which minerals should come to mind, where are they typically found, and what is the importance of this whole issue? To which other class of antibiotics (discussed elsewhere in this unit) do similar concerns and precautions apply?

4. In these troubled times, with concerns about bioterrorism, why has ciprofloxacin gotten so much attention in the news? Some have argued that the public at-large, or at least those with a higher-than-usual risk from this specific means of bioterrorism, receive ciprofloxacin. Give you thoughts about this concept.

5. What are some of the main similarities and differences between ciprofloxacin and the other fluoroquinolones identified in this chapter? Are all the drugs in this group so similar in basically all the clinically important effects that all you may need to look up in a reference book is the dosage (because of different potencies)?

6. According to many experts, metronidazole (given intravenously) is now a first-choice agent for managing antibiotic-associated suprainfection. In this role it has replaced a traditional antibiotic that for years was considered the first choice.

A. What is the main and usually most lethal condition seen in antibiotic-associated suprainfection? What is the main clinical presentation (signs and symptoms that lead to lethality or severe number 1 choice drug, which metronidazole has now replaced?

B. What was that number 1 choice drug, which metronidazole has now replaced?

C. Why has that previous first-choice drug become a second-choice agent? Is it because of lack of efficacy? Does that former "number 1 agent" play any role in managing this condition nowadays?

evolve To check your answers, go to http://evolve.elsevier.com/Lehne/ for Study Guide Comments from the author.

Antifungal Agents

KEY TERMS

azole antifungal
  (class of drugs)
candidiasis
dermatophyte
ergosterol
lozenge
mycosis (mycoses)
onychomycosis

opportunistic (or non-
  opportunistic) infection
polyene antibiotic
thrush
tinea (as a general name
  for dermatophytic
  mycoses)
troche

OBJECTIVES

After reading and studying this chapter you should
be able to:

1. Compare and contrast opportunistic and non-
   opportunistic infections (the general terms), particularly as they tell us about the patient
   populations most likely to acquire them. Name
   one type of infection for each category (prefer-
   ably, you will name the most common or most
   prevalent infection as identified in the text).
2. Identify the drug that is the agent of choice for
   most systemic mycoses; describe its main mechanism of antifungal action; state whether it is best
   used for minor or more serious fungal infections,
   and why.
3. Compare and contrast the basic biology, epidemiology, and treatment of fungi as opposed to bacteria. In your comparison, state why amphotericin
   B is effective against fungi but not against bacteria, and state why host-centered toxicity of
   amphotericin B is much greater and more prevalent than that of most antibiotics.
4. Discuss the main indications for intravenous
   amphotericin B; identify the drug's three most
   common adverse responses and the precautions
   that should be taken to minimize their effects.
5. Recognize what azole antifungal drugs are (give
   examples) and that when given systemically
   they can be a major cause of interactions with
   other drugs by inhibiting their hepatic metabolism.

CRITICAL THINKING AND STUDY QUESTIONS

1. Why do we care about ergosterol? What is its
   general significance in terms of the theme of this
   chapter and its specific importance with respect
   to the two main drugs or drug groups (amphotericin B and the azole antifungals) described in
   this chapter?

2. What are the most likely adverse responses (and
   signs and symptoms thereof) to intravenous
   infusion of amphotericin B. How in general do
   they occur, and how can they be minimized?

3. Given the main potential serum electrolyte
   abnormality (see above), what other class of
   drugs might aggravate this problem if they were
   administered concomitantly? There is one large
   group of drugs, commonly used, about which
   you should be thinking.

265

4. Several lipid-based amphotericin B formulations are available. What advantage(s) do they have over conventional formulations of the drug (i.e., amphotericin B deoxycholate [Fungizone intravenous])? Given the advantage(s), why aren't they used more often than they are? For now, ignore these points as they apply to topical administration of the drug.

5. When a patient is receiving a systemic (e.g., oral) azole antifungal agent and one or more other medications, what one thing must you check out (e.g., with a consult to a good reference book or a clinical pharmacist), and why?

6. While amphotericin B and ketoconazole are alike in many ways, as far as fungi are concerned, they differ in their mechanism of action. The azole antifungals inhibit steroid synthesis and so they have some potential for unique adverse effects in mammalian hosts. What are they?

7. Another difference between systemic amphotericin B and the azole antifungals is the main target of organ toxicity to the host. What, specifically, are we referring to?

8. Your text notes that itraconazole has negative inotropic actions that can decrease ejection fraction. What do those terms mean?

9. With the onset of summer and time to tan, a patient notices the development of "spots" on her upper arms and shoulders. They're small and of irregular shape and range in color from white (the patient's skin color when they weren't tanned) to pink to brown. What is a reasonable diagnosis and what are some of the approaches we might use to manage it?

10. What is thrush? What class of drugs (*Hint:* They are used to manage asthma in some patients.) can cause this side effect? How does it occur, and how can this drug-induced thrush be prevented?

CASE STUDY

Dana Throw is a 25-year-old woman who was recently diagnosed with acute myelogenous leukemia (AML). She is admitted for the induction phase of chemotherapy. Her platelet count is low and she has vaginal candidiasis.

The treatment of choice for her fungal infection is clotrimazole. It is essential that extreme care be taken in providing nursing care to Ms. Throw because she is at high risk for additional infections that could now be lethal. There are many areas to consider when combining the treatment for fungus with the numerous other physical problems faced by a patient with AML.

1. What are the side effects that Ms. Throw should know about when using intravaginal clotrimazole tablets for her vaginal infection?

2. Where are the most common sites of candida infections?

3. What is an oral troche?

4. Ms. Throw asks why she must use the vaginal tablets when she already has an IV for chemotherapy administration. What should you tell her?

Ms. Throw's fungal infection has advanced because of her severely compromised immune system. She now has systemic mycoses, which requires amphotericin B for treatment.

5. What system is typically affected adversely by amphotericin B, and is it relatively common or rare?

6. The amphotericin B is dispensed as a powder. This 50 mg of powder must be reconstituted using 10 ml of sterile water that does not contain a bacteriostatic agent, and then diluted with D_5W (5% dextrose in sterile water) to a concentration of 0.1 mg/mL for infusion. Why must the drug be mixed this way?

7. After Ms. Throw's test dose of amphotericin B, you are to give her 0.25 mg/kg of drug. She weighs 110 pounds. How many mg will you give her? Based on the information in question 6, describe exactly how much liquid you will have after reconstituting the drug and then diluting it.

8. What pretreatment medication would be used for mild versus severe reactions to amphotericin B?

evolve To check your answers, go to http://evolve.elsevier.com/Lehne/ for Study Guide Comments from the author.

Antiviral Agents I: Drugs for Non-HIV Viral Infections

KEY TERMS

cytomegalovirus (CMV)
DNA polymerase (and its inhibitors)
Guillian-Barré syndrome
herpes labialis
herpes simplex virus (HSV)
interferon(s)
neuraminidase (and its inhibitors)

obligate parasite
pegylation (as in long-acting interferons)
purine nucleoside
shingles
thrombocytopenic purpura
varicella-zoster virus (VZV)
zoster

OBJECTIVES

After reading and studying this chapter you should be able to:

1. Summarize the main similarities (and differences) between the way a typical antibiotic affects bacterial metabolism, with minimal or no effects on host cell metabolism, and the way antiviral drugs affect both the target organisms and the host more often than the typical antibiotics.
2. Consider acyclovir as the drug of choice for most herpes simplex and varicella-zoster viruses, and focus on its main actions, uses, and other key clinical pharmacologic properties.
3. Describe the adverse effects of acyclovir and ganciclovir, and how administration route affects those responses.
4. Compare and contrast hepatitis B and C, the two most common strains of viral hepatitis, in terms of prevalence, mode of transmission, incidences of acute and chronic disease, lethality, and prevention/management (vaccines, treatments for active disease).
5. Summarize some current guidelines or recommendations for prophylactic influenza vaccination. Identify high-risk populations who are most likely to benefit from prophylaxis. Explain why we seem to have to keep changing the vaccines from one flu season to the next.

CRITICAL THINKING AND STUDY QUESTIONS

1. It's pretty easy to kill or inhibit the growth of bacteria using suitable antibiotics, without affecting normal metabolic pathways of host cells. Are things similar for viruses and most antiviral drugs?

2. Viruses are described as obligate parasites. What does that mean, and what are the implications of that in terms of antiviral drug therapy now and in the future?

3. Both viruses and cancer cells, and drugs typically used to treat them, use chemicals and chemical pathways on which normal mammalian cells depend. Likewise, the drugs we use to treat these infections act on those chemicals and pathways. Are viruses and cancer cells therefore the same thing?

4. In this text (and many other references) and in common conversation, you'll encounter the word *zoster*. What's a zoster? You don't need to quote a dictionary. Just give me a reasonable definition.

C. What is apparently the most common reason or mechanism by which acyclovir-sensitive viruses become resistant to the drug?

5. Your text notes that acyclovir is much more effective against herpes simplex virus (HSV) than it is against cytomegalovirus (CMV). Show your knowledge of basic acyclovir pharmacology to explain why this is so. (**Hint:** Your answer needs to include some comments about metabolism of the drug, and basic concepts of enzyme-substrate interactions that you learned in biochemistry should be plenty good for the answer.)

8. A patient presents with what is diagnosed as an initial genital herpes infection (HSV-2). Topical acylcovir could be prescribed but the physician decides it's best to start therapy with the oral dosage form of the drug, even though this is the first infection. Why might that be done?

9. What recommendations regarding sexual intercourse should we give to patients with genital herpesvirus infections? Do the recommendations differ depending on whether the patient is a man or a woman? Do they differ for heterosexuals and homosexuals?

6. Here's a good time to call on your knowledge of basic pharmacologic terminology. Acyclovir has to be metabolically activated to exert its desired effects. What, then, can we call acyclovir?

10. Which administration route(s) for acyclovir are usually associated with adverse systemic responses? What are they, and how can we minimize them?

7. A. The text notes that herpes virus resistance to acyclovir is rare in immunocompetent patients. What does that term mean?

11. A somewhat cynical colleague, commenting on valacyclovir (Zovirax), comments, "Eh, it's basically the same stuff as acyclovir. What's the big deal with it?"

B. By implication, in what groups of patients or in what conditions are we more likely to encounter resistance to acyclovir or more severe consequences?

A. Please comment on why and how he is wrong... and right!

B. Your colleague, tossing around some basic pharmacology terms, says that valacyclovir is a prodrug's prodrug. What might he mean?

C. Given what you've said in response to parts A and B of this question, why in the world would a drug manufacturer want to develop, test, and market a drug that's basically just the precursor of a drug that's already on the market? That can cost millions of dollars.

12. There are only a few major types of influenza virus that account for the millions of flu cases worldwide each year: A, and B. Why then is there such a ruckus every year as we wait for drug companies to make new flu vaccines?

13. Most people who get flu vaccines are given an "informed consent" form. One of the common questions is, "Are you allergic to eggs or egg products?" What in the world does that have to do with influenza? A fellow student says that patients who have adverse (allergic or hypersensitivity) reactions to eggs or egg products are resistant to influenza and so don't need (and shouldn't get) a vaccine.

CASE STUDY

My wife, another nurse who was working with her on the same shift, and a physician, were inserting an intra-aortic balloon/ventricular assist device to support left ventricular dysfunction in a patient with a quickly and severely failing heart. They were spattered by blood during the procedure and among the concerns was the risk of hepatitis. This was several years ago, before we had most of the currently effective antihepatitis drugs available. And this is essentially a true story.

1. There are several hepatitis viruses: A, B, C, D, and G. Which of these viral strains can cause acute hepatitis?

2. Statistically, which strains of hepatitis virus are most common?

3. In our society today, HIV probably receives the most attention as "the most common and important viral infection." Do current statistics support that notion?

4. What "defines" acute hepatitis and what do we typically do therapeutically about it?

5. How do the viral strains for hepatitis B and C, the ones most commonly associated with chronic hepatitis, differ in a general sense (rough comparisons, not exact numbers) in terms of the following:
   • Annual acute infections in the United States
   • Frequency of acute infections that develop into chronic hepatitis
   • Number of annual deaths from chronic infection

• Availability of a vaccine

It may be helpful to make a simple list or table based on Table 89-2 in your text.

Nowadays, in a situation such as the one we described at the outset of the case study, we might prescribe interferon alfa for known hepatitis B or C infections. So let's go from the past to the present as we continue.

6. Your text notes that interferon alfa, which can be used for either hepatitis B or C, blocks viral entry into cells. The meaning of that should be quite clear. But the drug also blocks synthesis of viral messenger RNA (m-RNA). What's the deal with that?

7. A patient is to receive pegylated interferon alfa. A colleague, trying to act bright, states that pegylated interferon alfa is more potent and more effective than a "standard" alfa and that it works in a different and better way. Do you agree?

8. Now your colleague talks about oral ribavirin (Rebetol). He says that this oral drug doesn't work well by itself. It must be given with subcutaneous interferon alfa for managing chronic hepatitis C. Is he correct this time?

9. Now your colleague states that ribavirin might be a great and very effective adjunctive drug, as well as convenient to take because it's taken orally, but "watch out...SC injections of alfa interferon may be painful or annoying and they may cause some side effects, but occasionally ribavirin can prove fatal." Is he correct or not? Let's ignore pregnancy considerations for this.

evolve To check your answers, go to http://evolve.elsevier.com/Lehne/ for Study Guide Comments from the author.

Antiviral Drugs II: Drugs for HIV Infection and Related Opportunistic Infections

KEY TERMS

acquired immunodeficiency syndrome (AIDS)

acute retroviral syndrome

class-sparing (therapy of HIV/AIDS)

HAART (highly active antiretroviral therapy)

human immunodeficiency virus (HIV)

lactic acidosis

myelosuppression

nucleoside

nucleotide

opportunistic infection

polymerases

protease (and inhibitors)

retrovirus

reverse transcriptase

syndrome

viral load

virion

OBJECTIVES

After reading and studying this chapter you should be able to:

1. Be able to explain how AIDS and HIV are related, yet they are not the same things.
2. Define retrovirus in terms of the transcription of information between viral DNA and RNA. You should be able to compare the sequence of the basic events in retroviruses with what goes on in a typical host cell.
3. Recognize that helper T lymphocytes (CD4 cells) are the main target of HIV. Explain what CD4 cells do to and for the HIV, why they are important to the host (whether there's a viral infection or not), and how this relates to the opportunistic infections that accompany AIDS.
4. Describe the three phases of HIV infection and how CD4 and HIV levels are likely to appear in each. Explain why the changes in CD4 and HIV levels change as they do.
5. In simple terms, explain what the three main classes (and subclasses) of antiretroviral drugs do, biochemically, to impair viral replication or

function. Use zidovudine as the prototype nucleoside reverse transcriptase (NRTI), nevirapine as the prototype non-nucleoside reverse transcriptase inhibitor (NNRTI), saquinavir for the protease inhibitors, and enfuvirtide as the new HIV fusion inhibitor. If you understand what these drugs do, you'll have a good grasp of how retroviruses like HIV work to cause infections and cause damage to host cells.

6. Give a reasonable explanation of why HIV infection doesn't kill people directly, but rather it's the consequences of other events that develop when the infection turns into AIDS.
7. Briefly summarize the antiretroviral mechanism of action of the protease inhibitors. Recognize hyperglycemia (and its consequences), a pseudo-Cushing's syndrome (review Chapter 57 content if necessary), and hyperlipidemias as key adverse responses to these drugs. State the main monitoring methods or interventions for these adverse responses.
8. Explain what HAART is, and in your explanation indicate why multidrug therapy for HIV/AIDS is important. Give some reasonable explanation of how we go about selecting the drugs or drug classes that we should use and why we use combination therapy.
9. Recognize that the blood levels, effects, and toxicity of saquinavir (which we'll consider the prototype protease inhibitor) are very dependent on the level of activity of the liver's P450 drug-metabolizing system. Recognize that the proteases, in general, inhibit the P450 system. Be able to identify some of the key drugs that interact, therefore, with protease inhibitors by either inhibiting or inducing the P450 system, and predict the consequences of such interactions.
10. Compare and contrast the effects of saquinavir and of ritonavir on the P450 system. Explain the

272

general consequences of these effects when the patient is on multidrug therapy.

11. Identify the three main reasons for changing antiretroviral therapy, and summarize some reasonable guidelines for how we change treatment.

12. Identify some of the common opportunistic infections that we may encounter in patients with HIV/AIDS. Identify and describe some of the common treatment modalities for prophylaxis and treatment of these opportunistic infections.

13. Explain some of the main impediments to proper, optimal therapy of HIV/AIDS. Include in your explanation not only pharmacologic considerations but also economic and compliance factors.

14. What are the special therapeutic and preventive approaches for HIV/AIDS patients who are pregnant? for adolescents with active infection? for infected neonates and infants?

Note: Lehne's chapter is a comprehensive, holistic, and generally excellent compilation of information on HIV/AIDS—its treatment overall, and special considerations such as those that are important for pregnant women, children, or asymptomatic (and even non-infected) patients.

However, in order to keep things focused and manageable, I've tried to keep the study and case study items below targeted more towards general drug therapy concepts than to special circumstances. Be sure to ask your instructor what his or her expectations are.

You should have a good grasp of immune system function (see Chapter 63) before you start studying this chapter intensively. Also, because opportunistic infections are an almost inevitable consequence of AIDS, you need to be aware of the drugs and their actions for preventing or managing such things as *Pneumocystis carinii* and tuberculosis (virtually all the previous chapters in this unit). Although integrating that information might seem like an onerous task, it will really help you pull together the critical information, and in a way that hopefully will make sense.

CRITICAL THINKING AND STUDY QUESTIONS

1. You know that AIDS is an acronym for acquired immunodeficiency syndrome. What is the general definition of a syndrome?

2. What common malady does an initial HIV infection look like in terms of typical signs and symptoms? It's one that often leads the physician to miss the diagnosis of HIV and delay onset of treatment. It might be described as a "syndrome," but it might lead us to miss the diagnosis.

3. HIV infects and attacks two main cell types: CD4 T cells (helper lymphocytes) and macrophages (and those macrophages in the CNS that are given the special name microglia). What are the consequences of viral attack on these two cell types in terms of ultimate cell death and the clinical consequences of HIV infection?

4. Briefly go to your memory bank and summarize the main roles of CD4 cells. Why are they so important for immune system integrity?

5. What is a polymer, and what's a polymerase? Keep your explanation simple!

6. The text keeps mentioning reverse transcriptase. What's that? If there's a reverse transcriptase, there must be a "forward transcriptase" too. Is there? Where might we find it?

7. And the protease? What is its function?

8. The text describes the HIV reverse transcriptase as error-prone. In your own words, what does that mean, and what are the clinical implications of it? You might want to compare the action of HIV reverse transcriptase with how normal mammalian transcriptase (DNA-dependent RNA polymerase) works.

9. What information does following a patient's blood levels of HIV and of CD4 cells from initial infection on through the development of AIDS provide in terms of the "stage" of the infection and clinical disease?

10. Zidovudine can be considered the prototype NRTI. Explain what that means in your own words.

11. What are the main adverse hematologic effects of zidovudine? What are their consequences? What can/do we do about them?

12. The text notes that myelosuppressive drugs are among those that can increase the risk of hematologic toxicity to zidovudine and the NRTIs in general. What is, almost without question, the largest group of myelosuppressive drugs?

13. Nevirapine is classified as an NRTI. What does that mean in terms of its structure and mechanism of antiretroviral action? Compare these properties of the drug with those of zidovudine.

14. Is it correct to say that both NRTIs and NNRTIs can cause hepatic damage? Are the types (or signs or symptoms) of hepatotoxicity the same with both classes of drug? What's the "bottom line" with respect to hepatic consequences of antiretroviral therapy with these drugs?

15. What's the important take-home message about using just one anti-HIV drug for therapy?

16. Considering the group of protease inhibitors as a whole, how do these agents exert antiretroviral activity? A colleague says that they are just "another way" to inhibit viral DNA replication. Is he right?

17. You've learned that protease inhibitors, as a class, can significantly inhibit the activity of the liver's drug-metabolizing (P450) system. That's a major cause of drug-drug interactions. Ritonavir is a little unique. It can inhibit or induce (stimulate) the metabolism of some drugs.

A. Are all those interactions that involve inhibited metabolism by ritonavir "bad?"

B. Does ritonavir inhibit only the P450 system, in terms of metabolic rates of drugs? If not, what's the general clinical implication of this?

18. Give an ordinary, every-day (nonmedical) example of what "fusion" (as in fusion of HIV with a CD4 cell) means. That's important, of course, because the envelope surrounding a virion fuses with the membrane of a host cell, such as a CD4 cell.

19. What is unique (compared with reverse transcriptase inhibitors and protease inhibitors) about the mechanism of action of enfuvirtide (Fuzeon)?

20. What is the practical clinical utility of knowing that enfuvirtide is a synthetic peptide that contains 36 amino acids, has a molecular weight of 4492, and takes 106 steps to make?

CASE STUDY

Lance Gelding is a 30-year-old man who has been HIV-seropositive for 4 years. Until now he has never taken any antiviral agent. He is thin for his height (5 feet 8 inches and 115 pounds), but looks fairly healthy. Lance has multiple enlarged lymph nodes and a raised purple lesion (about 2 × 3 cm) on his left leg. His eye exam indicates several white retinal patches. He states that his vision is getting worse and he now has headaches and daily temperature elevations. He had been prescribed zidovudine (AZT), indinavir (Crixivan), and lamivudine (Epivir). With retinitis caused by cytomegalovirus (CMV), the treatment of choice is ganciclovir; however, its effects as a potent suppressor of hematopoiesis, especially combined with zidovudine, must be considered.

1. To understand the therapy being used for Mr. Gelding, you need to know the pathophysiology involved with HIV. Briefly describe what happens once a person is exposed to HIV. What are the typical phases of the infection and the subsequent development of AIDS?

2. Based on the information in the scenario, which phase of HIV infection is Mr. Gelding likely to be experiencing?
   You're discussing some critical things with Mr. Gelding about his HIV infection; what he can expect treatment- and outcomes-wise, and the like. You mention several key things (below). How would you explain these terms or concepts to Mr. Gelding?

3. He may develop opportunistic infections. What is an opportunistic infection? (***Hint:*** Think of what the general usage of the term *opportunity* means.)

4. You tell Mr. Gelding that he may develop "CMV retinitis." Explain in simple terms what that is, what it means to him.

5. Mr. Gelding has heard of PCP and that he might acquire it. He's familiar with PCP—phencyclidine—a hallucinogen. He asks whether he's going to start hallucinating. Explain this to him. Explain the preventive measures.

In the text (and it's particularly clear from Table 90-8), we see that an "established regimen" for initial treatment of established HIV infection should involve a combination of at least three drugs, such as a protease inhibitor and an NRTI "pair" such as zidovudine and didanosine.

In Mr. Gelding's case we choose as our protease inhibitors a combination of ritonavir and saquinavir. It's marketed as a fixed-dose combination product called Invirase. The NRTI combination that we'll use is zidovudine plus didanosine.

6. What is the purpose of including the ritonavir, which clearly has protease-inhibitory activity?

7. What's the general reason for using any two protease inhibitors together?

8. About 3 months after starting therapy Mr. Gelding reports excessive thirst and the urge to drink large amounts of "anything cold" (juices, water, pop). He reports urinary frequency. He seems to be urinating all the time; the urine volume seems unusually large; and the urine is clear and colorless. What is this most likely to reflect?

9. The text notes that we may be able to manage the diabetes with oral hypoglycemics. What does this tell you about the type of diabetes such a patient (anyone, not just Mr. Gelding) has? Is it type 1 or type 2?

When the text addresses the issue of managing protease inhibitor-induced diabetes mellitus with oral agents, it parenthetically mentions metformin (Glucophage) as the example. Recall that we're using not only protease inhibitors but also two NRTIs for this patient. When I read this in the text, two potential concerns popped into mind. (I am thinking "critically" and I hope correctly. Let's see if you can figure out the concerns.)

10. What adverse effect is shared by the NRTIs and metformin? (**Hint:** With metformin it's described as a "rare consequence, but one that is fatal about 50% of the time when it does occur.")

11. What other effect does metformin often cause? (**Hint:** It's one that's beneficial for many people with type 2 diabetes, but I wonder whether it might be unwanted for an HIV-infected patient.)

Now assume that our preferred protease inhibitor combination for Mr. Gelding is Kaletra: ritonavir plus lopinavir, formulated as the oral solution. Mr. Gelding develops clinical diabetes. The cost of therapy is getting high. The MD doesn't want to go with metformin as the oral antidiabetic drug (because of cost and possible added risks of lactic acidosis). She doesn't want to use one of the newer sulfonylureas (glipizide, glyburide) either, again because of cost.

12. The decision is made to add tolbutamide, an old, effective, yet inexpensive oral antidiabetic drug of the sulfonylurea class. What problems do you envisage with this?

13. Mr. Gelding wants to know whether it is safe to have sexual intercourse now that he is taking the antiviral agent zidovudine and ganciclovir. What is your response?

14. Mr. Gelding asks you when he can discontinue these medications. What is your reply?

evolve To check your answers, go to http://evolve.elsevier.com/Lehne/ for Study Guide Comments from the author.

Drug Therapy of Sexually Transmitted Diseases

KEY TERMS

chancre (syphilitic)
chancroid
chlamydia
condyloma acuminatum
  epididymitis
human papilloma virus
  (HPV)

nongonoccal urethritis
pelvic inflammatory
  disease (PID)
spirochete
syphilis

OBJECTIVES

After reading and studying this chapter you should be able to:

1. Give a simple but accurate definition of what a sexually transmitted disease... how the term encompasses more that one clinical presentation.
2. Make a reasonably accurate statement about the overall incidence of the individual STDs. Put this in the context of the question, "Given the incidence of these diseases, which am I likely to encounter in my clinical practice?"
3. Describe the various treatments and prophylactic measures for STDs. In your discussion, explain how and why previously effective antibiotic therapies have become outmoded because of resistance.
4. Describe the symptoms and time-courses of the "three main stages" of syphilis, and the typically recommended therapies for syphilis in adults and during pregnancy, and in newborns with congenital exposure to *Treponema pallidum*.
5. Summarize a reasonable (but general) drug plan for a patient with syphilis who also has a history of severe hypersensitivity reactions to a penicillin.
6. State the most common route by which neonatal gonoccal infections occur and the most common and handicapping consequence of that neonatal infection. In your comments, state what the usual precautionary (prophylactic) measure is and why it must be done.

Note: As your text indicates (*Key Points* at the end of the chapter), "all the drugs used to treat STDs have been introduced in other chapters." I have, therefore, put study and case study items on those medications in the respective chapters of this book. Refer to them as needed.

CRITICAL THINKING AND STUDY QUESTIONS

1. A 25-year-old woman who describes herself as very sexually active and sometimes promiscuous during her late teens and early 20s eventually gets involved in a monogamous relationship with a man. The man has absolutely no history of STD. Two years after they get married they attempt to have children but are unsuccessful. A thorough gynecologic work-up indicates she is sterile. Assume this woman did have an asymptomatic STD. Which one is most likely to account for her sterility, and why?

2. Gonorrhea (an infection by *Neisseria gonorrhoea*) is said to be easy to recognize in men but not in women. Why?

3. With primary syphilis, where does the initial chancre usually occur? Consider in your answer heterosexual men, homosexual men, and women (heterosexual or homosexual). Comment on how this may affect the early detection and treatment of this STD. (In some ways, this question parallels question 3 immediately above.)

4. The text notes that the incidence of syphilis increased during the 1980s but declined throughout the 1990s. Can you make a reasoned guess about what accounted for the decline, and which population generally benefited from this reduced incidence? Given what you may know about our society nowadays, can you speculate about the changing demographics of syphilis infections in the United States? Where and among whom do we find these cases?

5. With what are a high percentage of patients with a gonoccal infection co-infected, and what, if anything, do we do about it therapeutically?

6. A fellow student, studying for an exam on the treatment of STDs, is in a tizzy because he can't remember whether the preferred drug for genital herpes (*herpes simplex*) infections is a penicillin ("and which one," he pleads?), a fluoroquinolone, or a cephalosporin. Help the lad out with the simple answer to his dilemma.

7. You've read many chapters and other articles related to sexually transmitted disease and can't come to any conclusion about what to do. Overall, what is the effective way to prevent the spread of STDs?

evolve To check your answers, go to http://evolve.elsevier.com/Lehne/ for Study Guide Comments from the author.

Antiseptics and Disinfectants

KEY TERMS

antiseptic

aseptic

disinfectant

sanitation (sanitized)

sterile

tincture

OBJECTIVES

After reading and studying this chapter you should be able to:

1. State the main criterion that differentiates an antiseptic from a disinfectant.
2. Discuss what healthcare providers, using antiseptics and disinfectants, can do to protect patients, and themselves, from infections.
3. Describe the preferred treatments for established local cutaneous infections.

CRITICAL THINKING AND STUDY QUESTIONS

1. We almost always think of an antiseptic as a drug we place on the surface of the body, for example, the skin. Can you think of a situation for which we administer the antiseptic systemically? What group of drugs offers the best treatment?

2. Why is it arguably more important for healthcare providers to use proper antiseptics and antiseptic techniques than to use topical antiseptics on their patients? Consider this in the context of a patient who is about to undergo a "clean" surgery, such as thoracotomy for bypassing an occluded coronary artery. (The best way to define clean surgery is to state some examples of "dirty" surgery: repairs of tissues that have been traumatized or contaminated from such sources as motor vehicle accidents or falls, abdominal operations for a ruptured bowel, etc.)

3. Think of the last time you were "poked" with a needle by healthcare provider, whether it was a venipuncture for drawing blood or one for getting some type of injection. What do you recall about it in the context of what was done?

4. You pick up a bottle of topical anesthetic and note the word *tincture* on it. What does that mean by way of one of the ingredients and how you should (or shouldn't use) the product?

evolve To check your answers, go to http://evolve.elsevier.com/Lehne/ for Study Guide Comments from the author.

Anthelminthics

KEY TERMS

ascariasis
cestode
entcrobiasis
filiariasis
helminth (helminthiasis)

nematode
schistosomiasis
trematode
trichinosis

OBJECTIVES

After reading and studying this chapter you should be able to:

1. Summarize the main risk factor for helminthiasis, the main way to prevent such infestations, and why certain types of helminthiasis are endemic in certain regions of the world (as opposed to being prevalent on a more global basis).
2. Recognize the three major classes of parasitic worm and their "lay" descriptions: nematodes (roundworms), cestodes (tapeworms), and trematodes (flukes). State where these parasitic worms are generally found and the main way they infect human hosts.
3. Recognize the prevalence, importance, and consequences of helminthiasis. However, focus on the general issues (including main therapies) rather than attempting to memorize such things as genus, species, and class of the various parasites. Likewise, realize that your course deals with pharmacology. It is useful, but not necessary, to know the specific biochemical mechanisms by which the various anthelminthic drugs affect their parasites. Focus on the human consequences of administering (or not) these drugs to humans.

CRITICAL THINKING AND STUDY QUESTIONS

1. Without going into specifics, summarize the major sources of parasitic worms and the main routes by which they infect human hosts. By "source" we do not mean geographic locale; rather, we're asking about where, in the environment, these parasites typically reside.

2. In terms of symptoms and clinical outcomes, why in general can we be a little less concerned about intestinal nematode infestations than about those that are called extraintestinal?

3. What distinguishes thiabendazole (Mintezol) from most of the other antiparasitic drugs discussed in this chapter? What accounts for that difference?

4. Let's assume (or optimistically pretend) that your clinical practice will expose you only to patients who live in big city and suburban settings. Which helminth infestations are you most likely to encounter, and why? (An inelegant way to ask the question is, "Which helminth infestations are likely to be most important for you to know about?")

CASE STUDY

Ashley Clinton is a 3-year-old girl who attends Our So Very Precious Little Child Daycare Center in an upper-middle-class suburb.

Ashley has been restless and not sleeping well; she's been scratching her perineal area frequently and wetting the bed at night. During a parents' meeting, Ashley's mother talks to several other moms and learns that their kids have been exhibiting the same unusual behaviors. It seems to be more than mere coincidence.

Mrs. Clinton calls the pediatric nurse practitioner, who tells her to put a loop of transparent sticky tape in Ashley's anal area in the early morning before the child awakens. She's instructed to remove the tape later in the morning, put it in a plastic bag, and bring it to the office with Ashley.

1. Given the signs, symptoms, and ages of the patients, and what you should know about the epidemiology of helminth infestations, what is your first guess about the cause?

On examination of the tape sample, the pediatric nurse practitioner confirms the suspected diagnosis. She orders mebendazole for the entire family.

2. What is the probable mode of transmission of the parasite in this case? Can you tell whether the infection was acquired at school, at home, or somewhere else?

3. Is it necessary or wise to treat the entire family, not just Ashley? Why?

4. Approximately how long will it take before Ashley (or anyone on the treatment) starts to notice symptom relief which would indicate complete or near-complete removal of the parasites from the system?

5. If the infected patient has severe diarrhea during or because of the infestation, how might that affect the outcome of treatment? Would you be concerned about impaired systemic absorption of the drug because of it?

6. Ashley's mother wonders whether she should notify the daycare center of Ashley's condition. What are your thoughts?

evolve To check your answers, go to http://evolve.elsevier.com/Lehne/ for Study Guide Comments from the author.

Antiprotozoal Drugs I: Antimalarial Agents

KEY TERMS

blackwater fever
cinchonism (and
    cinchona alkaloid)
clinical cure (of malaria)
dormant (as in dormant
    parasites)
exoerythrocytic (form of
    malaria parasite)
falciparum malaria

parenchyma
    (parenchymal cells)
Plasmodium
    (*P. falciparum,*
    P. vivax)
radical cure (of malaria)
suppressive therapy (of
    malaria)
vivax malaria

OBJECTIVES

After reading and studying this chapter you should be able to:

1. Recognize automatically that discussions or comments about *Plasmodia (P. falciparum, P. vivax)* are focusing on common causes of malaria.
2. Compare and contrast vivax and falciparum malaria in terms of cause, prevalence, signs and symptoms (and severity of them), and overall management.
3. Summarize the usual appropriate drug and nondrug measures that should be implemented before a patient travels to an area where malaria is endemic.
4. State a rationale why you, as a student who is probably living in a rather civilized part of the world, should be concerned and knowledgeable about diseases such as malaria, which occur rarely here. Give your comments on why our ability to travel to distant parts of the world has such a dramatic impact on what you may need to know as a healthcare provider.
5. Summarize the main elements of drug therapy for malaria once it has developed. Your answer should demonstrate your understanding of the terms clinical cure, radical cure, and suppressive therapy as they apply to vivax malaria.

6. Discuss the adverse effects of the various drug therapies used for the different forms and stages of malaria.

Notes: Although you may never encounter a case of malaria in your clinical practice, you should gain a reasonable grasp of the disease's origins and transmission characteristics; common signs and symptoms; and the basic nature and stages of treatment, including the main drugs for nonresistant strains of Plasmodium. See study question 1 below.

Given the important role of quinine and quinidine in some cases of malaria, your instructor may wish you to review the pharmacology of these cinchona alkaloids in more detail. Given the more common use of quinidine for certain and common cardiac rhythm disorders, you will find that information in Chapter 47 (*Antidysrhythmic Drugs*).

CRITICAL THINKING AND STUDY QUESTIONS

1. Given the relative rarity of malaria cases acquired in the United States, why is knowledge of malaria and its prevention or treatment necessary?

2. Your text notes that in the human phase of the life cycle of Plasmodium, infected mosquitoes inject malarial sporozytes that invade "parenchymal cells." Just what are parenchymal cells?

3. Why do the main signs and symptoms of malaria typically have a fluctuating clinical course—peaking in severity, then becoming milder, worsening again, and so on? What is going on, what human cells are contributing to the cyclic course?

4. Whether malaria is caused by *P. vivax* or *P. falciparum,* hemolysis occurs. Given that common feature, what main clinical features differentiate between these main types of malaria? Your answer should focus on signs and symptoms (and their severity and lethality), potential for relapse (and why that is), and resistance to typical antimalarial drugs.

5. Focus on vivax malaria and explain why achieving a clinical cure with the appropriate drug(s) is no guarantee that the patient will not have symptom relapse. Why is this issue of relapse after clinical cure not an issue with falciparum malaria? (Assume we've removed the patient from all exposure to malaria-carrying mosquitoes.

6. Why was gin and tonic such a popular beverage years ago for the Europeans and other westerners who colonized malaria-endemic parts of the world?

CASE STUDY

Joseph Wright, 45 years old, has just taken a job with an international business conglomerate looking to get an economic foothold in a country that is known for its prevalence of malaria.

1. Assume Mr. Wright will not seek medical advice from a tropical medicine or infectious disease specialist. Instead he's sent to his company's general medicine doc. What is arguably one of the best resources for the physician, or any other healthcare practitioner, to consult about the risks of malaria (or any other geographically localized diseases) worldwide?

2. Mr. Wright has received all his immunizations, and now the MD needs to reduce Mr. Wright's risks of malaria. Which drug is generally considered the first-line agent for this? What factors might change the drug choice?

3. Mr. Wright, being not too diligent a chap, doesn't take the necessary prophylactic medication for malaria. About a month after arriving at his assigned destination he develops bouts of chills, fever, and sweating. He also reports feeling weak. A local doctor, knowledgeable in treating malaria, diagnoses vivax malaria. What is the likely medication to be given and what "type" of treatment is the physician trying to achieve?

4. In a matter of days, Mr. Wright feels back to normal. Assume that Mr. Wright has "had enough" of these "strange illnesses." He will travel back to "big-city USA," where there's no malaria, right away. Will therapy need to be continued or modified? He has had, after all, a clinical cure. Explain your reason(s).

5. Mr. Wright waits too long to receive primaquine upon return home. He has another bout of the erythrocytic phase (symptomatic malaria). Would it be reasonable to start primaquine therapy at this time? If we did, what would we expect?

6. Now assume that rather than return home after recovering from his *P. vivax* attack, he will stay on-site for several more months. He's done a little reading on the subject and knows that there are drugs for a permanent cure. He asks the physician whether he will now get the drugs to eradicate the parasites from his liver to avoid another bout of the illness. What is the MD likely to say, and why?

evolve To check your answers, go to http://evolve.elsevier.com/Lehne/ for Study Guide Comments from the author.

Antiprotozoal Drugs II: Miscellaneous Agents

KEY TERMS

amebiasis
Chagas' disease
disulfiram-like reaction
giardiasis

leishmaniasis
toxoplasmosis
trichomoniasis
trypanosomiasis

OBJECTIVES

After reading and studying this chapter you should be able to:

1. Describe the principal protozoal infections endemic to the United States and those we might see here because of world travel.
2. Discuss drug therapies for the various protozoal infections.
3. Discuss precautions that patients should take with the drug therapies for protozoal infections.
4. Discuss the fungal infection *Pneumocystis carinii pneumonia (PCP)*.
5. Discuss the drug therapies for PCP.

Note: Be sure to consult Chapter 87 for more information about the uses and adverse effects of metronidazole. Check Chapter 90 for more information on management of *pneumocystis carnii pneumonia* in the context of advanced HIV infection. Given the relative rarity of protozoal infections you'll see in your practice, you may not need to study this chapter in as much depth as others; you might simply use the information as a good reference when needed.

CRITICAL THINKING AND STUDY QUESTIONS

1. What is noteworthy about and amebiasis, giardiasis, and trichomoniasis?

2. What is noteworthy about metronidazole?

3. What are the main routes of exposure to and transmission of the following:

A. Amebiasis

B. Giardiasis

C. Trichomoniasis

Ectoparasiticides

KEY TERMS

ectoparasite   pruritis
nit   scabies
pcdiculosis

OBJECTIVES

After reading and studying this chapter you should be able to:

1. Give a short summary of the differences between scabies and the three main types of pediculosis in such a way that you can explain what these infestations are to a layperson.
2. Identify the common modes of acquiring and transmitting pediculosis and scabies, the characteristic signs or symptoms of these ectoparasitic infestations, and generally effective first-line approaches to managing them (both pharmacologic and nondrug).

CRITICAL THINKING AND STUDY QUESTIONS

1. Identify the common modes of acquiring and transmitting pediculosis (head, pubic, or body lice and scabies), the characteristic signs or symptoms of these infestations, and generally effective first-line approaches to managing them (both pharmacologic and nondrug).

2. The text notes that malathion is an organophosphate (acetyl) cholinesterase inhibitor. (Some of the other agents in the chapter work that way too.) What does that classification mean, and what does that tell you about how the drug kills the lice? The label instructions on malathion lotion (as well as labels for nearly all the other drugs in this chapter) say "For external use only. Do not swallow." What signs and symptoms would you expect if someone did swallow this drug in amounts sufficient to cause toxicity? What, if any, antidote might be helpful?

CASE STUDY

Joan is a 7-year-old in the second grade. For over a week she's been constantly scratching her head, so much that her very long hair is tangled and almost impossible to brush. Her scalp is bleeding. As the school nurse, you notice small white spots in her hair. You contact her mother to report these nits (or eggs), telling her it is probably Pediculus humanus capitis (head lice). The physician orders permethrin (Nix) shampoo.

1. Joan's mother is quite upset about the lice. She wants to know how the school could "allow" her daughter to get lice. She wants to know how to tell whether others in the family have them or if there's even a risk that they might acquire the lice from little Joan. What is your response?

2. Joan's mom snaps, "I don't have time to stop by our pediatrician's office to pick up the prescription for the Nix!" How might you allay her anger a bit?

3. Joan's mother calls you 2 days later to say she was told by a friend to cut all of Joan's hair to get rid of the lice. How would you respond to this?

4. Assume now that the lice-infested patient is not a 7-year-old girl, but an 18-year-old college freshman, and you're his mom. He calls home from his dorm room saying he has "all these bugs" in his head. With what important nondrug measure is this 18-year-old be unlikely to take, and why?

evolve To check your answers, go to http://evolve.elsevier.com/Lehne/ for Study Guide Comments from the author.

Basic Principles of Cancer Chemotherapy

KEY TERMS

adjuvant therapy (of cancer)
apoptosis
cell cycle
complete remission
cure (in the context of cancer chemotherapy)
debulking (of a solid tumor)
G_0 (phase of cell cycle)
growth fraction
invasive cell growth
Karnofsky Performance Scale

malignant
metastasis
mustard
neoplastic cells
oncogene
palliative treatment
persistent proliferation
P-glycoprotein
remission
selective toxicity
telomerase
vesicant

OBJECTIVES

After reading and studying this chapter you should be able to:

1. Describe why the three main treatment approaches to cancer—drugs, surgery, and radiation—can be considered and often are used as adjuvants (adjuncts) to one another. State the general types of cancer for which surgery and/or radiation therapy generally are not the primary approaches, and so we rely mainly on drugs.
2. Summarize the main states of the cell cycle (G_0, G_1, S, G_2, M) and give a brief comment on what is occurring during each stage. Comment on whether or why the state of the cancer cell's cycle affects its response to anticancer drugs. Explain how this relates to the concept of growth fraction and how, in general, solid tumors differ from disseminated cancers in terms of their responsiveness to cancer chemotherapy.
3. In general terms, compare and contrast the "typical" cancer chemotherapeutic drug with the typical antibiotic with respect to the concept of "selective toxicity" (to those cells we want to

destroy as opposed to host cells, which we don't want to damage).
4. Recognize that cancer cells tend to develop resistance to anticancer drugs by random mutations and that these mutations can have the following consequences in terms of the cancer cell's response to a specific drug. The cells...
   • become less able to take up the drug; or
   • become better able to pump the drug out of the cells; or
   • lose their ability to transform the drug into an active and cytotoxic metabolite; or
   • develop better or faster ways to repair the damage caused by the chemotherapeutic agent.
5. Summarize the basic principles and concepts that apply to how and why we often use multidrug therapy to treat cancers.
6. Give a succinct but accurate explanation of why (in most cases) drug therapy of disseminated cancers can be more successful than drug treatment of solid tumors. (For the purposes of meeting this objective, ignore metastatic disease and focus on the primary tumor.)

Notes: The text narrowly defines cancer chemotherapy as that which involves use of cytotoxic drugs, and so focuses on them. We will do the same here. Nonetheless, you should have an understanding of the use of hormones and hormone antagonists and of immunomodulating drugs, which are presented in several other chapters.

I expect my nursing students (sophomores and juniors in a BSN program) to understand the main mechanisms by which anticancer drugs work, the mechanisms by which resistance to their effects can develop, and the basic rationales for combining more than one drug. I do not expect them to memorize the specific mechanisms for each anticancer drug or class. There is too much to be learned (whether in this unit or in a course as a whole) that I don't think such memory-matching is helpful, constructive, or needed. But, I don't grade you. Be sure to check with your instructor to learn what his or her expectations are.

289

CRITICAL THINKING AND STUDY QUESTIONS

1. In simple terms, what's the main reason for using intermittent chemotherapy (repeated courses of drugs) rather than attempting to "blast" all the cancer cells at once with a whopping dose of the drug?

2. A biostatistician might say that "probability therapy" becomes important when explaining one of the reasons that combinations of anticancer drugs tend to be better in terms of not developing resistance than using just one drug. She says, "If you flip a coin, on average you have a 50% (1 in 2) chance of a head coming up. Flip two coins and the chance of two heads is 25% (1 in 4). That's sort of like what we're dealing with when we're talking about resistance to anticancer drugs." What might this mean?

3. Here's one to coerce you into recalling some "old" stuff and applying some general principles to what you're reading about and learning in the current chapter. When we're treating a patient with essential hypertension, it's quite common to prescribe two or three (maybe even more) drugs. Why do we do that, and how do we select our drugs? What do we hope to achieve, aside from just lowering blood pressure? (Think "general concepts.") How do those same principles apply to cancer chemotherapy? (I'm thinking about concepts other than drug resistance, so you can ignore the resistance issue for this question too.)

4. Some anticancer drugs cause "targeted toxicity" to a particular organ, and there are several sites of toxicity that are rather common with all these drugs. One of them poses particular dangers to the host. What is it?

5. A patient has heard of some magic potion (advertised on the Internet) that is claimed to "cure" cancer. Give us your understanding of the roles of our immune system in the self-regulation of cancer and our response to anticancer drugs. (For the purpose of this question, disregard the cancer drugs classified as immunomodulators.)

6. The oncologist with whom you're working tells a patient that cancer chemotherapy has caused a complete remission. By all subjective and objective measures, the patient is symptom free. There are no blood (or other) tests to detect markers of the cancer and no x-rays, MRIs, or other methods that might be used provide data consistent with the conclusion that the cancer is undetectable. Does this mean that the patient is cancer free? Have we cured the cancer? Why or why not?

7. We might say that blood flow to—and out of—a solid tumor is a mixed blessing: both good and bad. Free-associate and comment on this. What are some of the good—and bad—things about a tumor's blood supply?

8. There are three main adverse hematologic effects of anticancer drugs, owing to their effects on the bone marrow. What are they, and how (in general) do we assess for them?

9. What is the Karnofsky Performance Scale? Upon what is it based, and why is it important to your patient and to you as a care provider?

10. As you will learn in other chapters in this unit, some anticancer drugs are (and were derived from) nitrogen mustards that are classified as vesicants. What is a vesicant? Where, nowadays, might you encounter them outside the realm of cancer chemotherapy?

evolve To check your answers, go to http://evolve.elsevier.com/Lehne/ for Study Guide Comments from the author.

98

Anticancer Drugs I: Cytotoxic Agents

KEY TERMS

alkylating agent
antimetabolite
bifunctional (and
  monofunctional)
  alkylating agent
biologic response
  modifier
cell-cycle (phase)
  specific (and
  nonspecific)
  anticancer drug
extravasation (as of an
  administered drug)
G_0 (phase of cell cycle)

intercalation (as into
  DNA)
leucovorin (and
  leucovorin rescue)
metaphase arrest
microtubules
mitotic inhibitor
nitrogen mustard
purine(s)
pyrimidine(s)
scission (as of DNA
  strands)
topoisomerase
vinca (or vinca alkaloid)

OBJECTIVES

After reading and studying this chapter you should be able to:

1. Identify and describe the main classes of anticancer drugs in terms of their main mechanisms of action.
2. Differentiate between cell-cycle–specific and cell-cycle–nonspecific anticancer drugs in terms of their mechanisms of action on cell growth and replication. State the main advantages or limitations of drugs in these two "classes" in terms of general efficacy against cancer cells. In this regard, restate your general understanding of what the cell cycle is and how it affects responses to both cancer and host cells.
3. In the context of objective 2, summarize the main roles of DNA replication, transfer of DNA's genetic message to RNA and on to protein synthesis, and the role of mitosis and microtubular formation, as they affect cancer cell growth and reproduction.
4. Identify the side effects/adverse responses that are generally common to all anticancer drugs, and explain in simple terms why they occur.

5. Identify those anticancer drugs that cause selective toxicities that are not caused by many or any other anticancer agents. Focus on pulmonary, cardiac, renal, hepatic, and neurotoxicites (including such special neurotoxicities as ototoxicity).
5. Explain what leucovorin rescue is, the basic principle behind this approach, and the anticancer drug for which leucovorin rescue is used adjunctively.
6. State why xanthine oxidase (and its inhibition) is generally important in the setting of malignancies and treatment of malignancies. Identify the anticancer drug for which administration of a xanthine oxidase inhibitor might seem reasonable in concept but is actually deleterious in practice.

Notes: Be sure you're familiar with the general terms and concepts presented in Chapter 97 (*Basic Principles of Cancer Chemotherapy*). They are essential to understanding and applying information presented in this chapter, and the next, about specific drugs.

There are many dozens of anticancer drugs and uses for each. You could spend many hours memorizing which drug is used for which cancer. However, I don't think that's as important—at least now—as having a good grasp of how the drugs work to kill cancer cells by interfering with key aspects of cancer (and host) cell metabolism. I think it's wise and necessary for you to have a solid foundation of the biochemical actions of the anticancer drugs, particularly as they affect the biochemistry of cancer and host cells. I do not think it's necessary, however, for you to be able to recognize structures (you do need to recognize terms describing those structures) or sketch out all the steps and chemicals involved in such things as DNA replication or nucleotide synthesis. I also don't expect you to become a surrogate oncologist.

It's not so much what you memorize as what you understand and apply from what you read (present and past tense).

I have therefore tried to write the objectives to be in accord with my expectations. But, as always, you'd better check to see just what your profs want.

CRITICAL THINKING AND STUDY QUESTIONS

1. What is the basic rationale or principle behind using a combination of anticancer drugs, one that is cell-cycle-specific and one that is nonspecific? Include in your comment a simple discussion of what the cell cycle is (or represents) and the special importance of G_0.

2. You know by now that the main anticancer drugs are grouped according to their main mechanism(s) of action. What are the rationales behind using together two effective drugs that have the same mechanism of action? Do not consider this only in the specific context of anticancer drugs (although you need not ignore that altogether). Instead, think of this in terms of general pharmacologic principles with which you should be familiar through your prior learning throughout the course.

3. Why do we need to time the administration of a cell-cycle-specific drug properly, which often means infusing it by prolonged infusion?

4. The text notes that most alkylating agents work by interacting with a specific site on a guanine molecule in one or two DNA strands. One consequence of that is DNA strand scission. What does *scission* mean?

5. DNA cross-linking by an alkylating agent requires which type of alkylating agent? What type of chemical bonds are involved in the cross-link, and why is it important in a practical, cytotoxic sense? What might be considered the prototype alkylating agent?

6. The text considers cyclophosphamide (Cytoxan) as the prototype nitrogen mustard-type alkylating agent (and that's a great choice). It's not a vesicant, but other alkylating agents (e.g., the nitrosourea and carmustine [BCNU]) are. What should you know about the implications of the terms *nitrogen mustard* and *vesicant?*

7. The text notes that, among other adverse effects, cisplatin (Platinol-AQ) can cause tinnitus and high-frequency hearing loss. What general term is used to encompass those adverse effects? What other "ear problems" can be caused by some drugs with this type of toxicity? What is the main clinical significance of high-frequency hearing loss?

8. What is one of the most important pharmacokinetic properties of the nitrosourea class of alkylating agents, and what are the clinical implications of that?

9. The text notes that a special formulation of carmustine can be administered topically. Since you've probably worked your way through many parts of the book, and are certainly familiar with topical administration of drugs in general, what's your basic interpretation of what "topical administration" means or involves? How is topical administration of carmustine different?

10. The text notes that methotrexate and related drugs are antimetabolites. What does that general term mean in terms of mechanism of action. Can you think of another class of drugs (discussed in other units) that act as antimetabolites? One big group comes to my mind, and perhaps you've taken one yourself.

11. Assume a cell has limited ability to actively take up (pump in) a drug that we just must get into that cell in effective concentrations. Or imagine that a cancer cell that used to be able to actively accumulate a drug develops resistance by reducing the uptake process. What might we do to increase intracellular concentrations of that drug? With what anticancer drug do we often use this technique, and why?

12. A trade name for methotrexate ("MTX") is Rheumatrex. Although we don't like you to remember trade names (at the expense of learning generic names), the trade name of this particular drug should lead you to recognize another important use for this drug. What is it?

13. The text notes that when given to pregnant women MTX has been associated with fetal malformations and death. Does this relate to yet another use for the drug?

14. What is leucovorin and the principle or concept behind its use in leucovorin rescue?

15. For most anticancer drugs (and most other drugs in just about any class you can imagine), dosing instructions basically say "Don't give any more than [this amount] at any one time." For which anticancer drug are the instructions a little different from that, and how are they different? What is the main concern with ignoring this recommended maximum?

16. What are the "links" between the use of mercaptopurine (Purinethol)—the prototype purine analog—and allopurinol? What are the clinical implications of this link? How might not knowing about or forgetting about this important link, which might be viewed as an exception to the rule or at least an exception to common practice, pose problems for the patient? A colleague says that giving allopurinol to a patient who is receiving mercaptopurine will counteract the cancer drug's desired effects.

17. If we shouldn't give allopurinol to a patient who is being treated with mercaptopurine, what can we do to reduce the risk of gout and/or renal tubular damage or kidney failure from high uric acid levels?

18. Vinca alkaloids (e.g., vincristine [Oncovin]) and taxoids (e.g., paclitaxel [Taxol]) are said to be mitotic inhibitors that work by impairing microtubular assembly. What are microtubules, and why are they important to the cell? One of your classmates says that microtubules are the "small tubes or pores in cell membranes that allow the cells to take up important nutrients." Do you agree?

19. What toxicologic property does vincristine have (or not have), in comparison with most other anticancer drugs, that makes it a "good" drug, perhaps especially when used as an adjunct to other anticancer drugs for responsive cancers? Can you name another anticancer drug (it's in another class) that is similar to vincristine?

20. You've been studying this chapter very hard, and you need a break. You're at a party with a rather eclectic group of people, and you're talking about paclitaxel (Taxol). One partygoer is a botanist who says, "Yes, I know all about that stuff." Another is a huge advocate of alternative and herbal medicines who says, "See, all natural drugs are good drugs." What are they talking about? How might they know?

CASE STUDY

Kathy Turner is a 41-year-old woman admitted to the outpatient area of the hematology-oncology center for her first course of adjuvant chemotherapy for metastatic breast cancer. Four weeks ago Ms. Turner underwent a left modified radical mastectomy and axillary lymph node dissection for infiltrating ductal carcinoma of the breast. Two of 20 nodes sampled were positive for cancer.

Ms. Turner will be receiving standard dosage therapy of doxorubicin (Adriamycin), cyclophosphamide (Cytoxan), and fluorouracil (Adrucil) IV bolus. Premedications include intravenous ondansetron (Zofran) and dexamethasone (Decadron).

In addition, Ms. Turner will receive filgrastim (Neupogen) SQ daily for 10 days beginning 24 hours after chemotherapy completion. Ms. Turner is anxious and fidgeting as you begin your assessment.

1. Ms. Turner's several anticancer drugs are all targeted to destroy the same cancer but they don't all possess the same mechanism of action. Wouldn't it be more appropriate in terms of multidrug therapy to prescribe drugs that work in the same ways in terms of cellular responses to them?

2. What is the purpose of giving ondansetron (Zofran) and dexamethasone (Decadron) as premedications before chemotherapy?

3. We're giving Ms. Turner several very effective anticancer drugs. Why the need for the surgery?

4. What is purpose of giving filgrastim? A colleague states that it's to enhance the anticancer actions of the chemotherapy.

5. Ms. Turner is concerned about the possible side effects of her treatment, so requests specific information concerning the side effects of the medication she is receiving. Briefly discuss the information you will share with her.

6. What special consideration should be given to the doxorubicin now and in the future?

7. Cyclophosphamide is an alkylating agent. Briefly discuss the mechanism of action. Is Cytoxan cell-cycle–specific?

8. What kind of safety precautions should the nurse use in the administration of chemotherapy?

evolve To check your answers, go to http://evolve.elsevier.com/Lehne/ for Study Guide Comments from the author.

Anticancer Drugs II: Hormones, Hormone Antagonists, Biologic Response Modifiers, and Other Anticancer Drugs

KEY TERMS

aromatase
biologic response modifier
lymphoid tissue

selective estrogen
 receptor modifier
 (SERM)

OBJECTIVES

After reading and studying this chapter you should be able to:

1. Compare and contrast the basic mechanisms of action, clinical indications, and general toxicities of anticancer drugs discussed in this chapter with those discussed in the previous chapter, that is, the cytotoxic agents.
2. Summarize the likely benefits of glucocorticoids, not merely as anticancer drugs *per se,* but also as useful adjuncts in management of cancers with other drugs or nondrug modalities. Consider the main systemic adverse responses that almost always occur along with the beneficial effects.
3. State the precautions and related risk factors that should go into a decision about whether to administer tamoxifen either to prevent or to treat estrogen-sensitive breast cancers in women.
4. Summarize the desired and unwanted effects of antiestrogens and selective estrogen receptor modifiers when used to treat cancer.
5. Explain the paradoxical effects of leuprolide on androgen-dependent advanced prostatic cancer, and state what adjunctive intervention we might use to prevent the drug's unwanted effects on the cancer.

Notes: Be sure you're familiar with the general terms and concepts presented in Chapter 97 (*Basic Principles of Cancer Chemotherapy*). They are essential to understanding and applying information presented in this chapter, and the next, about specific drugs.

Be sure you have a fundamental grasp of the main concepts about glucocorticoids—their actions, mechanisms, adverse effects, and uses—as described in Chapters 57 and 68. Do the same for estrogen. You will find pertinent information in not only Chapter 59, but also in Chapter 60, which deals with estrogens as contraceptives. Finally, be sure to know the basic actions and uses of the bisphosphonates, which are widely used for such common disorders as osteoporosis. Bisphosphonate actions and uses are quite strongly related to the uses and actions of estrogen, so be sure you understand and appreciate the connections.

CRITICAL THINKING AND STUDY QUESTIONS

1. Why are the hormone and hormone-antagonist drugs discussed in this chapter used mainly for breast and prostate cancers? How does this account for the similarities, or differences, in the typical spectrums of toxic responses in the host (host cells) compared with a cytotoxic agent?

297

2. Why is it misleading, if not inaccurate, to refer to the selective estrogen receptor modulators (SERMs) as antiestrogens?

3. What is the main biochemical mechanism by which tamoxifen, toremifine, and raloxifene exert desired effects on responsive breast cancer cells? What characteristic must those breast cancer cells possess in order to respond to these drugs?

4. What are the main *adverse* effects that SERMs can cause via estrogen-receptor activation?

5. What are the main factors that should go into the decision of whether we use tamoxifen for prophylaxis of breast cancer, or avoid it?

6. What seems to account for the growing use of anastrozole (Arimidex) and the simultaneously declining use of tamoxifen, especially for postmenopausal women with breast cancer?

7. What is aromatase, and why aren't aromatase inhibitors as effective or useful in women who have not begun or completed menopause?

8. A man with advanced prostate cancer is given leuprolide (Lupron). Should he be told that if we give him ordinarily effective dosages of the drug, he will be cured?

9. A colleague is debating with you. He says that giving leuprolide for prostate cancer is stupid. He correctly mentions that leuprolide *mimics* the effects of gonadotropin-*releasing* hormone (GnRH), which ultimately increases production of testosterone, a substance that is supporting the growth of the androgen-responsive tumor. Do you agree that this approach is stupid? Why or why not?

10. In the preceding question, we stated that your colleague is correct about the ultimate testosterone-stimulating effects of leuprolide. When the drug is first given, it does increase testosterone release and so may temporarily stimulate growth and replication of prostate cancer cells. That's not good. So what do we do about that until the "chemical castration effect" of the leuprolide develops and the prostate cancer is deprived of stimulation?

11. Why use leuprolide as an alternative to surgical castration for a man with advanced prostatic carcinoma?

12. The text notes that biologic response modifiers such as interferons alfa-2a and alfa-2b are generally more effective against hematologic cancers than against solid tumors. Why might this be? (**Hint:** The answer lies in a main action of the biologic response modifiers, and that's what I'd like you to recall.)

CASE STUDY

Let's go back to the case study of Kathy Turner, whom we introduced in the case study in the previous chapter.

To refresh your memory, Ms. Turner is 41 years old and has metastatic breast cancer. She had a modified radical mastectomy and axillary lymph node dissection (2 out of 20 lymph nodes were positive for cancer). She will receive doxorubicin (Adriamycin), cyclophosphamide (Cytoxan), and fluorouracil (Adrucil) IV bolus. Premedications include intravenous ondansetron (Zofran) and dexamethasone (Decadron).

1. We said that we'd give Ms. Turner dexamethasone as part of a regimen to suppress chemotherapy-related nausea and vomiting. After reading this chapter, can you envisage other benefits that might come from giving the dexamethasone?

2. If Ms. Turner also had diabetes mellitus, would you have any added concerns? Why?

3. If Ms. Turner also had asthma, would you expect the glucocorticoid to worsen it? Why or why not?

Now we learn that Ms. Turner also has metastatic bone cancer.

4. What main serum electrolyte abnormality would you expect to find? Why?

5. A colleague who thinks he's a "good study" on osteoporosis notes that estrogen is commonly used for some women with osteoporosis. "It hinders bone breakdown and increases formation of new and healthier and stronger bones." We should use it for Ms. Turner. Do you agree?

6. Someone says, "We should provide a bisphosphonate [e.g., alendronate (Fosamax)] for Ms. Turner." Would you agree in principle?

Given this new information, we might consider alternative chemotherapy. For now, the MD is thinking about either tamoxifen or raloxifene.

7. Ms. Turner is 41. Other factors aside, does that alone contraindicate tamoxifen use?

8. If Ms. Turner has risk factors for endometrial cancer, would your preference be for tamoxifen or for raloxifene? Why?

Drugs for the Eye

KEY TERMS

angle-closure glaucoma
(narrow-angle
glaucoma)
carbonic anhydrase (and
its inhibitors)
cycloplegic (drug or
effect)
glaucoma(s)
miotic (drug or
effect)

mydriatic (drug or
effect)
ocular hypertension
photophobia
primary open-angle
glaucoma
Schlemm canal
tonometry
trabeculae (trabecular
network of eye)

OBJECTIVES

After reading and studying this chapter you should
be able to:

1. Compare and contrast open-angle glaucoma and
   angle-closure glaucoma in terms of etiology,
   prevalence (including demographic/ethnic factors), and management.
2. Summarize how the sympathetic and parasympathetic branches of the autonomic nervous system
   control pupil size, and why pupil size is important
   for narrow-angle glaucoma; state the classes of
   autonomic drugs that cause miosis; cause mydriasis; explain whether the effects of these drugs
   are beneficial or harmful for glaucoma, and why.
3. State the very simple, fundamental mechanism by
   which all drugs that have been shown to be effective for managing glaucoma, regardless of their
   mechanism of action or class, are beneficial for
   this eye disorder.
4. Give a general and accurate description of how
   the following may help lessen IOP: adrenergic
   agonists, muscarinic agonists, acetylcholinesterase inhibitors, carbonic anhydrase inhibitors,
   and PGF$_2$ alpha or its analogs.
5. State comorbidities that might be aggravated by
   stated drugs or drug groups that are suitable for
   managing glaucoma. Conversely, name some
   drugs or drug classes, and the main indications
   for their use, that might raise IOP and aggravate
   glaucoma.

6. State whether topical ophthalmic administration
   of drugs for glaucoma (as opposed to administering by, say, the oral route) will ensure that no systemic side effects occur, and explain why;
   identify what administration techniques can be
   used to minimize systemic problems.

Be sure to review pertinent information about
adrenergic and cholinergic agonists and blockers,
and about acetylcholinesterase inhibitors. Drugs in
these classes play important therapeutic roles, or
cause significant problems, for patients with glaucoma and many other relatively common disorders.
You will find this information in Chapters 14, 15,
17, 18, and 19.

CRITICAL THINKING AND STUDY QUESTIONS

1. A patient has a thorough exam of both eyes and
   another eye exam 6 months later. Intraocular
   pressure is 25 mm Hg. Both exams reveal no
   visual changes, nor any changes in the optic disk
   (retinal vessels, optic nerve endings in the retina).
   Is this glaucoma? If not, what is this condition
   called, and what is its relation to glaucoma?

2. Can you make a sweeping—and correct—statement that drugs that affect the size of the pupil
   have beneficial (or adverse) effects on glaucoma?
   Give some examples to support your conclusion.

300

3. For what pre-existing medical condition are beta-adrenergic blockers, muscarinic agonists (e.g., pilocarpine, carbachol, ACh itself), and cholinesterase inhibitors (e.g., demecarium, echothiophate) all contraindicated, particularly if given systemically (by mouth or parenterally)? Would these medications or drug groups pose a risk for glaucoma patients with this disorder, but who use these meds as topical ophthalmic preparations (e.g., eye drops)? Why or why not?

4. Name some *prescription* drugs or drug groups, and their main non-ophthalmic uses, that might aggravate narrow-angle glaucoma. State the common mechanism by which this worsening of glaucoma is likely to occur.

5. In educating a patient with recently diagnosed narrow-angle (angle-closure) glaucoma, you need to prepare a list of OTC medications that the patient should avoid. What drugs and drug classes would be on your list, and in what types of OTC products are they typically found? What are the untoward actions of these drugs or products that would make them candidates for your "avoid these" list?

6. A friend tells you she has glaucoma but doesn't know which "type" (open-angle or narrow-angle). She's complaining of some seasonal allergies and wants to take an antihistamine periodically. In terms of OTC products, which would you recommend, knowing that regardless of the type of glaucoma she has, an antihistamine is not likely to aggravate her eye disorder?

7. How is acetazolamide classified, and how does it apparently provide relief in glaucoma?

Drugs for the Skin

KEY TERMS

actinic keratosis
atopy (as in atopic
    dermatitis)
comedone
keratolytic (drug or
    effect)

psoriasis
salicylism
seborrheic dermatitis
    (seborrhea)

OBJECTIVES

After reading and studying this chapter you should be able to:

1. Summarize the basic etiology (and pathophysiology of the skin) of common acne. Explain the benefits and limitations of, and indications for, the main drugs used for acne: cleansers and drying agents, benzoyl peroxide, antibiotics, and vitamin A derivatives.
2. Identify the main drugs or other factors that can increase risk of local or systemic toxicity of topical retinoic acid derivatives (e.g., tretinoin) and of isotretinoin (oral).
3. Summarize the main adverse responses associated with isotretinoin therapy and the precautions that should be taken to avoid them or deal with adverse responses that might occur. Be sure to include comments on the drug's common adverse effects, the potential for psychiatric depression, pregnancy- and breast feeding-related matters, and interactions with other drugs and vitamins (as described in the text).

Notes: Be sure to review pertinent material (see Chapters 57 and 68) on the glucocorticoids. Some of the study questions below also encourage your recall of antihistamines (see Chapter 66) as topical medications for certain types of dermatitis.

CRITICAL THINKING AND STUDY QUESTIONS

1. An adult visits his physician for a routine physical and comments that he has a couple of plantar warts (common warts, *verruca vulgaris,* on the soles of the feet) and one on one knuckle of a finger. Each wart is 2–3 mm in diameter (less than 1/8 inch). The physician examines them and is satisfied that there is no underlying neoplasia or other worrisome pathology. The doctor offers to remove the warts (at some expense), but says "sure" when the patient asks if he can try some relatively inexpensive OTC wart remover.

   The patient chooses a liquid that contains, as the active ingredient, 17% salicylic acid. The patient applies the medication sparingly (one or two drops) to each wart, as directed on the bottle's label.

   A. When salicylic acid is used for this purpose, what is its main mechanism of action?

   B. What nondrug strategy might enhance the desired effects of this OTC medication?

   C. When used as directed, is salicylic acid likely to cause systemic side effects (e.g., salicylism) or outright systemic toxicity? After all, the text says that it is readily absorbed through the skin.

D. You probably haven't used salicylic acid for warts or any other skin conditions. However, you have almost certainly "put some salicylic acid into your system" on many occasions. Any idea what I'm talking about?

E. Imagine that the man who is using the wart-removing liquid that contains the salicylic acid leaves the bottle of medication (it's actually quite small) in an unsafe place in his home. His 6-year-old son finds the bottle, opens it up, and swallows some of the medication. What is the most serious initial adverse response you can imagine from this? Your colleague says it would be salicylism—systemic toxicity from the drug. Do you agree? Why?

2. You and two colleagues are discussing the case of a young adult man with severe nodulocystic acne vulgaris that hasn't responded to OTC medications or to such prescription drugs as tetracyclines. He will be started on isotretinoin (Accutane) soon. Each of you starts thinking about the possibility of psychiatric depression while the patient is taking the drug.

A. One colleague suggests that perhaps the doctor ought to start the patient on an antidepressant for prophylaxis. What are your thoughts on this?

B. The other colleague suggests instead that now's not the time to start an antidepressant. It can be started at the time depression signs and symptoms are diagnosed. Do you agree with this approach?

3. The text mentions eczema and calls it by its more proper name, atopic dermatitis. You know what the general term *dermatitis* means?

A. What does the adjective *atopic* (or the noun from which it is derived, *atopy*) mean?

B. Given what you now know about atopic dermatitis (eczema, if you prefer), comment on whether topical products that contain an antihistamine (H_1 blocker) as one of the ingredients (or the only active ingredient) might be useful. After all, histamine is an important substance in allergic responses. If one should use a topical antihistamine-containing product on a long-term basis, what clinical responses might you expect? Why? To keep things simple, assume that the topical product you're considering *does not contain a glucocorticoid*.

C. Now, use your knowledge to predict whether a topical glucocorticoid or a topical antihistamine-containing product might be more efficacious for eczema. Give some insight about why you reached that conclusion. (Yes, you may need to refresh your basic pharmacology knowledge about histamine and histamine-receptor blockers. That's in Chapter 66.)

4. A man who has hypertension but has his blood pressure well controlled with an oral medication (assume his BP at rest is 114/76) has male pattern baldness. He wishes to use an OTC topical minoxidil preparation (Rogaine). A colleague insists he should avoid the topical minoxidil. "After all," she says, "minoxidil was originally developed as an antihypertensive drug—and it's a very effective one, at that. If he uses the Minoxidil, he's likely to lower his blood pressure too much and cause hypotension." Do you agree? Why?

5. The text notes, quite correctly, that both isotretinoin (Accutane, for severe, refractory acne) and finasteride (Propecia, for hair loss) are quite teratogenic. That's not good at all, is it? Heck, all a pregnant woman needs to do is handle crushed or broken finasteride tablets early in the gestational period and if things don't go well and she's carrying a male baby, fetal deformities can occur. Given this information, can these drugs be purchased over the Internet without a complete and proper work-up by a physician who has actually seen the patient?

6. Given the teratogenic risks of isotretinoin (Accutane), is legitimately getting a prescription for it from a personal physician, and getting the prescription filled by a walk-in pharmacy, a relatively simple matter? Please visit the website of the U.S. manufacturer (*http://www.rocheusa.com/ products/accutane*) and take a look at the information about "getting" the drug. (At that URL you'll find a document listing the complete information for patients and healthcare providers. It's a PDF, and it's long. Don't print it out. Just scan the document and you'll be able to answer my question.)

Drugs for the Ear

KEY TERMS

cerumen
Eustachian tube
mastoiditis
otalgia
otitis externa (incl.
  nccrotizing)
otitis media (acute,
  chronic)
otitis media with
  effusion

otomycosis (fungal otitis
  externa)
otorrhea
prurulent (as might be
  used to describe
  otorrhea)
"swimmer's ear"
tympanic membrane
tympanostomy
  (myringotomy)

OBJECTIVES

After reading and studying this chapter you should be able to:

1. Compare and contrast acute otitis media (AOM), otitis mcdia with effusion (OME), and antibiotic-resistant otitis media in terms of the most common pathogenic causes (epidemiology), typical signs and symptoms, and treatment.
2. Comment on the pros and cons of routinely treating all (or even most) causes of acute otitis media with antibiotics, as opposed to holding off with antibiotic therapy for a short time and seeing whether the signs and symptoms of the condition resolve spontaneously ("prescribe and wait").
3. Comment on the use of antibiotic prophylaxis for recurrent otitis media in children. Imagine you are talking to a mom who has brought her daughter into your pediatrics office three times in the last year with an ear infection; she wants a prescription, for antibiotics, to prevent another infection.

Be sure to review pertinent information about the general pharmacology of the antibiotics, particularly the penicillins, that are discussed in this chapter.

CRITICAL THINKING AND STUDY QUESTIONS

1. Your text notes that otitis media affects about 95% of children by the age of 12; more than 5 million cases are diagnosed each year. It goes on to note that "antibiotics are used routinely [for ear infections and] ...in fact OM is the most common reason for giving these drugs to kids." Based on your reading of the chapter, is such widespread antibiotic prescribing justified?

2. When "resistant" acute otitis media needs to be treated, the preferred approach is to use high doses of amoxicillin-clavulanate. Just what is clavulanate, and what does it do? Is it an antibiotic, *per se?*

3. The risk of mastoiditis—clearly a serious condition that can be a consequence of nontreated or poorly treated otitis media (especially with effusion)—has been cited as a reason to prescribe antibiotics at once (as soon as the diagnosis is made) for most children with middle ear infections. Comment on whether the data support this contention—whether this is a good reason, a wise thing to do.

305

CASE STUDY

Samantha Samson brings her 7-year-old daughter, Emily, to your peds office. Emily has been tugging at her ears and not sleeping well for several days. When you check her, Emily is crying occasionally. Pulse and respirations are normal. Body temperature is 99.8° F. Emily sobs a little, but she's a good trooper despite obviously feeling not well at all.

Mrs. Samson tells you that ear infections "have been going around" Emily's class at school. You look at Emily's chart and see that this is the third visit for an ear infection in the last 12 months.

1. You check Emily's ears and comment, "Looks like she has ear infections." Mrs. Samson gets irritated. "The doctor isn't doing something right. After all, she's had these infections twice before." How would you explain the situation to Emily's mom?

2. Peeking at Emily's ears with your ototoscope, you note that her eardrums are inflamed but not bulging. What does this finding usually mean, given the other signs and symptoms? In contrast, what is the usual clinical significance of finding bulging tympanic membranes that present with otalgia and the other signs and symptoms?

3. You check Emily's chart again. Each time she's had an ear infection she's been prescribed amoxicillin-clavulanate, even though there was no evidence of acute bacterial otitis media (i.e., no bulging eardrums, no prurulent discharge). Here she is, back for her third ear infection in a year. Does this indicate that Emily has developed resistance to the antibiotic? What information would help you decide whether she did? How helpful would information in Emily's office chart be in terms of answering this question?

As you wrap things up with Emily and her mom, you instruct mom to administer an acetaminophen pediatric formulation at the usual dose, saying it should relieve the discomfort. You write another prescription for amoxicillin-clavulanate, but tell Mrs. Samson to wait 3 days. If Emily is still having significant discomfort, she should get the prescription filled promptly and administer it to Emily per written directions. Otherwise, just discard the prescription form.

4. Mrs. Samson wants to know why she shouldn't get the 'script' filled and start giving it to her daughter right away. She now backtracks from her initial position and says, "If it worked before, won't it work again?" You comment by speculating that Emily's prior ear infections may have gotten better despite the antibiotic, not because of it. What might you mean by saying this?

5. Now Mrs. Sampson asks again about what to do with the antibiotic prescription if she doesn't need it this time. Can she just get it filled and hold on to it until Emily gets another ear infection?

6. Mrs. Samson knows several parents of kids with recurrent ear infections. They've taken their children to an eye-ear-nose-throat (EENT) specialist, who has inserted "tubes" (myringotomy or tympanostomy tubes) into the kids' ears. Mrs. Samson asks what they are, why they're used, and whether she should take Emily to an EENT specialist right away. Explain things.

7. Several months have passed since the episode described above. Emily is now back to the office for a scheduled well-child visit in late September—not long after school started, not far away from another spread of ear infections among the class. Emily's ears are fine, but Mrs. Samson wants a prescription for antibiotics to prevent the ear infections for the next year. Instead you recommend a flu shot for the upcoming influenza season. She gets irritated, saying she's concerned about the ear infections; her child has never gotten the flu. How would you respond?

103

Miscellaneous Noteworthy Drugs

Note: In general nursing practice you will encounter drugs used for erectile dysfunction, benign prostatic hypertrophy, and cancer chemotherapy more often than you will drugs used for other conditions discussed in this chapter. Therefore, we will focus on what we consider the more common "priority" content.

DRUGS FOR ERECTILE DYSFUNCTION (ED)

KEY TERMS

cyclic GMP

CYP3A4

erectile dysfunction (ED)

nitric oxide

phosphodiesterase (PDE)

priapism

OBJECTIVES

Note: Given the widespread use and availability of sildenafil (Viagra), moreso than any other current drugs(s) used for erectile dysfunction, you should focus your studying on it.

Be sure to review Chapter 49 (*Drugs for Angina Pectoris*) to refresh your memory about the pathology of the three major forms of angina; the mechanisms by which antianginal drugs such as nitroglycerin exert beneficial (or adverse) effects; and drug-related and other (physiologic) factors that can worsen or precipitate angina. Be sure to hit the highlights about the actions and uses of other antianginal drugs, specifically beta-adrenergic blockers (their basic pharmacology is presented in Chapter 18) and calcium channel blockers such as verapamil and diltiazem (basic pharmacology of these is covered in Chapter 43).

After reading and studying this section of the chapter you should be able to:

1. Identify the main patient-related conditions, or other applicable factors, that contraindicate use of sildenafil. You should be able to describe the main systemic hemodynamic effects of the drug. The main concerns involve the cardiovascular system, so focus on that.

2. State the likely consequences of administering sildenafil with drugs that inhibit the liver's cytochrome P450 system. The text notes the specific enzyme, CYP3A4. Identify the main groups of those drugs.

3. Discuss guidelines or recommendations about the use of sildenafil by a patient who is taking nitroglycerin or any other nitrate vasodilator/antianginal drug; describe the likely outcome(s) if these recommendations are ignored.

CRITICAL THINKING AND STUDY QUESTIONS

1. Sildenafil can be purchased easily via orders placed on the Internet or by calling a toll-free phone number. At best, some places selling this drug offer "free consultations" with a medical professional of some sort. Given what you've learned about the potential adverse responses of this drug and precautionary or contraindicating conditions, comment on the sale of this medication over the 'Net. (Before you answer this question, you might want to skip ahead and try to answer the rest. Doing that will probably give you the answer and plenty of good reasons to support your position.)

2. The text cautions against use of sildenafil by "men taking nitroglycerin or any other drug in the nitrate family." What is the main reason for which nitroglycerin is used? How can combined use of sildenafil and nitroglycerin alter the response(s) to nitroglycerin or the medical condition for which it has been prescribed?

3. The text lists *unstable angina* as a contraindication to sildenafil. What is unstable angina?

4. What are the other main types of angina? Is sildenafil OK for patients with those other types of angina? Does it depend on which antianginal drug(s) they're taking?

5. Two of the conditions that contraindicate sildenafil use are resting hypotension (BP < 90/50 mm Hg) and resting hypertension (BP >170/110). Both hypotension and hypertension? Seems contradictory, no? Explain what the concern(s) is/are for each, if we were to ignore the precautions and take this drug for ED.

6. The chapter identifies several prescription drugs or drug classes that can alter the responses to a given dose of sildenafil. What are they? How, in general, do they interact and what are the likely outcome(s) of the interaction(s)?

7. Are any of the key interactants available OTC? If so, what alternative drug(s) might you recommend to patients who wish to take that particular medication?

DRUGS FOR BENIGN PROSTATIC HYPERPLASIA

KEY TERMS

5-alpha-reductase (and its inhibitors)
dynamic obstruction (of/by an enlarged prostate)
mechanical obstruction (of/by an enlarged prostate)
prostate specific antigen (PSA) saw palmetto

OBJECTIVES

Review Chapter 18 (*Adrenergic Antagonists*) to refresh your memory about alpha-adrenergic blockers, including the prototype, phentolamine, with a focus on mechanisms of action, the expected effects of these drugs, and related side effects and precautions.

After reading and studying this section of the chapter you should be able to:

1. Describe the pathologic changes in benign prostatic hyperplasia (BPH) in terms of how they contribute to common signs and symptoms (describe them).
2. Compare and contrast finasteride and a drug such as prazosin in terms of how they alter BPH signs and symptoms, their main side effects, and the basic mechanism(s) by which they occur.

CRITICAL THINKING AND STUDY QUESTIONS

1. By what mechanism does finasteride (Proscar) work to alleviate signs and symptoms of BPH?

2. Before finasteride is prescribed, what specific lab test must be conducted? Why?

3. Although it's not listed in this chapter, there's another approved use for finasteride. Do you know what it is? If not, look it up; hop on the Web, if you wish. (**Hint:** It's related to testosterone metabolism and what might be described as a "cosmetic" problem for many men as they get older.) And no, it has nothing to do with the prostate or the male genitalia (or how that body part works).

4. By what mechanism do doxazosin, prazosin, and tamsulosin alleviate signs and symptoms of BPH?

5. In terms of profiles of activity, how does tamsulosin differ from doxazosin and prazosin? What are the clinical implications of this?

6. A patient with essential hypertension is being treated with, and responding very well to, an angiotensin-converting enzyme inhibitor (e.g., captopril; see Chapter 42). A couple of years later he develops BPH and the physician decides to prescribe prazosin, saying, "This drug will not only have a good chance of helping the BPH, but it will also further lower the patient's blood pressure." Would you agree that this drug is a good choice?

DRUGS FOR NEONATAL RESPIRATORY DISTRESS SYNDROME

KEY TERMS

neonatal respiratory distress syndrome

surfactant

OBJECTIVES

Review Chapter 57 (*Drugs for Disorders of the Adrenal Cortex*), Chapter 68 (*Glucocorticoids for Nonendocrine Disorders*), and Chapter 62 (*Drugs That Affect Uterine Function*); the content of this section of this chapter relates directly, in one way or another, to what you'll find there.

After reading and studying this section of the chapter you should be able to:

1. Recognize respiratory distress as the main cause of illness and mortality in premature infants.
2. Discuss the main physiologic roles of lung surfactant and the main consequences of surfactant deficiency in terms of lung mechanics (alveolar surface tension, lung compliance or elasticity) and blood oxygenation.
3. Recognize that cortisol production by the fetus is a main stimulant for surfactant production, that this process starts around month 8 of gestation, and that peak effects don't develop until about weeks 34–36 (close to full term). Relate this information to the critical role of administering glucocorticoids antenatally (to the mother) in the setting of premature labor and delivery.
4. Recognize that the use of uterine relaxants (e.g., ritodrine; see Chapter 62) to slow premature labor and delay delivery of a premature fetus does not eliminate the need for proactive and proper therapy for neonatal RDS.

DRUGS FOR CYSTIC FIBROSIS

KEY TERMS

chloride channel

cystic fibrosis

OBJECTIVES

After reading and studying this section of the chapter you should be able to:

1. State the mechanism and nature of the nutritional defects typically seen as cystic fibrosis develops. In your explanation be sure to consider altered pancreatic secretory activity (what secretions are involved?) and its consequences on absorption (or lack thereof) of key nutrients.

2. State the mechanism and characteristics of the pulmonary problems typically seen as cystic fibrosis develops. In your explanation be sure to consider how it affects lung hydration, mucus volume and viscosity, and lung mechanics.

3. Explain the roles and expected beneficial effects of administering pancreatic enzymes and vitamins A, K, E, and D. Explain why those vitamins, as opposed to others, are the ones that need to be given.

4. Explain the roles and expected beneficial effects of administering dornase alfa to CF patients.

5. Explain the need for such antibiotics as tobramycin in the management of CF. Include in your explanation comments on the statement that "cystic fibrosis is *not* an infectious disease, even though drugs typically used for infections may become important."

DRUGS FOR SICKLE CELL ANEMIA

KEY TERMS

hemoglobin S (HbS)   sickle (sickled) cell

OBJECTIVES

After reading and studying this section of the chapter you should be able to:

1. Give a general and generally accurate overview of the epidemiology, incidence, and transmission of sickle cell disease.

2. Explain how anatomic and functional changes in the sickled erythrocyte contribute to key signs and symptoms of the disorder.

3. State the mechanism(s) by which analgesics (opioid or otherwise) can benefit patients with sickle cell crisis. Explain whether those drugs target the disease itself or merely the symptoms of it.

DRUGS FOR HYPERURICEMIA CAUSED BY CANCER CHEMOTHERAPY

KEY TERMS

purines (and purine   xanthine oxidase
  degradation pathway)

OBJECTIVES

Be *sure* to review Chapter 69 (*Drug Therapy for Rheumatoid Arthritis and Gout*) with a focus on the drugs used for gout (hyperuricemia). Much of the information in that section of that chapter relates to the proper use of allopurinol. Unit XVII (*Cancer Chemotherapy*) provides good information on how cancers, and treatment of them, can lead to hyperuricemia and its consequences.

After reading and studying this section of the chapter you should be able to:

1. Explain how some cancers, and their treatment with suitable chemotherapeutic agents, lead to hyperuricemia.

2. Discuss the main endogenous source of uric acid—the substance(s) from which it normally arises during cell metabolism and breakdown. In your discussion, identify the enzyme that's responsible for the formation of uric acid and its immediate precursor, hypoxanthine.

3. State the main mechanism by which excesses of uric acid cause their adverse effects. For example, is it due to uncoupling, inhibition, or stimulation of some key enzyme in the body?

4. Explain the rationale for using allopurinol rather than other drugs traditionally used in the management of hyperuricemia and gout.

CRITICAL THINKING AND STUDY QUESTIONS

1. How do rasburicase (Elitek) and allopurinol (Zyloprim) differ in their mechanisms of action? A simple answer will do.

2. The text notes that rasburicase is a very new drug; allopurinol is a very old one. Is the newer one better? Preferred? Comment on the statement, "This is one of those instances when going with an old agent is probably a better idea than going with the new kid on the block." (To answer this, you may have to go back to previous chapters, which give more information on allopurinol and other drugs for hyperuricemia.)

3. Probenecid is a drug that increases renal excretion of uric acid, and does that very well. Why not use it instead of allopurinol or rasburicase to manage hyperuricemia associated with cancer and cancer chemotherapy?

GAMMA HYDROXYBUTYRATE FOR CATAPLEXY IN PATIENTS WITH NARCOLEPSY

KEY TERMS

cataplexy   narcolepsy

OBJECTIVES

Review Chapter 38 (*Drug Abuse: Opioids, Depressants, etc.*) for more information on GHB. Chapter 35 (*Central Nervous System Stimulants*)

will provide a good refresher on other drugs that can be used for narcolepsy. In Chapter 20 (*Introduction to Central Nervous System Pharmacology*) you'll also find important relevant information on the neurotransmitter, gamma hydroxybutyric acid (GABA). It relates to what's covered below too.

After reading and studying this section of the chapter you should be able to:

1. Explain why the availability of GHB for use in management of cataplectic attacks is so limited. In your explanation, state the more common and illicit use of the drug.
2. Explain how GHB, a CNS depressant, is useful in managing narcolepsy and cataplexy, both of which are very obvious consequences of CNS depression.
3. Comment on why the drug form of GHB should not be used in patients with heart failure, hypertension, or renal dysfunction.

evolve To check your answers, go to http://evolve.elsevier.com/Lehne/ for Study Guide Comments from the author.

Herbal Supplements

KEY TERMS

adulterant
alternative medicine
decoction
dietary supplement
Dietary Supplement
   Health and Education
   Act 1994 (DSHEA)

extract (fluid, solid)
German Commission E
herbal medicine
infusion (type of herbal
   drug preparation)
tea
tincture

OBJECTIVES

After reading and studying this chapter you should
be able to:

1. Give "working definitions" of the terms *herbal
   supplement* and *nutritional supplement.* Do this
   in terms of drug action (what *is* a drug?) and the
   legal/regulatory matters discussed in the chapter.
2. Recognize that herbals usually do contain active
   ingredients, some of which can cause desired
   effects and some that can cause serious adverse
   effects or can interact beneficially or not with
   prescribed FDA-approved drugs.
3. List and describe the main reasons why we may
   turn to herbal medicines, as either supplements or
   alternatives to traditional medicines and medical
   practice.
4. Recognize what the German Commission E is as
   it applies to herbals. (When you read the literature you will often read such statements as, "This
   herbal medication is listed by the German
   Commission E." You ought to have a clue about
   what that means.
5. Summarize what the Dietary Supplement Health
   and Education Act (DSHEA-1994) permits (and
   doesn't) in the way of manufacturing, advertising, and labeling herbals.
      Compare and contrast the general criteria that a
   manufacturer of a prescription medication must
   prove before the drug can be marketed.
      Compare those criteria and the overall
   approval and safety-monitoring procedures for
   them with those for herbal medicines (as encom-
   passed by DSHEA 1994). As a healthcare profes-

sional (future or current), comment on the question "What's wrong here?" with respect to the
disparities between regulatory controls over prescription and herbal medicines.
6. Explain how calling a product a dietary supplement rather than a drug allows the manufacturers
   of these products to circumvent standards of
   purity, efficacy, and safety that apply to FDA-
   approved drugs, and discuss how that ability to
   skirt more stringent regulations and requirements
   can harm us.
7. Recognize that if you took an array of ostensibly
   the "same" herbal medications, prepared and sold
   by various individuals or companies, you are
   likely to find very large differences in the
   amounts of active substance, impurities, and
   adulterants, such that you will conclude that there
   is little uniformity.
8. State the main reasons that some practitioners of
   "traditional Western medicine" are skeptical of
   herbals and nutritional supplements.
9. Summarize, according to your personal beliefs
   and your factual knowledge (as gained from this
   chapter), the major benefits and risks of using
   herbal medicines instead of or in addition to prescription drugs. Then be able to translate those
   beliefs and the facts (as we know them) into
   advice you would give to someone (friend, family
   member, or patient) who wishes to use an herbal.
   Your advice should be as objective as possible; it
   should include general issues that apply to virtually all herbal medicines and specific information
   that applies to the several herbals you can select,
   as suggested in the following *Notes.*

Note: You will have to check with your instructor to
learn just what he or she expects you to learn from
this chapter. If I were your instructor I'd rather you
focus on general concepts than details about specific
herbal remedies (you can always look that up). I
therefore formulated my objectives to address more
general (but very important) points.
   I think it would be appropriate (and a good learning experience), however, to have you select three or
four herbal supplements that are familiar to you
(whether through personal use or use by someone

313

you know, or perhaps one that you've seen or heard advertised heavily). For each herbal, state the main reason(s) it is used, summarize the known information about efficacy and safety (including known adverse responses, as noted in your text), and identify the main interactions with prescription drugs with which they may be involved.

CRITICAL THINKING AND STUDY QUESTIONS

1. Contrast the provisions of DSHEA 94 as they apply to the manufacture and sale of nutritional supplements with the rules and regulations that apply to prescription drugs. Focus on the issues of efficacy and safety... and cost.

2. Now that you have an idea of what DSHEA allows, can you speculate about some of the reasons that the bill was proposed and eventually became law? (You've gathered enough information through this text, through various courses, and through being even casually familiar with government to be able to make an educated guess about this.)

3. Some manufacturers of herbal supplements are very reliable and trustworthy. They analyze their products to standardize the doses of the active ingredients from lot to lot; they use state of the art manufacturing techniques; they make sure there are no impurities or adulterants in their products. Their reputations are impeccable.

   But other companies *don't* do that. Why not?

4. Why don't more manufacturers of nutritional supplements do the necessary clinical trials to prove safety and efficacy?

5. A friend is taking a nutritional supplement (herbal medicine) and swears it works. Just by chance you're doing some web surfing and find several articles indicating that the particular brand of medicine he's taking—the very same product—has been tested thoroughly. Chemical analysis reveals no active substance in it, and there's good evidence that the manufacturer has been selling this active ingredient–free stuff for many years.

   A. What probably explains your friend's claim that the stuff works?

   B. Might your friend actually be better off taking a product that was shown to contain no active ingredient than one that did?

   C. Your friend gets a little miffed at what you found. He logs on to the manufacturer's web site with you and scrolls down to the "testimonials" section. "See," he says, "right there it says that this product has been clinically proven to be *just as effective* as placebo. And I know," he says, "that drug companies compare their drugs with placebos all the time." How would you try to explain things to him?

   D. Not liking the possibility he's been confronted with information that doesn't fit him impressions or beliefs, he calls you (the "practitioner of Western medicine" [the term *Western* often meaning evil]) a snooty and arrogant college grad. How might you reply (politely), should you wish to waste your breath at all?

6. Someone you meet at a party (not a patient) engages you in conversation and sort of thumbs her nose at you because occasionally you take "nasty chemicals"—prescription drugs. They're artificial substances that are "bad for you," she exclaims. She takes herbals, saying they're "better for you because they're 'all natural.'" How might you reply?

7. According to some who follow trends (in the United States) of the rising use of herbal medicines, one factor more than any other is responsible for their growing use. Do you have an idea what that is? Some would say it's seeking better health. Some would say it's dissatisfaction with traditional medicine. Others claim it's our desire to be "all natural." None of those seem to be the main reason. So, what is?

8. Does the FDA regulate the accuracy of labels on packages of herbals that are sold in the United State—for example, statements about the use(s) of the product or the ingredients that are or aren't in it? If not, what is the loophole the manufacturer can use in terms of claims or other label information?

9. Does the government (i.e., the FDA) ever get involved and investigate?

10. If I were to "require" you to become very familiar with the "clinical pharmacology of just one of the herbal supplements discussed in this chapter," (in its broadest context), I would pick ephedra (ma huang). Why?

11. Why would it be correct (and not merely a pun) to say that the roots of "traditional" medicine are plants?

12. Someone with a fascination for herbal medicines, and who is taking them, recognizes that a plant with the "active substance" is growing nearby, right in her backyard. She wants to make the drug herself. Is it a matter of "just grab the plant" and make a tea? Steep it in some alcohol? Grind it up and eat it? The whole thing?

13. A patient is taking a prescribed medication that is known to cause a severe disulfiram-like reaction. What is that reaction? What drug causes the interaction, and how (in simple terms) does it occur? What are its major signs and symptoms? What type of oral herbal formulation is likely, therefore, to cause adverse responses in a patient who's taking this prescription drug too?

evolve To check your answers, go to http://evolve.elsevier.com/Lehne/ for Study Guide Comments from the author.

105

Management of Poisoning

KEY TERMS

adsorb
antidote
chelator (chelation)
petroleum distillate

poison
toxicant
toxicologist (toxicology)
Wilson's disease

OBJECTIVES

After reading and studying this chapter you should be able to:

1. Describe the five basic common elements of effective poisoning management, regardless of what the poison is.
2. Identify five mechanisms for reducing the absorption of toxicants. Comment on the pros and cons, benefits and limitations, and settings for appropriate use of each.
3. Describe methods (including drugs) that can be used to accelerate the removal of *absorbed* poisons.
4. Discuss the general mechanism(s) of actions by which chelating agents work; why no one chelator is effective for all heavy metal poisonings; and other properties that they should have to cause their desired effects.
5. Be able to recognize poisoning syndromes that involve muscarinic agonists and acetylcholinesterase inhibitors, antimuscarinic drugs, benzodiazepines, and opioids. You should be able to describe not only the typical clinical presentations of these syndromes but also the antidotes and the likely additional measures to prevent a lethal outcome.

Notes: There is much good information in this chapter about management of poisoning with nondrug measures. However, we will consider this in the domain of medical-surgical nursing and focus largely on pharmacologic approaches.

Table 105-1 (Specific Antidotes Discussed in Previous Chapters) is one small part of this chapter, but it's very important. Why? Because if you look at the list of toxic/overdosed substances you'll find many drugs or drug classes you will encounter, and

often administer, in clinical practice. So you need to know the antidotes (and other aspects of management) for them. We'll also coerce your recall of this information with some Critical Thinking and Study Questions.

CRITICAL THINKING AND STUDY QUESTIONS

1. If a person who ingested an unidentified poison arrives at the emergency room, what is the first thing to do after checking and beginning to correct vital signs (symptomatic, supportive care)?

2. If you and your staff are unsure about the diagnosis of the poisoning or what to do about it, what should you do?

3. What are you likely to face when a patient is brought to the emergency department who falls into one (or more) of these categories: took the medication in a suicide attempt; was consuming large amounts of alcohol; was at a party and didn't seem to take anything but alcoholic beverages (perhaps only a small amount of alcohol); is known to be an abuser of illicit drugs.

4. What should be administered routinely for patients who have coma of unknown etiology?

5. Your text notes that "if convulsions develop [in a patient with a known or suspected overdose], IV diazepam is the treatment of choice." I disagree with that. Argue with me... convince me.

6. The text notes that such analytic procedures as gas chromatography/mass spectrometry can provide qualitative and quantitative information about the identity of a poison. They do. But there's one assumption, and a potential problem, with this comment. What might that/they be? (You don't have to be an analytic chemist or toxicologist to answer this. However, I admit that this might be a bit above your everyday knowledge. Nonetheless, thinking about this should be instructive.)

7. You almost certainly know the definition of *ab*sorption, one of the four main processes that contribute to the pharmacokinetic properties of drugs (unless the drug is given intravenously). What then is *ad*sorption? Just a unique type of absorption?

8. What's the fundamental problem with inducing emesis in a patient who has swallowed a very caustic or corrosive substance such as an acid or drain cleaner (lye)? Keep your explanation simple, but that's all that's needed. And if we don't induce vomiting in one of these cases, what *do* we do?

9. A colleague is debating with you about not inducing vomiting in a patient who has swallowed gasoline, cleaning fluid, or some other petroleum-based liquid. He says, "Heck, these things aren't caustic or corrosive! Why *not* induce vomiting?" Give a correct response to your colleague. What *is* the real risk?

10. What are the essential prerequisites before we administer (or advise a parent or other caregiver to administer) syrup of ipecac?

11. The text notes that administration of sodium bicarbonate (orally or IV, as dictated by the actual scenario) alkalinizes the urine and facilitates excretion of some drugs, particularly those that are weak acids (e.g., aspirin). Consider aspirin as the cause of the poisoning. Just what does "decreases the passive absorption [of aspirin]" mean in terms of what's going on in the kidneys? Just what are we trying to do?

12. Bonus question: What other drug might we give to an aspirin-poisoned patient to increase salicylate excretion even more? It works by further alkalinizing the urine.

13. We have a patient who has taken an overdose of a drug with no prior hepatic metabolism that is eliminated mainly in the urine. Its chemical and physical properties are such that alkalinizing or acidifying the urine won't do much to speed excretion. There are no other agents that will either speed up renal tubular secretion or reduce tubular reabsorption. What, then, might we administer to hasten excretion of the drug?

14. Your text notes that dimercaprol, an antidote used in treatment of poisoning with several heavy metals. What are those metals? The text also notes parenthetically that this heavy metal antagonist is known as BAL in oil. Do you have any idea of what BAL means, or stands for? (Yes, this is a bit of a history lesson, but it's still applicable.)

15. In Table 105-1 you'll see that pralidoxime (Protopam) is the antidote for organophosphate cholinesterase inhibitors.

    A. Where are you most likely to find that class of poison?

    B. What essential element of managing organophosphate cholinesterase inhibitors—aside from symptomatic, supportive care—was not mentioned in this part of the table? Why is it so critically important to use this drug also?

16. Quick hits: A patient who is an IV opioid abuser gets a batch of "uncut" (extremely potent) heroin and shoots up. He has, therefore, an acute opioid overdose. You give naloxone (Narcan), as noted in Table 105-1.

    A. How does naloxone work?

    B. What is the one expected response to this antidote, the one for which you give it?

    C. How is its duration of action likely to compare with the duration of action of the heroin? Why is that important?

    D. If you do give an effective dose of the naloxone, what other effect—probably one you really don't want to cause—is almost inevitable?

Potential Weapons of Biologic, Radiologic, and Chemical Terrorism

KEY TERMS

cholinergic crisis
dirty bomb
eschar
mustard (e.g., sulfur
  mustard)
nerve agents

plague (bubonic,
  pneumonic)
ricin
tularemia
variola

OBJECTIVES

After reading and studying this chapter you should be able to:

1. Identify the main bioterrorism agents (as discussed in this chapter) and the common properties that make this diverse group of agents suitable for their malevolent uses.
2. Discuss the controversies surrounding the prophylactic use of antibiotics for anthrax by the general population, who is not likely to be exposed to the causative bacterium.
3. Describe the signs, symptoms, and typical times to onset (after exposure) of cutaneous and inhalational anthrax. Summarize the general approaches to treating the infection and preventing the spread to others.
4. Identify the agents for which toxicity can be transmitted from person to person via exposure to body fluids, thereby constituting an "infectious disease."
5. Discuss the controversies surrounding the issue of vaccinating healthcare workers and first responders against smallpox. Include in your discussion some concept of the estimated risks from the vaccination itself, and compare and contrast them with the risks of being exposed (or having to care for an exposed patient) but not being vaccinated beforehand.

CRITICAL THINKING AND STUDY QUESTIONS

1. We have a variety of specific antibodies or other types of pharmacologic treatments for many of the bioterrorism agents. They're all effective, if used properly and early enough.

   However, there are two main limitations that should cause us concern if there is a mass attack with one of those bioweapons. What might they be?

2. A classmate proclaims that the current concerns over threats of an anthrax attack are just "government hype and scare tactics." He says, "After all, you know that the anthrax bacteria simply can't survive outside the body." Comment on this.

319

3. A neighbor, William Jefferson, lives and teaches high school in your small town in northern Vermont. Mr. Jefferson is "concerned" about a mass anthrax attack and has heard that ciprofloxacin is indicated as a preventive measure. He wants to get a prescription for the antibiotic and start taking it. Mr. Jefferson's physician states that taking the ciprofloxacin (or another antibiotic that might be effective) is unwarranted.
   A. If Mr. Jefferson can't get the ciprofloxacin from his personal physician, how might he obtain the drug?

   B. Regardless of who prescribes or supplies the antibiotic, what is/are your major concern(s) for Mr. Jefferson's long-term use of this antibiotic, regardless of whether he might ever be exposed to anthrax?

4. The text notes that smallpox vaccine shouldn't be administered to people with eczema or atopic dermatitis. What is atopic dermatitis? Specifically, what does the term *atopic* mean?

5. Symptoms and signs aside, why is pneumonic plague more of a health risk than the bubonic form of the plague?

6. The text notes that experience suggests that smallpox vaccinations pose significant risks: "If one million people were vaccinated, 1,000 would experience a serious adverse effect.... And, from 14 to 52 vaccinated people would develop a life-threatening condition (response), and 1 or two recipients of the vaccine would die."
   It's important to put the numbers into a proper perspective, so use those data and calculate the *percentage* of vaccinees who would do the following:
   A. Experience a severe adverse effect.

   B. Develop a life-threatening response. You can use 50 vaccinees, a worst-case scenario based on what's stated in your text, as your number for calculation.

   C. Die. Let's go with worst-case scenario and assume we have two deaths per million.

   D. You've now calculated some of the risks associated with mortality and morbidity from smallpox vaccinations. Now speculate about why some healthcare professionals are reluctant to get vaccinated against smallpox before such an attack occurs. Does knowing that the smallpox vaccine "may be effective when given within a few days after exposure" allay your concerns about what might happen should there be an actual attack? (Comment on this from the perspective of a healthcare provider/recipient of the smallpox vaccine and from the perspective of a potential victim who requires care.)

7. Jeb Clampett, 18, and his wife of 2 years, live in a very rural area. A real "back-woodsy" place. Mr. Clampett is brought to the emergency department with severe flu-like signs and symptoms. Auscultation of the chest and chest x-rays reveal significant congestion from pleural effusion. His lymph nodes are swollen. His blood pressure is low and falling.

   The medical team is puzzled about the etiology of Mr. Clampett's illness until his wife mentions that he went camping and hunting a week ago. "He ain't never gone huntin' for varmints before," his wife says. "Jeb sez he got him a bunch of rabbits and squirrels, gutted 'em, and made him a real good stew to eat."

   What might this information provide in the way of a clue about Mr. Clampett's illness?

8. In the spring of 2003, U.S. and British troops found large stores of castor beans in an "unfriendly" Middle Eastern country. The locals stated that these were going to be used to manufacture castor oil. That's used as an additive to certain lubricants and an important ingredient in the manufacture of certain paints, inks, and cosmetics. Castor oil also is still quite widely used as an oral cathartic, to evacuate the bowel.

   Why were the troops skeptical about this stockpile of castor beans? What compound, discussed in this chapter, is a by-product of castor oil processing?

9. The text notes that botulinum toxin, in adequately toxic doses, inhibits acetylcholine release from cholinergic nerves. Let's see what you remember from your basic pharmacology learning.

   A. Considering only the peripheral nervous systems, what *are* the cholinergic nerves that are important in this setting?

   B. When ACh release is blocked by botulinum toxin, muscles are affected such that their inactivity is the main cause of death. Which branch(es) of the peripheral nervous systems controls the activity of those muscles?

   C. Which pharmacologic antagonist or antidote other than botulinum antitoxin can be life saving in such a poisoning?

   D. Given the lethality of botulinum toxin, how can that agent be used therapeutically, as it certainly is used nowadays? And what is that current use?

10. Sulfur *mustard* (mustard gas) is described as an *alkylating agent* and *vesicant*. Where have you heard very similar information in earlier chapters of this text? What other drugs—and quite useful ones, at that—have virtually the same properties?

11. A. How are the "nerve gases" classified pharmacologically?

    B. Do they have any therapeutically useful counterparts, and for what uses are they given?

C. Where, aside from a bioweapons lab or stockpile or a hospital pharmacy, are you likely to encounter drugs classified as "irreversible" cholinesterase inhibitors?

F. Which responses, identified above, would *not be affected at all* by administration of atropine? Why is atropine's lack of effect on those structures so important, or isn't it important at all?

D. Aside from decontamination of the patient and his or her clothes, what are the three main approaches to treating exposure to a nerve gas?

12. In the context of responding to attacks using radiologic weapons, what is the main rationale for administering potassium iodide? What is its main limitation?

E. A chemical worker is accidentally exposed to a nerve gas. He arrives in the emergency department for evaluation and treatment. Based on the mechanism of action of the poison, what signs and symptoms of exposure would you predict?

13. Why might you be skeptical about the comment in the text that "a dirty bomb will not release iodine-131, and so taking potassium iodide won't help."

evolve To check your answers, go to http://evolve.elsevier.com/Lehne/ for Study Guide Comments from the author.